Microsurgical Procedures

Published volumes in this series

The Interphalangeal Joints
William H. Bowers

The Paralysed Hand
Douglas W. Lamb

Unsatisfactory Results in Hand Surgery
Robert M. McFarlane

Fractures of the Hand and Wrist
Nicholas Barton

Dupuytren's Disease
D. A. McGrouther, Robert M. McFarlane, M. H. Flint

Management of Pain in the Hand and Wrist
C. B. Wynn Parry

Volumes in preparation

Fingertip and Nailbed Injuries
Guy Foucher

The Thumb
James W. Strickland

Joint Replacement in the Upper Limb
William A. Souter

Congenital Malformations of the Hand and Forearm
Dieter Buck–Gramcko

Skin Cover in the Injured Hand
David M. Evans

Tumours of the Hand and Upper Limb
G. Bogumill and E. Fleegler

For Churchill Livingstone:

Publisher: Simon Fathers
Design: Design Resources Unit
Production: Neil A. Dickson
Editorial Co-ordination: Editorial Resources Unit
Copy Editor: Joanna Smith
Sales Promotion Executive: Louise Johnstone

THE HAND AND UPPER LIMB Volume 7

Microsurgical Procedures

Edited by

Viktor E. Meyer MD
Professor of Surgery; Director, Division of Hand, Plastic & Reconstructive Surgery, Department of Surgery, University of Zurich Medical School, Zurich, Switzerland

Michael J. M. Black FRCS
Consultant Plastic Surgeon, Royal Victoria Infirmary, Newcastle upon Tyne, UK

CHURCHILL LIVINGSTONE
EDINBURGH LONDON MELBOURNE NEW YORK AND TOKYO 1991

CHURCHILL LIVINGSTONE
Medical Division of Longman Group UK Limited

Distributed in the United States of America by Churchill Livingstone Inc., 1560 Broadway, New York, N.Y. 10036, and by associated companies, branches and representatives throughout the world.

First published 1991

ISBN 0-443-03463-X

British Library Cataloguing in Publication Data

A catalogue record for this book is available from the British Library.

Printed and bound in Great Britain by
Butler & Tanner Ltd, Frome and London

Preface

'Even the most successful operation never gave me the absolute joy and contentment that I felt in working with a microscope.'

Theodor Billroth

The operating microscope was, of course, used by otologists and ophthalmologists long before hand surgeons. The first clinical use in our field was for nerve repairs in the early 1960s. Its use became particularly important in the development of nerve grafting techniques. It was, however, the development of clinical applications of microvascular anastomosis that opened up new possibilities for hand surgery as well as general reconstructive surgery. Replantation and free skin flap surgery soon led on to more and more ambitious free tissue transfers.

This book brings together contributions from many of the pioneers of these advances. All aspects where the use of the microscope is currently useful are covered, and in the final chapter a tantalising look into the future is presented.

The editors express their sincere thanks to all the contributors, but wish to pay tribute especially to our dear friend and esteemed teacher Professor Jacques Michon who sadly died in March 1989 without seeing his contribution in print.

Zurich and Newcastle
1991

V.E.M.
M.J.M.B.

Contributors

Robert D. Acland MD
Director, Microsurgery Laboratory, University of Louisville, Louisville, Kentucky, USA

Christian Bour MD
Assistant, Department of Plastic and Reconstructive Surgery, Nancy Medical School, Jeanne d'Arc Hospital, Toul, France

Roberta Brockman MD
Orthopaedic/Hand Surgeon, The Hospital for Special Surgery, New York, USA

Gregory M. Buncke MD
Fellow, Microsurgical Transplantation/Replantation Department, Ralph K. Davies Medical Center, San Francisco, California, USA

Harry J. Buncke MD
Chief, Microsurgical Transplantation/Replantation Department, Ralph K. Davies Medical Center, San Francisco, California, USA

F. Brunelli MD
Attaché Service des Brûlés, Hôpital Cochin; Institut Français de la Main, Paris, France

G. Brunelli MD
Professor and Director, Division of Orthopaedic & Traumatic Surgery, University of Brescia, Brescia, Italy

Robert A. Chase MD
Emile Holman Professor of Surgery, Stanford University Medical School, Stanford, California, USA

François Dap MD
Associate Professor, Department of Plastic and Reconstructive Surgery, Nancy Medical School, Jeanne d'Arc Hospital, Toul, France

Paul R. Ellis JD MD
Senior Fellow, Christine M. Kleinert Fellowship in Hand Surgery, University of Louisville School of Medicine, Louisville, Kentucky, USA

Jill S. Forster MD
Formerly Hand Fellow, Division of Orthopaedic Surgery, Duke University Medical Center, Durham, North Carolina, USA

Guy Foucher MD
Hand Surgeon in Charge, SOS. Main, Strasbourg, France

Manfred Frey MD
Professor, Division of Hand, Plastic and Reconstructive Surgery, University Hospital, Zurich, Switzerland

Alain Gilbert MD
Former Clinical Chief of Paris Hospitals, Institut Français de la Main, Paris, France

Helmut Gruber MD
Professor, Institute of Anatomy, University of Vienna, Vienna, Austria

Michael E. Jabaley MD
Clinical Professor of Plastic & Orthopaedic Surgery, University of Mississippi Medical Center, Jackson, Mississippi, USA

Joseph E. Kutz MD
Clinical Professor of Surgery, University of Louisville School of Medicine, Louisville, Kentucky, USA

P. C. Leung MS FRACS FRCS
Professor and Chairman, Department of Orthopaedic and Traumatic Surgery, The Chinese University of Hong Kong, Hong Kong

Ralph T. Manktelow MD FRCS(C)
Professor of Surgery, University of Toronto, Toronto, Canada

Michel Merle MD
University of Nancy, Dommartin-Les-Toul, France

Viktor E Meyer MD
Professor of Surgery; Director, Division of Hand, Plastic & Reconstructive Surgery, University Hospital, Zurich, Switzerland

Jacques Michon MD (deceased)
Formerly Professor of Plastic Surgery, University of Nancy, Dommartin-Les-Toul, France

Robert W. H. Pho FRCS
Professor, Department of Orthopaedic Surgery, Singapore General Hospital, Singapore, Malaysia

Colin Rayner MD FRCS FRCS (Ed)
Senior Lecturer in Surgery, University of Aberdeen; Consultant Plastic Surgeon, Grampian Health Board, Aberdeen, UK

Joseph M. Rosen MD
Assistant Professor of Surgery, Division of Plastic & Reconstructive Surgery, Stanford University Medical School, Stanford, California, USA

Tsu-Min Tsai MD
Associate Clinical Professor of Surgery, University of Louisville School of Medicine, Louisville, Kentucky, USA

James R. Urbaniak MD
Professor and Chief, Division of Orthopaedic Surgery, Duke University Medical Center, Durham, North Carolina, USA

Frederick A. Valauri MD
Fellow, Microsurgical Transplantation/Replantation Department, Ralph K. Davies Medical Center, San Francisco, California, USA

E. F. Shaw Wilgis MD
Chief, Division of Hand Surgery, Union Memorial Hospital; Associate Professor of Orthopaedic and Plastic Surgery, Johns Hopkins University, Baltimore, Maryland, USA

Contents

H. J. Buncke, G. M. Buncke and F. A. Valauri

1 The history of microsurgery

Microsurgery is now a well-established discipline with a variety of applications in several surgical specialities. With the advent of a small, sturdy microsurgical needle and the operating room microscope, the microsurgeon's reconstructive potential has become limitless. The origins of microsurgery are from surgical fields as diverse as its current applications: plastic surgery, vascular surgery, neurosurgery, ophthalmology and otolaryngology surgery all made contributions to the development of microsurgery.

The early work of Murphy (Murphy 1897), Carrel (Carrel 1902), and Guthrie (Guthrie 1908) demonstrated the feasibility of vascular anastomoses with predictable patency rates. Using their famous triangular vascular repair, Carrel and Guthrie were able to perform autoreplantation experiments of the dog leg, kidney and scalp (Carrel 1906). Carrel credits Hopfner (Hopfner 1903) of Germany for having performed the first of such operations. Carrel went on to receive the Nobel Prize in 1912 for his work in organ transplantation. Unfortunately, Guthrie received little recognition for his contribution to this monumental work. After Carrel and Guthrie separated, Guthrie moved to the University of Pittsburg and there continued his work in transplantation. In 1908, he successfully transplanted an entire dog head to the neck of another dog, and was able to demonstrate lid function and salivation in the transplanted head (Guthrie 1908).

In spite of the monumental technical achievements in the first decade of this century, very little progress was made in the field of human organ transplantation, because the rejection phenomenon was poorly understood and remained untreatable. Not until 1964, when Joseph Murray of Boston transplanted a kidney between identical twins (Murray 1964a), and then between unrelated donors (Murray 1964b), was there a renewed interest in the field of organ transplantation. Murray's work led others to review the earlier work of Hopfner and Carrel.

Clifford Snyder (Snyder & Knowles 1960) at the University of Florida, Gainesville and Lapchinsky (Lapchinsky 1960) in Russia were instrumental in stimulating interest in the field of limb replantation and transplantation. In 1960, Lee successfully transplanted a rat kidney orthotopically, thereby developing the first small animal model for laboratory investigation of the rejection phenomenon and modification of the immune response (Fischer & Lee 1965).

The appearance of the historical articles by Siedenberg (Siedenberg et al 1958) on small vessel repair (3–5 mm) and free intestinal transplants for oesophageal reconstruction marked the beginning of reconstructive microsurgery. The 3 mm-vessel barrier had been conquered; however, further progress with smaller-diameter vessels was stymied by the lack of small-diameter needles, suture material and instruments. Utilising these microsurgical techniques, clinical limb replantation became a reality when Malt (Malt 1964 replanted a completely severed arm. The Chinese (Chen 1963, 1965) soon followed, in 1963, with a rapidly expanding series of upper and lower limb salvaging procedures. With the exception of the pioneering work of Douglas (Douglas 1959) and Ladanyi (Ladanyi 1970), most digits did not survive without vascular anastomosis. In November, 1962, Harold Kleinert anastomosed a digital artery with 7/0 silk in a devascularised crush injury of a thumb, thereby saving the thumb (Kleinert et al 1963). In reporting this case, Kleinert recommended that magnification be used in the future to improve the accuracy of such small vessel anastomoses. The first complete digital replant was that of a thumb by Tamai on July 22, 1965 (Komatsu & Tamai 1968), and was performed with the operating microscope.

Reconstructive plastic surgeons have struggled for centuries with the problems associated with transplanting large blocks of tissue by the use of flaps and tubed pedicles. In 1957, Tom Gibson of Glasgow, Scotland pioneered a new method. He postulated that one might be able to transplant a large flap immediately by supporting its circulation with a temporary, small, extracorporeal pump oxygenator while neovascularisation occurred at the edges of the flap. Unfortunately, this project was plagued by haemolysis attributed to the pump, and inadequate funding. However, he suggested that in order to avoid haemolysis, direct hook-up between a flap vessel and a recipient vessel might be performed (Gibson 1986).

To become a reality, a technique for the anastomosis of 1 mm vessels had to be developed.

Inspired by this concept, experimental work was begun on 1 mm vessels prepared in the animal laboratory at the University of California, San Francisco, in the autumn of 1958. The first experimental model was developed using the rabbit ear, mobilising the entire ear on a single pedicle and transferring it to the opposite side (Buncke & Blackfield 1963). Teflon tubes were then used as intraluminal stints, hoping to preserve patency of the vessel long enough to permit peripheral revascularisation. These vessels universally thrombosed within a few hours, and the rabbit ear subsequently underwent necrosis. A vascular cuff device, a modification of the Peyers technique of 1903 that brought intima in contact with intima, was next tried but with limited success.

Working on 1 mm vessels without a microscope was technically difficult, and results were poor overall. Nylen of Sweden was the first to introduce the microscope for clinical use in 1921 (Nylen 1954). Jules Jacobson (Jacobson & Suarez 1960) of the University of Vermont pointed out the value of the microscope in suturing small vessels. While working with R. M. P. Donaghy, a neurosurgeon, Jacobson successfully removed clots from intracranial vessels, 2 mm in diameter, in acute stroke victims. The procedure was performed through a longitudinal incision that was then closed with sutures under the operating room microscope. The term 'microsurgery' first came into use during the same period.

Jacobson's instruments were large, and too clumsy for 1 mm-vessel anastomoses. Micromanipulative techniques and instrumentation were borrowed from the jewellery and micro-assembly industry. The Japanese Trade Center in San Francisco provided the first source of suture material. A single strand of silk from a cocoon was rendered blue with Tintex dye, and a small needle was made by hand drilling a hole of 25 μm in stainless steel wire 75 μm in diameter (Fig. 1.1). Armed with these threaded needles, a rabbit's ear was amputated and replanted by anastomosing 1 mm-vessels end-to-end, possibly the first successful

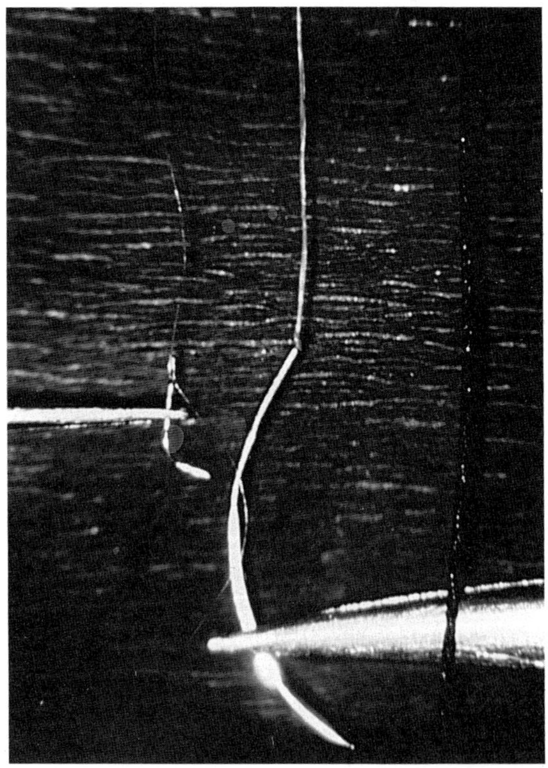

Fig. 1.1 Left: 25 μm hole in 75 μm diameter needle. Note the threaded single strand of silk. Right: 7/0 nylon. Middle: 6/0 silk.

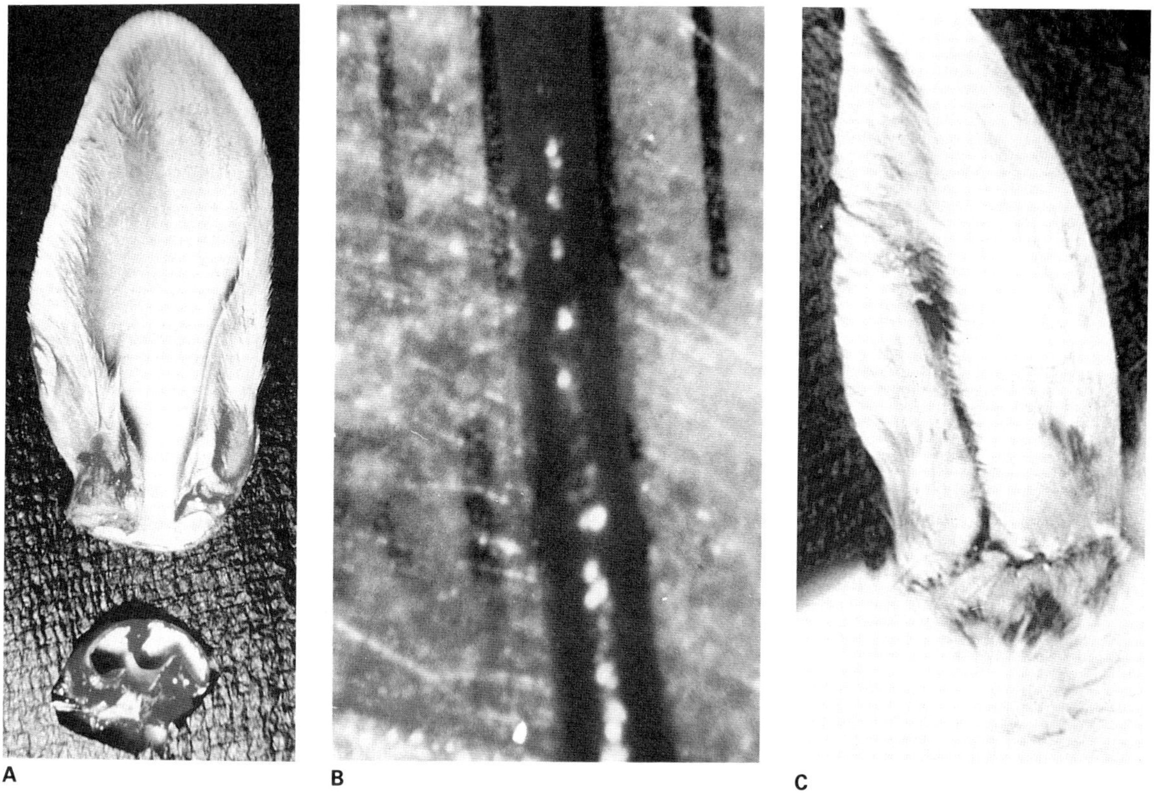

Fig. 1.2 A. Amputated rabbit ear. B. 1 mm microvascular repair. C. Successful replantation of rabbit ear.

replant of its kind (Fig. 1.2) (Buncke & Schultz 1966). However, considerable bleeding was frequently noted at the suture line, and attributed to the large holes produced by the needles. Werner P Schultz of the Stanford Linear Accelerator Laboratory solved this problem by electroplating the end of a 5 μm single nylon strand, thereby forming a needle. Acland (Acland 1972) of the United Kingdom, working with the Spingler-Tritt Company of Germany, eventually developed a commercially available needle of satisfactory diameter and sharpness. Soon, microneedles were available throughout the world. Progress in microsurgery accelerated at a rate directly related to the increase in the supply of microsutures and needles.

With the new equipment, experimental work was continued on primates. In the Rhesus monkey, successful replantation of a thumb and an index finger was performed in 1965 (Buncke & Schultz 1965). Angiographic documentation of patency of the anastomosed vessels proved to be a difficult challenge. Angiograms were surreptitiously performed at night in a San Mateo, California hospital with the cooperation of the radiology staff. The next successful procedure involved the transplantation of the large toe to the thumb in the Rhesus monkey, short-cutting the technique of Nicolandoni (Fig. 1.3) (Buncke et al 1966). These experiments were performed at the Asiatic Animal Import Company, a commercial firm that imported Rhesus monkeys for the development of the Salk polio vaccine. Unfortunately, Stanford Gulock, the owner of the Asiatic Import Company, became critically ill, and experiments had to be continued in the garage of Harry Buncke.

Robert Chase then invited Harry Buncke to move his equipment to Stanford University in order to help set up a microsurgery laboratory. A detailed prospectus for an NIH grant was submitted in 1965 to continue the work in digital replantation and transplantation, and to develop neurovascular and osteocutaneous flaps for transplantation to various parts of the body. One

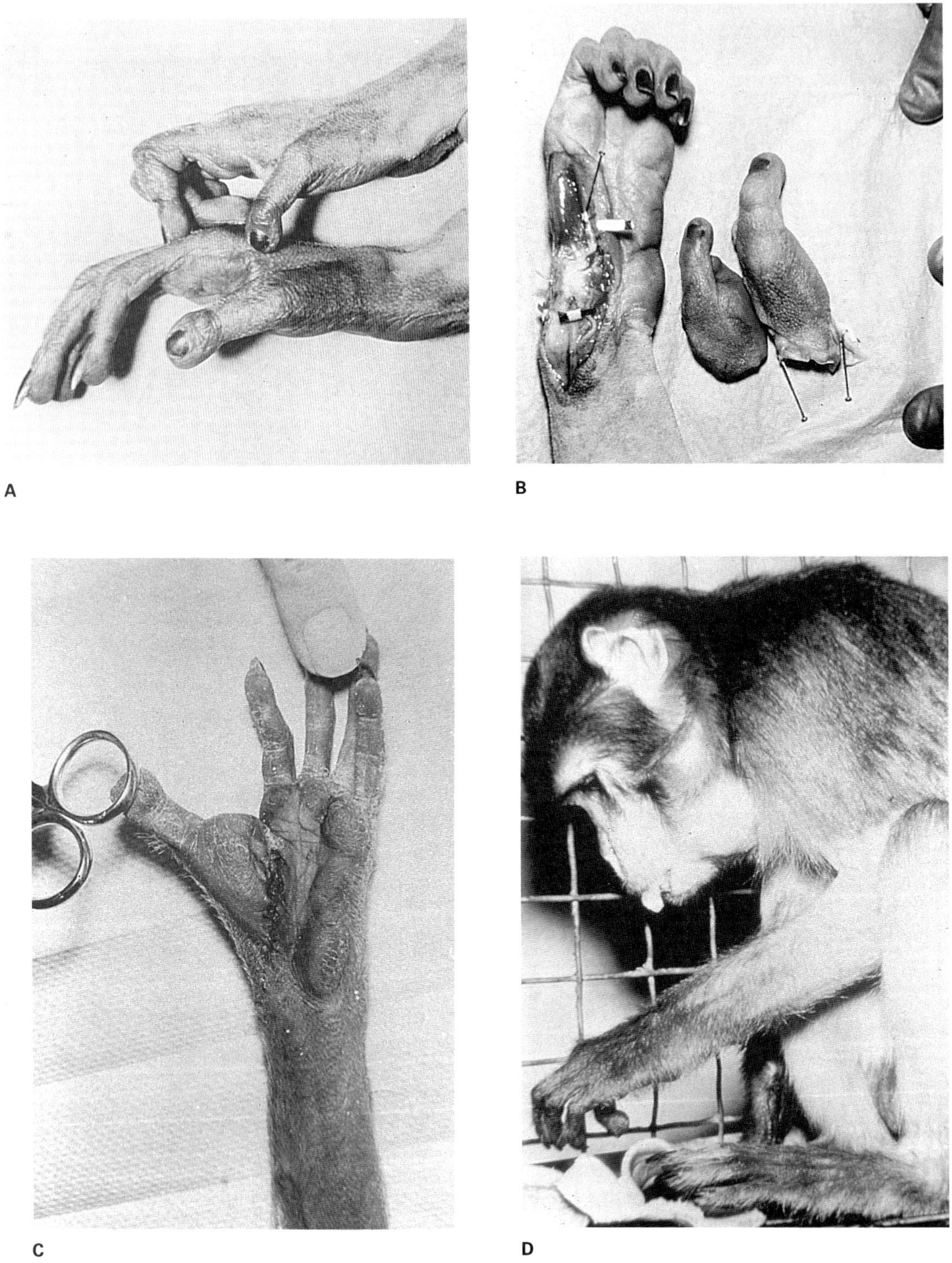

Fig. 1.3 **A.** Large toe-to-thumb transfer in Rhesus monkey. Figure shows the hand (top) and foot (bottom) before the operation. **B.** Amputation of toe and thumb. **C.** Successful toe-to-thumb transfer. **D.** Monkey using transplanted toe to eat.

procedure outlined in this grant, so-called homo-zoo-storage, involved the transplantation of human parts into primate host, hoping to alter the antigenicity of the part during the storage phase. Although the grant was turned down, Buncke and others have subsequently completed all its objectives, except the homo-zoo-storage. This concept may still have some application. The Baby Fae baboon heart transplant might be considered somewhat analogous. Perhaps a more logical process would be to store the human heart in a primate host for later replantation back into a carefully matched human recipient.

The diploscope at the Stanford laboratory became the training instrument for many microsurgical residents who subsequently made significant contributions on their own. While at Stanford, Avron Daniller (Daniller 1971) perfected kidney transplantation using end-to-end repairs, rather than the end-to-side repair described by Lee. Strauch and others modified the Krizek dog model (Krizek et al 1965), transplanting the groin flap to the neck of a rat (Strauch & Murray 1967). While working as a fellow for R. M. P. Donaghy, Gazi Ysargil came to Stanford for a short period of time. He learned, and eventually mastered, the end-to-end repair of 1 mm vessels. After returning to Vermont, he and Donaghy put together the first microsurgical symposium in 1964 (Donaghy & Ysargil 1967).

Parallel developments were taking place in the transplantation of blocks of composite tissue on isolated pedicles, established from an anatomical standpoint by Stuart Milton (Milton 1967, 1969, 1970, 1971). He described axial subcutaneous vascular patterns, and was able to show that skin flaps could be longer than their base if an axial vessel was included in the flap. His work opened the door to the development of direct cutaneous, musculocutaneous, fasciocutaneous, and microvascular free flaps. Goldwyn (Goldwyn et al 1963) and Krizek (Krizek et al 1965) were able to transplant abdominal flaps based on a simple large vessel. However, because of the use of large needle and suture material, Goldwyn's results were less than encouraging. Krizek had greater success in transplanting the abdominal flap to the neck of the dog, using Carrel's cuff end-to-side technique (Carrel 1906) with conventional suture material, bypassing the use of the operating room microscope.

From the mid 1960s to the present, microsurgery has been expanding at an exponential rate. Cobbett successfully performed the first toe-to-thumb transplant (Cobbett 1969). Buncke and Kaplan, in June, 1969, successfully transplanted a groin flap to the anterior portion of the floor of the mouth (Kaplan et al 1973). Although the flap was lost three weeks postoperatively, arteriograms performed shortly before that time showed patency of the vessel. Buncke and McClean, in 1969, performed the first successful clinical composite tissue transfer (Fig. 1.4) (McClean & Buncke 1972), when omentum was successfully revascularised to cover a large scalp defect. In January, 1973, Daniel and Taylor (Daniel & Taylor 1973) reported the first successful transfer of a vascularised cutaneous flap for reconstruction of a severely traumatised lower extremity. Harii, Ohmori and Ohmori (Harii et al 1974) soon followed with a series of dramatic microvascular transplants, describing the free scalp flap and free deltopectoral flap. In 1974, Harii, Ohmori and Torii (Harii et al 1976) also described the free gracilis transplant for facial paralysis.

The bottleneck was thus cleared. The reconstructive surgeon was no longer bound by attached vascular pedicles, and could therefore explore any part of the body for potential free flap donor sites.

Several innovative microsurgeons from different countries and disciplines made significant contributions with their anatomical descriptions and clinical use of a variety of free flaps. In the mid 1970s, Ian Taylor described the vascular fibular transplant (Taylor et al 1975), the vascularised nerve transplant (Taylor & Hann 1976), and the osteocutaneous groin transplant (Taylor & Watson 1978).

The free sensory cutaneous flaps of the arm were studied by many authors. In 1978, Yang of Peking introduced the radial forearm fasciocutaneous flap based on the radial artery (Yang et al 1981). The lateral arm free flap was described by Song of Peking (Song et al 1982) and Katsaros of Louisville, Kentucky (Katsaros et al 1984). The medial arm flap was originally described by R. K. Daniel (Daniel et al 1975).

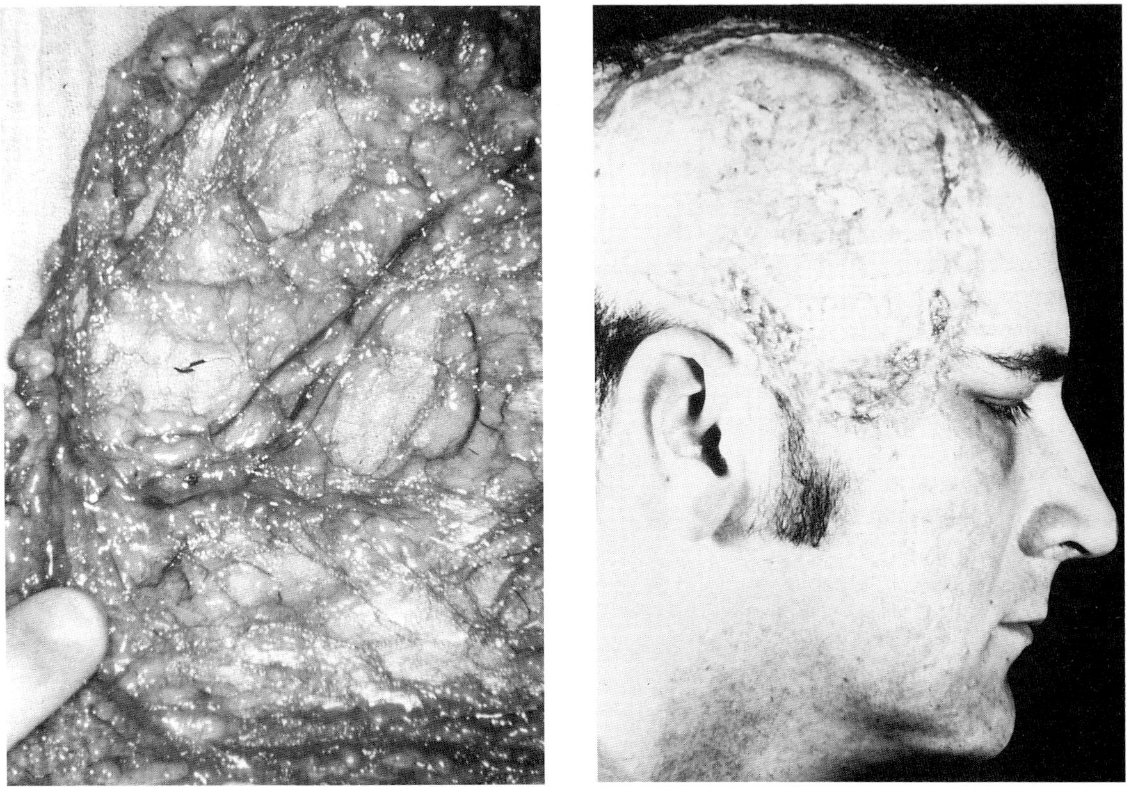

A B

Fig. 1.4 **A.** Omentum. **B.** Free transfer of omentum and split-thickness skin graft covering cranial defect.

Other sensory cutaneous flaps were identified in the foot by McGraw and Furlow (McGraw & Furlow 1975). Many authors, including Buncke (Buncke 1974), Daniel (Daniel et al 1975, 1976), Ohmori and Harii (Ohmori & Harii 1976), and May (May et al 1977), took this information one step further, describing various neurovascular island flaps of the foot. The use of the extensor digitorum brevis muscle, based on the dorsalis pedis artery, was reported by O'Brien in 1977 as a small free muscle transfer (O'Brien et al 1977).

The subscapular trunk in the axilla served as the vascular pedicle for many cutaneous, osteo-cutaneous, musculocutaneous and muscle free flaps. The cutaneous scapular flap, described by dos Santos (dos Santos 1984) and utilised by Gilbert (Gilbert & Teot 1982), as well as the osteo-cutaneous scapular flap described by Teot (Teot et al 1981), are both based on the circumflex scapular artery and serve many reconstructive needs. Baudet (Baudet et al 1976) of Bordeaux, France, introduced the free latissimus dorsi musculocutaneous flap, which he called the thoracodorsal axillary flap. Both Maxwell (Maxwell et al 1978) and Godina (Godina 1979), who popularised the use of the latissimus dorsi musculocutaneous flap, give Baudet credit for this important discovery. The use of the serratus anterior as a free muscle transplant was described by Buncke (Buncke 1982), and as a functional muscle transplant for unilateral facial nerve paralysis by Buncke and Milliken (Milliken & Buncke 1986).

Other muscle and musculocutaneous flaps of the abdomen, thigh and buttocks have been described for a variety of uses. Breast reconstruction, using the superior gluteal musculocutaneous free flap, was originally described by Fujino (Fujino et al 1975), and further studied and improved by Shaw (Shaw 1983). The tensor fascia lata musculo-cutaneous flap was described by Nahai (Nahai et al 1978) as both a rotation flap and a free flap. The rectus abdominis musculocutaneous flap based on the superior epigastric artery has been well known in the plastic surgical literature as a reliable rotation flap for breast reconstruction. More recently, however, as described by Taylor (Taylor et al 1983) of Australia, the rectus muscle based on the inferior epigastric vessel can be used successfully as a free flap with a large cutaneous paddle.

The need for thin, soft tissue free flap coverage was met when Smith (Smith 1980) described the free temporoparietal fascia free flap based on the superficial temporal artery. His discovery has opened the door to the exploration of other free fascial flaps.

At present, new flaps and innovative techniques for microsurgical reconstruction continue to be promulgated throughout the world. Microsurgery is no longer an expensive, time-consuming technique feared by the reconstructive surgeon. The ability to perform one-stage reconstructive operations makes microsurgical procedures cost-effective when compared to multi-stage, conservative measures. Thanks to the timeless, innovative work of many individuals, a fascinating addition to the armamentarium of the reconstructive surgeon has been elucidated and given practical application.

REFERENCES

Acland R 1972 New instruments for microvascular surgery. British Journal of Surgery 59: 181

Baudet J, Guimberteau J, Nascinemto E 1976 Successful clinical transfer of two thoracodorsal axillary flaps. Plastic and Reconstructive Surgery 58: 680

Buncke H J 1974 Panel Discussion. American Association of Plastic and Reconstructive Surgery Meeting. Seattle, May, 1974.

Buncke H J 1982 Free flap surgery: scope and technique. Scandinavian Journal of Plastic and Reconstructive Surgery 31: 353

Buncke H J, Blackfield H M 1963 The vasoplegic effects of chlorpromazine. Plastic and Reconstructive Surgery 31: 353

Buncke H J, Buncke C M, Schultz W P 1966 Immediate Nicoladoni procedure in the Rhesus monkey. British Journal of Plastic Surgery 19: 332

Buncke H J, Schultz W P 1965 Experimental digital amputation and replantation. Plastic and Reconstructive Surgery 36: 62

Buncke H J, Schultz W P 1966 The total ear replantation in the rabbit utilizing micro-miniature vascular anastomosis. British Journal of Plastic Surgery 19: 15

Carrel A, 1902 The operative technique of vascular anastomosis and transplantation of organs. Lyon Medical 98: 859

Carrel A, Guthrie C C 1906 Complete amputation of the thigh with replantation. American Journal of Medical Sciences 131: 297

Carrel A, Guthrie C C 1906 Anastomosis of blood vessels by the patching method and transplantation of the kidney. Journal of American Medical Association XLX11: 1648

Chen C W, Ch'en Y C, Pao Y S 1963 Salvage of the forearm following complete traumatic amputation: case report. Chinese Medical Journal 82: 632

Chen C W, Ch'en Y C, Pao Y S, Lin C T 1965 Further experience in the restoration of amputated limbs. Chinese Medical Journal 3: 225

Cobbett J R 1969 Free digital transfer. Journal of Bone and Joint Surgery 518: 677

Daniel R K, Taylor G I 1973 Distant transfer of an island by microvascular anastomosis. Plastic and Reconstructive Surgery 52: 111

Daniel R K, Terzis J N, Schwartz G 1975 Neurovascular free flaps. Plastic and Reconstructive Surgery 56: 13

Daniel R K, Terzis J N, Midgley R 1976 Restoration of sensation to anesthetic hand by free neurovascular flap from the foot. Plastic and Reconstructive Surgery 57: 275

Daniller A I 1971 Prolonged renal allograft survival in the rat. Plastic and Reconstructive Surgery 47: 168

Donaghy R M P, Ysargil M G 1967 Microvascular surgery. C V Mosby, St Louis

dos Santos L F 1984 The vascular anatomy and dissection of the free scapular flap. Plastic and Reconstructive Surgery 73: 599

Douglas B 1959 Successful replacement of completely avulsed portions of the fingers as composite grafts. Plastic and Reconstructive Surgery 23: 213

Fischer B, Lee S 1965 Microvascular surgical techniques and research surgery. Surgery 58: 904

Fujino T, Harashina T, Aoyagi A 1975 Reconstruction of aplasia of the breast and pectoral region by microvascular transfer of a free flap from the buttock. Plastic and Reconstructive Surgery 56: 178

Gibson T 1986 Forward. In: Webster M H C, Soutar D S (eds) Practical guide to free tissue transfer. Butterworths, London

Gilbert A, Teot L 1982 The free scapular flap. Plastic and Reconstructive Surgery 69: 601

Godina M 1979 Preferential use of the end-to-side arterial anastomosis in free flap transfer. Plastics and Reconstructive Surgery 64: 673

Goldwyn R M, Lamb D L, White W L 1963 An experimental study of large island flaps in dogs. Plastic and Reconstructive Surgery 31: 528

Guthrie C C 1908 Some physiologic aspects of blood vessel surgery. Journal of American Medical Association 51: 1658

Harii K, Ohmori K, Ohmori S 1974 Hair transplantation with free scalp flaps. Plastic and Reconstructive Surgery 53: 410

Harii K, Ohmori K, Ohmori S 1974 Free delto pectoral skin flaps. British Journal of Plastic Surgery 27: 231

Harii K, Ohmori K, Ohmori S 1974 Successful clinical transfer of 10 free flaps by microvascular anastomosis. Plastic and Reconstructive Surgery 53: 259

Harii K, Ohmori K, Torii S 1976 Free gracilis muscle transplantation with micro-neurovascular anastomosis for the treatment of facial paralysis. Plastic and Reconstructive Surgery 57: 133
Hopfner 1903 Arch. F. Klin. Chir. IXX: 417
Jacobson J H, Suarez E L 1960 Microsurgery in anastomosis of small vessels. Surgical Forum 9: 243
Kaplan E N, Buncke H J, Murray 1973 Distant transfer of cutaneous island flaps in humans by microvascular anastomosis. Plastic and Reconstructive Surgery 52: 301
Katsaros J, Schusterman M, Beppu M, Bannis J C, Acland R D 1984 The lateral upper arm flap: anatomy in clinical applications. Annals of Plastic Surgery 6: 489
Kleinert H E, Kasdan H L, Romero J L 1963 Small blood vessel anastomosis for salvage of severely injured upper extremity. Journal of Bone and Joint Surgery 45A: 788
Komatsu S, Tamai S 1968 Successful replantation of a completely cut off thumb. Plastic and Reconstructive Surgery 42: 374
Krizek, Tassboro T, Desperez Q O, Kiohn, C L 1965 Experimental transplantation of composite grafts by microvascular anastomosis. Plastic and Reconstructive Surgery 36: 358
Ladanyi I J 1970 Trapianto dell falange del dito. Minerva Medica 61: 71
Lapchinsky A G 1960 Recent results of experimental transplantation of preserved limbs. Annals of the New York Academy of Sciences 87: 539
McLean D H, Buncke H J 1972 Auto transplantation of omentum to large scalp defect with microsurgical revascularization. Plastic and Reconstructive Surgery 49: 268
McGraw J B, Furlow L T 1975 Dorsalis pedis arterialized flap. Plastic and Reconstructive Surgery 55: 177
Malt R S 1964 Replantation of severed arms. Journal of American Medical Association 189: 114
Maxwell G, Stueber K, Hoopes J 1978 A free latissimus dorsi myocutaneous flap. Plastic and Reconstructive Surgery 62: 462
May J W, Chait L A, Cohen B E, O'Brien M S 1977 Free microvascular flap from the first web of the foot in hand reconstruction. Journal of Hand Surgery 2: 387
Milliken R, Buncke H J 1986 Serratus functional muscle transplant for unilateral facial nerve paralysis. Plastic and Reconstructive Surgery (In press)
Milton S H 1967 Survival of experimental pedicle skin flaps. PhD Thesis. Oxford University
Milton S H 1969 The effects of delay on survival of experimental pedicle skin flaps. British Journal of Plastic Surgery 22: 244
Milton S H 1970 Pedicle skin flaps—the fallacy of length/width ratio. British Journal of Surgery 57: 502
Milton S H 1971 Experimental studies of island flaps. The surviving length. Plastic and Reconstructive Surgery 48: 574
Murphy J B 1897 Resection of arteries and veins injured in continuity—end-to-end suture: experimental and clinical research. Medical Research 51: 73
Murray J E 1964a Current evaluation of human kidney transplantation. Plastic and reconstructive Surgery 34: 93
Murray J E 1964b Human kidney transplantation conference. Transplantation 2: 147
Nahai F, Silverton J S, Hill H L, Vasconez L O 1978 The tensor fascia lata musculocutaneous flap. Annals of Plastic Surgery 1: 372
Nylen C-O 1954 The microscope in aural surgery, its first use and later development. Acta Otolaryngology Supplement 116: 226
O'Brien B, Mac C 1977 Microvascular free muscle transfer. In: Microvascular reconstructive surgery, Churchill Livingstone, London
Ohmori K, Harii K 1976 Free dorsalis pedis sensory flap to the hand with microvascular anastomosis. Plastic and Reconstructive Surgery 58: 546
Shaw W 1983 Breast reconstruction by superior gluteal microvascular free flaps without silicone implants. Plastic and Reconstructive Surgery 72: 490
Siedenberg B, Hurwitt E S, Cavtor C A 1958 The technique of anastomosing small arteries. Gynecology and Obstetrics 106: 743
Smith R A 1980 Free fascial flap. Plastic and Reconstructive Surgery 1980
Snyder C C, Knowles R P 1960 Auto transplantation of extremities. Clinical Orthopaedics 29: 113
Song R, Song Y, Yu Y, Song Y 1982 The upper arm free flap. Clinics in Plastic Surgery 9: 27
Strauch B, Murray D E 1967 Transfer of a composite graft with immediate suture anastomosis of its vascular pedicle measuring less than 1 millimeter in diameter. Plastic and Reconstructive Surgery 40: 325
Taylor G I, Miller G, Ham F 1975 The free vascularized bone graft: a clinical extension of microvascular techniques. Plastic and Reconstructive Surgery 55: 533
Taylor G I, Hann F J 1976 The free vascularized nerve graft. Plastic and Reconstructive Surgery 57: 413
Taylor G I, Watson N 1978 One stage repair of compound leg defects with free vascularized flaps of the groin skin and iliac bone. Plastic and Reconstructive Surgery 61: 494
Taylor G I, Corlett R, Boyd J B 1983 The extended deep inferior epigastric flap: a clinical technique. Plastic and Reconstructive Surgery 72: 751
Teot L, Bosse J P, Moufarrege R, Papillon J, Bauregard 1981 The scapular crest pedicle bone graft. International Journal of Microsurgery 3: 255
Yang G et al 1981 Forearm free skin flap transplantation. National Medical Journal of China 61: 139

R. D. Acland

2 Technical prerequisites and training in microsurgery; technique of small vessel anastomosis

The surgeon newly in training often receives his first taste of microsurgical work under the most discouraging conditions. Late at night, he will be called to the operating room to assist with a replant or free flap procedure that has already been running for many hours. All at once, he is met with a bewildering set of demands. He is asked to irrigate, mop, hold a stay suture, cut threads, hold a vessel edge, keep his hands out of the light, refrain from shaking the table or the microscope — all this while dealing with his view being out of focus, his neck three inches too short, his hands entangled in an external fixation device, his knees in combat with an immovable part of the operating table, and the principal surgeon becoming more and more short-tempered.

For the average surgeon newly in training, exposure to such conditions is not directly educational. The main effect of such an experience is to deter him from seeking to attain competence in this useful and interesting field.

To pave the way for a more painless introduction to microsurgery, this chapter addresses some of the central issues in learning to do good microsurgical work, and provides a review of the essential aspects of microvascular technique.

Firstly, the role of the teaching laboratory should be briefly discussed. A microsurgery teaching laboratory exists to provide the ideal setting in which the trainee can rapidly overcome the early difficulties which microsurgical work presents; and where he can learn the habits of thought and action which will make his clinical work successful. Anyone wishing to acquire microsurgical skills should spend a short period of time in an efficiently run laboratory: to do otherwise wastes an inordinate amount of time. In the laboratory, the trainee will quickly learn that the central issues in microsurgical skill concern parts of the body and of the mind that are altogether remote from the fingertips.

The basic principles of microsurgical technique are learned most thoroughly when the trainee can spend several consecutive uninterrupted days in the laboratory, rather than have his practice sessions broken up and scattered over a long period of time.

THE PRECONDITIONS OF MICROSURGICAL SKILL

Peace of mind

The first precondition of good microsurgical work is a quiet mind. Some fortunate individuals have quieter minds than others. This does not automatically make them more skilful in microsurgery, but it does enable them to learn more quickly and to perform under a wider range of stresses than those whose inner peace is readily disturbed. For those less fortunate (but still determined), the following points, gained from personal experience, may prove helpful.

Do not work for too long at a stretch without taking a break. After an hour of continuous active learning work at the microscope, take a break of five minutes, and notice how much more skilful you are when you resume. The learned ability and willingness to take breaks should persist into clinical work, although the intervals between breaks can be longer once the specially stressful early learning period is left behind.

Fight the habit of neglectfully allowing desperation to overtake you. Desperation comes from allowing difficulties to accumulate. Difficulties should be seen for what they are — finite and identifiable obstacles to success which we must either remove or avoid. In a microsurgical practice session, the difficulty might be: an unfocused eyepiece; a malfunctioning clamp; a needle hooked at the point; poor access to the vessels; blood in the wound; a pain in one's back; or not quite knowing what to do next. It is easy idly to allow each of these difficulties to persist uncorrected, and to allow them to accumulate one upon another until a state of desperate malfunction is reached. It is not the number of difficulties, nor their severity, that is the root cause of desperation. The root cause is an act of omission — the fact that one allowed the difficulties to accumulate unchecked.

The habit of mind to learn in the laboratory, and carry over into clinical work, is that 'difficulties' should be identified promptly and removed at the earliest opportunity so that orderly work can continue. With increasing experience, one's difficulties become predictable. They thus become, with careful thought and action, almost entirely preventable. The surgeon who, by careful forethought, keeps his avoidable difficulties to a minimum, will work with well-earned peace of mind. He will have *set himself up for success.*

Comfort

The second major precondition of microsurgical work is comfort. Surgeons commonly think of comfort as a luxury; but, in microsurgery, comfort relates directly to success. The deliberate process of getting comfortable before getting started is an integral part of a good microsurgeon's technique. To leave comfort out of consideration, and to allow discomfort to erode one's skill and patience, should be regarded as an act not of heroism, but of bad technique.

A position of working comfort is one which can be maintained with the least amount of muscular exertion, and in which every joint in the body is somewhere close to the middle of its working range.

The arrangement of comfort is achieved by sitting down and thinking about one's body position from the floor upward. Comfort begins at floor level. Both feet are placed out in front of the stool, not beneath it; all obstacles to this, whether they are at knee or floor level, must be removed. The feet should be apart, not together, so that if looked at from above, the seat and the two feet would be seen to form an equal-sided triangle. The back should incline slightly forward, so that the line running straight down from one's centre of gravity falls within the load-bearing triangle that exists at floor level. This being so, the weight of the body is borne fully by the seat and the feet. The exact, balanced position of the head and pectoral girdle is maintained by unnoticeable actions of the leg and back muscles. A specially important aspect of this three-point support, balanced-body sitting position is that one does not lean on one's elbows for body support: the hands and forearms take no part in supporting the weight or forward thrust of the body. With the upper extremities bearing no weight except their own, arms and forearms are free to relax fully and to take part in the making of fine voluntary movements, rather than in the production of tremor.

The task of sitting comfortably is made harder by the harsh presence of the operating microscope and the unyielding measurements which surround it and the operating table beneath it. It is worthwhile understanding this in terms of ergonomics — the science whereby the body and the task are accommodated to one another.

When the surgeon is sitting, there is an almost unalterable vertical distance between his eyes and his knees. The surgeon's natural eye-to-knee distance can be increased a little by sitting up straighter, or tilting the head upward, or by forcing one's ischial tuberosities up off the stool. Each of these actions, if sustained, is uncomfortable.

The surgeon, whatever his eye-to-knee distance may be, must fit himself into his working situation with his eyes level with the eyepieces of the microscope, and his knees beneath the underside of the operating table. Clearly, the vertical distance between the eyepieces above and the underside of the table below, which we can jokingly call the 'painful' distance, is critical to the surgeon's comfort. The 'painful' distance has four components: the height of the microscope head; the focal length of the objective lens; the thickness of the part of the body being operated on; and the thickness of the operating table.*

Provided that the surgeon's eye-to-knee distance is greater than the 'painful' distance, he can gain a satisfactory working position by the following simple sequence of adjustments. He sits down, brings the underside of the operating table down close to his knees, brings the microscope to its working position and adjusts his stool to bring his eyes level with the eyepieces; he is then ready to work in comfort.

By contrast, if the 'painful' distance is greater than the surgeon's eye-to-knee distance, discomfort is unavoidable. When this is the case, the surgeon must pay serious attention to reducing one or more components of the 'painful' distance, listed above. Clearly, such adjustments cannot be made at the last minute, and need to be carefully thought out, well before the start of the procedure.

Control of unwanted movement

The third major precondition of microsurgical skill is control of unwanted hand movements, known collectively as tremor. The control of tremor lies not in the avoidance of specific vices, as is commonly supposed, but rather in the thoughtful adoption firstly of a comfortable posture as described above and secondly of a *fully supported hand position*.

All unwanted movement occurring at the fingertips is derived from muscle activity somewhere in the body. No muscle acts quite smoothly: all muscle contraction is a little unsteady, and this unsteadiness, sometimes increased by recent exertion, present fatigue, or mental distress, is the cause of 'tremor'. The muscles which cause almost all microsurgical tremor are those whose work counteracts the force of gravity whenever the upper extremity and the hand are foolishly suspended in mid air. The more the weight of the upper extremity and the hand are laid down to rest, the fewer muscles need to be busy in keeping the extremity still.

* The various distances are described here for simplicity as though they were simply vertical. In reality, many of them have important horizontal components.

When the effort is made to hold the whole of the upper extremity motionless in mid air, the deltoid, trapezius and supraspinatus muscles all must be sustained in a state of balanced tonic contraction in the effort to keep the limb from moving at the shoulder. The unsteadiness of these muscles' activity is transmitted directly along the unsupported limb to the fingertips. If the elbow is simply placed on a firm surface, the weight of the arm and thus the action of the shoulder muscles is put to rest, and much of the large-amplitude random hand movement disappears at once. Severe fine tremor persists, however, because other muscles are still busy, keeping the unsupported forearm and hand up in the air. To keep them there, biceps, brachioradialis and pectoralis major (as external rotator) muscles must remain in tonic contraction. However, if the wrist is laid down on a firm supporting surface, these muscles too will lose the need to act, and the amount of tremor will at once become less. Even so, some small, rapid vertical movement persists, because the hand itself, by no means a light object, is still in mid air. It is kept there by contraction of the radial wrist extensors. If the ulnar border of the hand is finally laid to rest, then the wrist extensors too will at last fall quiet, leaving the fingertips completely motionless.

Three simple actions thus eliminate tremor: resting first the elbows, then the wrists, then the ulnar borders of each hand on firm but comfortable surfaces. The microsurgeon's instrument is then held in a chuck grip, as in holding a pen, with the thumb, the index, and the middle fingers. Nothing moves — except the fingertips.

Note that freedom from unwanted fingertip movement is arrived at deliberately by comfortably immobilising every part of the body, except the fingertips themselves. Note in particular that a forward leaning posture, which thrusts support of the body weight onto the elbows and forearms, must be avoided since it makes muscles in the upper arm undesirably busy.

Every microsurgical working situation is a little different, and in every new situation the surgeon must spend some time and thought arranging good hand and arm support both for himself and for his assistant. This is best done by a thoughtful piling up of folded sheets, towels and gowns to make a slightly pyramidal mound on which to rest the hands and forearms.

The habit of using firm hand support needs to become firmly established, otherwise its value will be lost when it is needed most — at times of stress and difficulty. At such times, muscle tension tends to mount; and if the surgeon's habit of firm hand support is not well ingrained, his hands will tend to rise from their support surfaces and erupt into unwanted movement, greatly increasing his existing difficulties.

Understanding the microscope

The fourth precondition of microsurgical skill is the ability to use the microscope. The surgeon who uses a microscope needs to acquire a certain small body of knowledge about operating microscopes in general, and about the microscope he is using in particular, in order to get the best possible use from it.

He must know how to set the distance between the eyepieces accurately to match his own interpupillary distance, and thus provide himself with a stereoscopic view. He must also know how to set the individual focus adjustment on each eyepiece, in order to obtain optimal focus and parafocality (sharpness at all magnifications) for both eyes. He should be able to recognise whether the lighting system is working properly or not. He should know what a perfectly clear view looks like, and know as though by instinct when he is looking at something with other than the best clarity of vision that the microscope can give him.

The surgeon needs to be completely familiar with all the controls affecting focus, magnification, X–Y shift, and lighting: and with all adjustments and locks which affect the height, swing, tilt and mobility of the microscope head. The middle of a procedure is no time to be exploring these matters.

Knowing how to exercise the microscope to the full gives the surgeon the ability to see what he is doing, all the time, without thinking about it. As the saying goes in microsurgery, 'You can only do it if you can see it'.

Instruments

The fifth major precondition of microsurgical skill is insistence on the use of good instruments.

Instruments are a fine extension of the surgeon's hand; their tips are his final point of impact on the patient. The quality of a surgeon's work is determined by the state of the tips of his instruments; this in turn is determined by how well they were made, how well chosen, and how well cared for.

When choosing instruments for microsurgery, have an operating microscope ready at hand to inspect their tips, since important details cannot be checked by one's unaided vision.

Instruments made of high-grade stainless steel should be used. Those made of softer, antimagnetic materials, including titanium, should be avoided since their tips do not stand up to normal use. Instruments should be of a suitable length for the work to be done; this depends on the size of the surgeon's hand and the depth below the surface at which the work lies. Instruments 13 cm long are right for surface work in a normal sized hand. To work comfortably in a wound 5 cm deep, instruments 5 cm longer are needed.

Almost all microsurgical instruments are spring-handled, and the strength of the spring is of critical importance. If the spring is too weak, the instrument tips will close completely as soon as the instrument is held in the hand; and the instrument will tend to fall out of the hand whenever the grip is relaxed enough to make the tips separate. If the spring is too strong, the thenar muscles will quickly become fatigued.

In inspecting instrument tips under the microscope, note carefully how the tips of forceps meet. There should be no cross bite or over-bite, the tips should meet at a 2° angle, and this angle should close progressively as more pressure is applied, with no re-opening at the tips. With scissors, as the instrument is slowly closed, the two cutting edges should maintain perfect contact right up to the tip. A single wet cotton fiber is a good test material for scissors. The very tip must cut the fiber perfectly, not just bend it. Needle holder jaws should have a 45° curve for versatility. The gripping surfaces should be flat and parallel, and free of sharp places where a thread could become caught. Clamps should be chosen of various sizes, suitable in size and closing force for the vessels that are likely to be worked on. Large clamps on small vessels tend to do unnecessary damage; small clamps on large vessels tend to fall off.

The best principle for avoiding damage to microsurgical instruments is personal ownership, and a firm refusal of any request to borrow. The instruments should reside in the rack of an instrument box and should remain there, except when they are in the surgeon's hand, or are being cleaned. Their tips should never come in contact with another metal object. For cleaning, microsurgical instruments should be soaked in enzyme detergent, then vigorously rinsed in water, then air dried before being put back in their case. Autoclaving should be done immediately before use, to avoid prolonged dampness.

PRELIMINARY ASPECTS OF SURGICAL TECHNIQUE

Access

When a microsurgical procedure is said to have been 'very difficult', it can be seen in almost every case that the surgeon produced a difficulty of his own choosing by not having good enough access. The surgical wound often needs to be extended, and the patient's position altered, in order to allow full access to the vessels being worked on. The willingness to work hard to make a difficult task easy is a positive virtue, not an exhibition of weakness.

Haemostasis

A high level of haemostasis is a precondition of all microsurgery. Absence of blood in the wound increases the surgeon's assurance and precision, both in fine dissection and in vessel anastomosis. Good haemostasis also reduces the risk of vasospasm, since freshly shed blood in contact with the outside of the vessel wall is known to be a potent source of vessel constriction. Haemostasis must be complete at every step of the procedure, the first step being the skin incision. Small bleeders cannot be left to 'take care of themselves'; they must be ligated or coagulated.

The bipolar coagulator is the most effective instrument for microsurgical haemostasis. Its power setting must be frequently changed throughout the procedure, to match the size of the vessel being coagulated.

The bipolar coagulator is intended to produce heat damage only within a very small area close to the instrument tip. Still, the heat can sometimes spread. To guard against this when coagulating the branches of an important small vessel, it is best to grip the branch with plain jeweller's forceps right at the point of origin of the branch; then apply the bipolar forceps to the branch close by, and coagulate it. The plain jeweller's forceps, acting as a heat sink, prevent spread of heat to the main vessel.

Haemostasis is aided by good irrigation. While mechanically powered irrigators are available, none matches a 10 ml syringe for accuracy, versatility, and power when needed. A short 25 gauge needle gives the most vigorous splash — without undue flooding.

When a tourniquet is to be used in a procedure involving fine vessel dissection, it is best not to exsanguinate the limb too vigorously, for it then becomes impossible to see minute vessel branches, and many will be divided unknowingly. The best conditions for fine vessel dissection are obtained by simply elevating the limb for 30 seconds prior to inflation of the tourniquet. Enough blood then remains in the vessels for every small branch to be seen clearly.

In cases where it is impossible to obtain total haemostasis, it is useful to have an ultrafine suction catheter sutured in place at the lowest point in the wound at which blood can accumulate.

Small vessel dissection

The key to straightforward small vessel dissection is to work in the easy perivascular plane between the vessel and its vascular sheath. Once the sheath is divided, it is drawn away from the vessel by gentle traction, and the few fibres which attach the vessel to the sheath are divided using scissors with rounded tips. In tissue that has been heavily traumatised in the past, the perivascular plane becomes obliterated by fibrosis, and dissection close to the vessel is then unsafe. If it is essential to proceed with a vessel dissection in previously traumatised tissue, the dissection should proceed outside the vascular sheath.

For effective traction on the vessel or its sheath during dissection, Pierse forceps are preferred because of their powerful, yet atraumatic, grip. It is unwise to use a branch of a vessel as a handle with which to pull the main vessel aside. Such traction easily leads to internal disruption of the vessel wall at the point of branching.

Whether to make progress in fine vessel dissection with knife or with scissors is sometimes debated, but both are unsatisfactory to the author. Both instruments call for frequent halts, as vessels are encountered which need coagulation. The author's own preference is to use neither knife nor scissors, but, rather, to use the bipolar coagulator as the principal cutting instrument throughout a vascular dissection, using it to divide not only vessels but also all other soft tissues. Bipolar dissection can be done very close to important vessels, provided that care is exercised in regulating the power setting. Bipolar dissection provides a field so bloodless that observers express amazement. After a flap-raising dissection has been done under tourniquet using bipolar dissection technique, and the tourniquet then released, the wound remains bloodless enough for good photography for upwards of 30 seconds.

Choice of vessels

In deciding which vessel to use, and which point on it to choose as the site of anastomosis, the dominant concern for success is the need to work on normal healthy vessels. Traumatised vessels have a stiff, inelastic wall with a strong tendency to vasospasm, and they seem to lack the natural anti-thrombotic endothelium of normal vessels. Vessels which lie within a zone of trauma, whether the trauma be recent or remote in time, should be avoided unless very serious considerations dictate their use.

Good guides to the suitability of a vessel are its appearance when first seen, and the ease with which it can be dissected from its vascular sheath. A healthy vessel has a normal complement of vasa vasorum, can be dissected readily from its vascular sheath, has a soft wall, and is abundantly pulsatile. A vessel which proves upon dissection to be densely adherent to its vascular sheath, has few vasa vasorum, has a thick wall, and transmits no pulsation, gives the surgeon abundant warning that he should not be using it. Whenever we ignore these warnings, we imperil the success of the procedure.

With the chosen vessel dissected out, clamped and divided, blood is irrigated out and the inside of the vessel carefully inspected. Several findings may dictate that the vessel be cut back further, to secure conditions favorable for anastomosis. If any adherent clot or thrombus is seen, or if the intima is not perfectly clean, the vessel end must be cut back. In veins, if a valve lies close to the vessel end, the end should be cut back. In addition, if a major ligated branch lies immediately next to a vessel end, the vessel should be cut back beyond it.

As the surgeon cuts further and further back in search of normal vessel, a second vital concern tends to weigh increasingly on his mind, namely the need to make the anastomoses without tension. This should be a secondary concern, because any gap whether large or small can be overcome at once with a vein graft. Vein grafting should be kept in mind as a procedure of first, not last, resort. If the surgeon is guided by the false idea of 'getting away without a vein graft', he will constantly be distracted from the real priority, which is to obtain healthy vessel ends to work on. Thus, he will produce for himself the worst of all possible conditions: tight anastomoses on bad vessels.

Vasodilatation and vasodilator agents

Good blood flow is a precondition of success in microvascular surgery, and vessel dilatation is a precondition for good blood flow. The importance of vasodilatation applies not only to the small vessels which lie in view under the operating microscope; it applies also to the large recipient vessels which lie out of sight proximally and, most of all, to the tiny vessels of the microcirculation which lie out of sight distally. Through these vessels, the blood which runs past the surgeon's anastomosis must ultimately find its way.

Vessels that the surgeon touches will constrict in response to the trauma of dissection, and will constrict additionally if blood is spilled on them. Following dissection, a vessel will usually regain its natural diameter within 20 minutes if it is left alone, with blood running through it, in a wound that is warm and bloodless. If spasm persists, a topical vasodilator is needed. Lignocaine in 2% concentration has been used for many years: only recently has its use in higher concentration been recommended. Lignocaine 20% is an extremely potent topical vasodilator, but the possibility of systemic overdosage must be watched.

With regard to the microvasculature, the most effective measures for maintaining maximum dilatation are to maintain extremely good hydration and to keep the patient's core temperature above 36°C (97°F). To maintain full hydration, lactated Ringer's i.v. is used, starting when the patient's preoperative fasting period begins, and continuing throughout the procedure. Urine output is monitored for an output above 75 ml per hour. In patients with poor cardiopulmonary reserve, the risk of hypervolaemia is checked using a pulmonary artery catheter beginning at the start of the procedure. To maintain core temperature, several steps are important. The patient must be kept warm in transit to surgery; the operating room should be at 24°C (75°F). A table warming blanket should be in use. The wet chilling episode of skin prepping should be minimised. Extra layers of drapes should be applied, and the inspired gases should be warmed. Warming the inspired gases is the most useful single measure; by comparison, the effect of warming the i.v. fluids is slight. The author's experience is that, in maintaining dilatation of the microvasculature, respectful attention to normal physiology is of much more value than the use of any number of pharmacological agents.

The seasoned microsurgeon, having read thus far, would no doubt agree that fully three-quarters of everything that needs to be described regarding microsurgical technique, has been touched on already in this chapter. What follows, regarding the intimate details of vessel anastomosis, is a relatively small, though central, part of the microsurgeon's overall technical capability. His principal capability, as described above, is his ability to set himself up for success in what now follows.

ANASTOMOTIC TECHNIQUE

End-to-end anastomosis

In setting up the vessel ends in an approximator clamp, any heavy handling of the vessel with the clamp should be avoided. A length of vessel end equal to one vessel's width should project from each clamp. If the clamp is to be turned over during anastomosis, a further length of vessel should be dissected free between the outer edge of the clamp and the undissected tissue. This must be done before the clamp is applied; it allows for twisting of the vessel without undue trauma. The clamps are approximated until the gap between the vessel ends is about one-quarter of the total gap between the clamps. The slight separation ensures a small degree of tension on the vessel ends as the sutures are placed and tied. This tension helps to orient the tissue into a clearly recognisable form.

Any blood in the open vessel ends is removed before it has time to clot, using either heparinised Ringer's irrigation, or a vented sucker larger than the vessel. Adventitia is pulled away from the vessel end and carefully trimmed off with scissors. Only adventitia which actually overhangs the vessel end, or which can be made to do so by gentle pulling, need be trimmed off. In trimming the adventitia, the scissor blades must be safely slanted so that they do not endanger the media. Lastly, in preparing each vessel end, a smooth-tipped vessel dilator should be passed a short way into the lumen and opened guardedly, overstretching the vessel wall for a moment by about 50%.

The principal suturing faults which lead singly or in combination to failure of a small blood vessel anastomosis are tearing, leaking, narrowing, through-stitching and inclusion of adventitia. Before considering further each of these errors of needle-point detail, we should remember that all such errors have one major cause in common — failure to attend to the basic preconditions of microsurgical skill. These preconditions, as the diligent reader will recall, are peace of mind, comfort, avoidance of unwanted movement, command of the microscope, and good instruments.

Tearing at a suture site is caused first by taking too small a bite and/or by pulling the needle through the tissue roughly. Tearing is more common when too large a needle is used. Tearing is also caused by trying to tie the knot when the clamps are set too far apart (an approximator clamp set wrongly can be a 'distractor clamp'). Tearing is more likely when there is already some small nick in the media caused, perhaps, when the vessel was divided or the adventitia trimmed. In addition, tearing will occur whenever the needle tip has been passed repeatedly through the same, or almost the same, spot — as often happens when things are already going slightly wrong.

Leakage is seen: wherever there is a needle-hole tear; or where there is too great a gap between two sutures; or where a suture has been placed so obliquely that one edge gapes open; or, sometimes, where a tiny cut branch lies close to the anastomotic site.

Narrowing of the lumen is caused by taking oversized bites of tissue; or by passing sutures with wildly varying obliquity; or by entangling knots with one another; or by tying a running suture without countertraction.

A *through-stitch* is made when the tip of the needle picks up the far wall of the vessel and drags it across the lumen toward the near wall. Through-stitching is caused by a combination of the following errors: failure or inability to see where the needle tip is going; having the needle pointing downward into the lumen rather than along the vessel; having the unsutured back wall snug up against the front wall; and having adventitia hanging off the edge of the back wall.

Inclusion of adventitia within the lumen can only happen when trimming of the adventitia has been incomplete. Adventitial inclusion is sometimes caused by through-stitching an adventitial frond which belongs to the back wall; sometimes by a loose adventitial tag dropping into the lumen between sutures; but most often by mistakenly picking up just adventitia, rather than media, when making the entry or the exit bite.

From this survey of possible errors, it follows that the essence of good small vessel technique lies in full control, a sense of purpose, avoidance of unnecessary actions and insistence on seeing with every stitch exactly what the needle tip is doing. Hoping one can see, thinking one can see, and wishing one could see, are all poor substitutes for the real thing — which is to see that one can see.

For a clear view of the vessel edge as the needle goes in and out, the field must be bloodless and the visual background dark. The microscope must be brought to high magnification and clear focus during the essential moments when the needle tip is passed through the tissue.

For complete control of the needle as it is passed, the tip of the needle itself should be set up for success. The needle tip should be pointing in exactly the direction of its intended travel through the tissue before the movement of making the entry bite is begun. Its exact direction is determined by arranging the right combination of two relative positions, the position of the needle in the needleholder, and the position of the needleholder in the hand. The position of the hand itself must also be changed in some extreme situations, to point the needle where it is going.

With regard to suture size, the diameter of the needle should always be less than one-tenth the natural diameter of the vessel, and preferably less than one-fifteenth. The ratio between the diameter of the needle and the diameter of the thread should be less than 4:1.

Certain critical dimensions and proportions surround the correct placement of sutures. These measurements, learned by experience and judged by eye, become part of the surgeon's intuition. The bite size, or distance from the cut vessel edge to the point where the needle goes through, is determined by one of two factors, either the thickness of the vessel wall or the diameter of the needle, whichever is the greater. If the vessel wall is thicker than the needle, the bite size should be between one and two times the wall thickness. If the needle is thicker than the vessel wall, the bite size should be between one and two times the needle diameter.

The distance between each adjoining suture is predetermined by the total number of sutures which the surgeon aims to place. Since each stitch does some harm as well as some good, the aim is to use the smallest number of sutures which will give an almost leakproof vessel anastomosis. This number varies, depending not on the diameter of the vessel, but on whether it is thick walled or thin walled. The thickest walled vessels need as few as six sutures; the thinnest need as many as 12. The reason for this difference lies in the fact that the leakproof wad of coapted tissue made by each suture is not only deeper when the vessel wall is thicker, but is also wider. This is due to the stiffness of the tissue that the vessel wall is made of, and to the larger bite size that is taken when the vessel wall is thicker.

Returning now from geometry to action, the

needle tip is passed in and passed out at wisely chosen spots. The tissue which the needle penetrates must be the vessel wall, the whole vessel wall and nothing but the vessel wall. What the histological layers may be is unimportant at the moment of action, since the surgeon cannot see the cells. What ultimately matters is that the needle goes through meat, not fluff.

With the needle tip passed through the tissue, the shaft and the thread-end of the needle, followed by the thread, are drawn through with care to avoid enlarging the needle hole by any careless tweak of the needle or drag of the thread.

With monofilament nylon, the first half knot should be made with a double throw so that it can be tightened in a controlled way without springing open. Tightening should be done progressively, guided by eye, not by feel. Tightening should stop at the moment when the vessel's edges touch, while there is still a visible circle of thread within the coapted tissue. When tightening is overdone and the circle of thread within the tissue disappears, the needle holes are enlarged by the cheese-wire action of the tightening thread, and the suture line becomes leaky and also weak.

Once the knot has been completed with two further half hitches, the ends are cut short with care to avoid their entry into the lumen.

The first and second sutures are placed as stay sutures one-third of the way round the vessel from each other. This time-honoured manoeuvre divides the vessel edge circumference into recognisable sections, and makes the proper placement of all the following sutures much easier to judge. This one-third placement of the stay sutures gives a short front edge and a long back edge, supposedly protecting the back edge from the danger of through-stitching. This works well, but only when there is some little longitudinal tension on the vessel ends so that the loose back edges hang not only down but also away from each other. The stay sutures can be held either in a suture-holding device, or by a reliable assistant. They can even be held one at a time in one's own other hand, but this lessens their usefulness since only one stay can be so held; besides, this means that the hand is tied up when it could be helping passage of the needle.

Whether to use a third stay suture on the back wall depends on how recognisable the proportions of the two back edges are, once the vessel is turned over. A third stay is quite useful if the vessels are thin walled and floppy, or if they are unequal in diameter. Under such conditions, the surgeon needs all the help he can get in judging precise coaptation.

The seasoned microvascular surgeon might interject impatiently, 'But I do without approximator clamps, stay sutures, arithmetic and geometry, and my anastomoses are always perfect'. To which I would reply, 'I do without them myself sometimes, and mine are almost perfect often enough. But how did you learn? And how do you teach?' Let us proceed. These details are important to anyone learning.

As the regular, in-between sutures are placed and tied, the wide-open gap between the stay sutures closes up and it becomes hard to see what the tip of the needle is doing. To maintain an open view of the vessel edges, it is best to leave the last two or three stitches untied until they are all in, then tie them all. Any open gap which can still be seen between sutures once all the intended sutures are tied, should be closed with a partial thickness suture. Once all suturing seems complete, one clamp is released momentarily to check for leakage. Any leak where blood jumps clear of the vessel should be repaired with another stitch — with the clamp reapplied and with blood cleared away. If a serious leak issues from a battered zone, where one more closely-placed stitch might only make matters worse, a loosely and widely-placed muscle patch stitch will often save the situation and relieve the necessity to redo the anastomosis. A minute piece of freshly cut muscle taken from somewhere nearby is impaled on the needle and run back along the thread. The entry and exit bites are made well wide of the hole and, as the suture is tied, the muscle patch, with its freshly cut side toward the vessel, is manoeuvred over the hole.

Post-anastomotic care

With all leakage stopped, any heparinised irrigating solution is chased out of the wound with plain Ringer's solution, and the clamps are finally released, first from the artery, then from the vein. The surgeon is responsible for establishing that his anastomoses are patent before closing the wound, but he should wait awhile before doing so, since 'immediate' thrombotic occlusion takes some minutes to develop. Thirty minutes, which is twice the time it usually takes for thrombotic occlusion to become complete, is a good interval to leave between releasing clamps and assessing patency. During this time, the best treatment of the vessels, other than controlling any bleeding which spills blood on them, is to leave them warm, moist and undisturbed.

Patency can often be confirmed by simple inspection. If true expansile or wriggling pulsation is seen distal to the arterial anastomosis, or within the tissue perfused by it, the artery is patent. Beware of being misled by longitudinal pulsation, or 'kicking' at the anastomosis, which is a sure sign of blockage.

Venous patency too can be ascertained simply by inspection in most cases. The vein is carefully watched as the clamps are taken off it, the arterial clamps having been released shortly before. Once reflow begins to distend the anatomically distal vein, the clamps are taken off one at a time — the upstream one first, then the downstream one. If the anastomosis is good, the anastomotic site will distend to more than its natural diameter and will start to leak vigorously the moment the upstream clamp is released. If venous outflow is unimpeded, the diameter of the anastomotic site will subside to normal, and leakage will almost stop as soon as the downstream clamp is released.

Close observation will give continued evidence of venous patency. Following a good start, the vein can be assumed to be patent if 1) it stays the same diameter above and below the anastomosis; 2) its colour shows a progressive and sustained change from dark to a natural venous red; and 3) the tissue drained by it remains a natural colour with normal capillary refill. A steady acceleration of capillary refill, with a progressive deepening of shade of the tissue, are sure signs of venous obstruction. It should be noted that steadiness of tissue colour and capillary refill cease to be dependable signs of good venous return if there is much haemorrhage from the tissue drained by the vein. A flap that is leaking profusely from uncontrolled haemorrhage may have good colour and refill, but the leaks may be its only outflow. All leaks must be stopped, otherwise the anastomosed vein has no chance either to do its job or to show its patency.

If there is any doubt about through flow, one simple test is often enough to check the whole system: a clamp is applied to the vein just downstream from the anastomosis, kept on for 30 seconds, then released. During this time, the condition of the vein upstream from the anastomosis is closely observed, especially at the moment of clamp release. If applying the clamp causes the vein progressively to distend, and removing the clamp makes the vein instantly deflate, then it is certain that both the artery (distension) and the vein (deflation) are patent. If serious doubt persists after using this test, the traumatic but dependable empty-and-refill test must be done just one time, on whichever vessel is in doubt.

Two good pairs of jeweller's forceps, capable of closing the vessel without doubt but without undue harm, should be used for the empty-and-refill test. The test is begun at least one vessel-width downstream from the anastomosis, to avoid dislodging any thrombus that may be there. The first pair of forceps occludes the vessel. The second pair is applied distal to the first, is slid along the vessel in the natural direction of flow, emptying it completely, and is then closed to occlude the emptied vessel. Then the first pair of forceps, the upstream pair, is released, permitting the emptied segment to refill in the natural direction of flow. The result of a careful empty-and-refill test, performed with clear intent, and accompanied by willingness to learn the truth, is seldom in doubt. However, the deceptive simplicity of the empty-and-refill test gives us many opportunities to deceive ourselves if we so choose. These include: doing the test upstream from the anastomosis; doing the emptying backwards; doing the refilling backwards; performing the test in a blood-filled wound or with an insufficient view; and accepting a committee decision on the result. These are obvious dangers, but the real danger is that the surgeon may be only partly willing to learn what the test may tell him, and to act on that information.

End-to-side anastomosis

End-to-side anastomosis is called for whenever the

vessels to be joined are of disproportionate size, and whenever it is important to preserve the continuity of the recipient vessel. In addition, end-to-side arterial anastomosis provides direct access to a higher and more certain pressure head than does end-to-end anastomosis. Furthermore, in the previously damaged extremity, the problems of arterial retraction and vasospasm, often serious with end-to-end anastomosis, are minimal with the end-to-side method.

Several major considerations in end-to-side anastomosis come before suturing. These include: the angle of anastomosis; the avoidance of twisting of the small vessel; the position of the arteriotomy around the large vessel; and the method of cutting the arteriotomy.

The angle between the main vessel and the branching vessel at the anastomosis is not an important determinant of blood flow. The rate of blood flow that is possible in the branching vessel depends on two principal factors: the available head of pressure in the main artery; and the peripheral resistance of the vascular tree to which the branching vessel leads. Narrowing of the effective lumen at the anastomosis, whether from kinking, twisting, bad suturing or thrombus formation, is an added and important determinant of flow. Compared to these factors, the importance of the anastomotic angle is negligible. Therefore, the anastomosis can safely be made at whatever angle best suits the branching vessel, taking into account any unusual obstacles and respecting the need to avoid twisting, tension, compression and kinking. The only steps needed to establish a particular anastomotic angle are to cut off the end of the branching vessel obliquely at the chosen angle, and then to make the arteriotomy of a size matching that of the obliquely cut end.

Twisting of the branching vessel can produce occlusion of the anastomosis. There is a special danger of producing a twist at the moment when the end of the branching vessel is cut off obliquely. The aspect of the branching vessel which is cut off is obliged to end up facing the main vessel. If the branching vessel lies in an unseen twist at the moment when this is done, the twisting will persist, and will haunt the finished anastomosis most incurably. To be sure that the cutting is done on the correct aspect of the branching vessel, its end should be brought to lie against the main vessel in a distinctly untwisted state. Then the corner of the branching vessel closest to the main vessel should be picked up and cut off at the appropriate angle.

Regarding the siting of the arteriotomy around the main vessel, it should be planned so that it lies on the aspect of the main vessel which most directly faces toward the branching vessel's line of travel. This avoids putting a sideways kink on the branching vessel as it leaves the anastomotic site. The chosen site for the arteriotomy may lie far around the main vessel from the point of view of surgical convenience. To bring it within easy view, the main vessel, having first been well mobilised, must be rotated so that the site of arteriotomy faces the surgeon. The rotation is best managed with a Satinsky clamp, which should have a generous curve to encompass the anastomotic site.

There is no one best method for making an arteriotomy, though there are plenty of unsatisfactory ones. Whatever shape of cut is made in the vessel, the resulting hole will become pretty much elliptical once the anastomosis is completed, because of tissue retraction and the moulding effect of intraluminal pressure. What matters in making the hole is that it should end up neatly cut without ragged corners and without weak spots where different scissor cuts have intersected. Scissors, in fact, generally make a poor arteriotomy, since their squeezing and shearing action tends to push the layers of the vessel wall apart from each other. The author's preference is to excise an ellipse of vessel wall with a number 11 scalpel blade. The ellipse to be excised is grasped in the rounded tip of a clamp made for this purpose, and the blade is run around the tip of the clamp to produce the smoothest possible elliptical arteriotomy.

Regarding the suturing of an end-to-side anastomosis, it is best to put in the two end stitches at the 'heel' and the 'toe' first. This makes it easy to judge the placement of the rest of the stitches. Each stitch of the anastomosis, whether interrupted or running, must be passed in a direction radial to the centre of the arteriotomy, not at right-angles to the main vessel. Radial suturing, especially near the heel and the toe, is most important to avoid leakage.

Often, the main vessel wall is so much thicker than that of the branching vessel that simple sutures will not produce good approximation of intima to intima. When this difficulty is foreseen, the heel and toe sutures should be passed in half-mattress fashion, going in through the whole thickness of the main vessel edge, then from within out through the whole thickness of the branching vessel edge, then out again through part of the thickness of the cut edge of the main vessel. These half-mattress sutures draw the end of the branching vessel down into the depths of the arteriotomy. With this position established, it is possible to complete the anastomosis with regular through-and-through stitches, using perhaps another half-mattress halfway along each side as a further guarantee of good intimal coaptation.

Sometimes, both sides of the anastomosis are equally accessible for suturing and it does not matter which side is sutured first. At other times, there is distinctly a near side and a far side to be sutured, and which side to do first becomes an important question. The author prefers to take one of two approaches, depending on whether or not it will be possible to bring the far side into clear view by suitable rotation of the main vessel and by suitable retraction of the branching vessel. If this will clearly be possible, the near side is sutured first, then the far side. If the main vessel cannot be turned around to make the far side accessible, or if the branching vessel is too short to allow effective retraction, then the back side is done first using a continuous running suture, doing the suture from within the open arteriotomy. This is simple to do, and is preferable by far to the struggle which occurs when a blind far side is left to last.

It should always be remembered in microvascular surgery that to struggle is to invite disaster! The ability to avoid a struggle by careful thought and preparation remains the cardinal virtue in microsurgical technique.

M. Merle, F. Dap and C. Bour

3 Digital replantation

It is the spectacular procedure of digital replantation that has contributed most to the dissemination of knowledge of the new field of microsurgery.

Since 1965, when Komatsu and Tamai (Komatsu & Tamai 1968) succeeded in performing the first replantation of a thumb, in a 28-year-old patient, many surgical teams have performed thousands of digital replantations throughout the world.

Replantation has become routine, and has therefore wrongly ceased to attract the interest of senior microsurgeons, who prefer to focus their attention upon free flaps for reconstructive surgery. The waning of interest may in part be explained by the uncertain functional results of replantation for proximal digital injuries, but this fact has highlighted the success of more distal replantations, where every replantation distal to the proximal interphalangeal (PIP) joint gives the patient at least a useful range of motion.

In this chapter, we would like to stress the technical points that seem important to us, in order to achieve acceptable results for digital replantation at the proximal phalanx or through the PIP joint. We will discuss separately the problems that are specific to the thumb, and we will conclude with an evaluation of functional results.

COURSE OF ACTION IN DIGITAL AMPUTATION

First aid

The amputated digit should be kept in a sponge soaked in physiological saline, sealed in a waterproof plastic bag and placed on ice. If the digit is refrigerated at 4°C, replantation may still be successful even after 17 or 18 hours have elapsed.

Unfortunately, too many general practitioners, nurses and first-aid workers do not undertake these simple steps. In spite of an information campaign in the industrial field, we still encountered an error rate of 5–10% in the transportation of amputated parts leading to a survival failure rate of 75% following replantation.

It is essential to make X-ray examinations both of the hand and of the amputated digits, because, for example in injuries due to machine tools, the level of amputation may vary from digit to digit in relation to joints. (Figs 3.1 and 3.2).

Whilst the anaesthetist is performing an axillary block, the surgeon begins dissection of the amputated digit using magnifying loupes. The best exposure of the neurovascular bundles is via mid-axial incisions, allowing dissection of the arteries and nerves for 1.5 cm. Inspection of the vessel wall with the microscope will reveal any evidence of damage due to avulsion, or of intimal damage as such (for example the ribbon sign). Depending on the level of amputation, it is possible to shorten the skeleton by between 3 and 5 mm, but the more it is shortened, the more deficient the function of the flexor tendons will be. It can be useful to locate the dorsal venous system before attaching the digit. Although this is also done with the aid of magnification, experience has shown that it is not always the vein with the best appearance at this stage that necessarily shows the best flow after revascularisation.

The examination of the injured digits has also

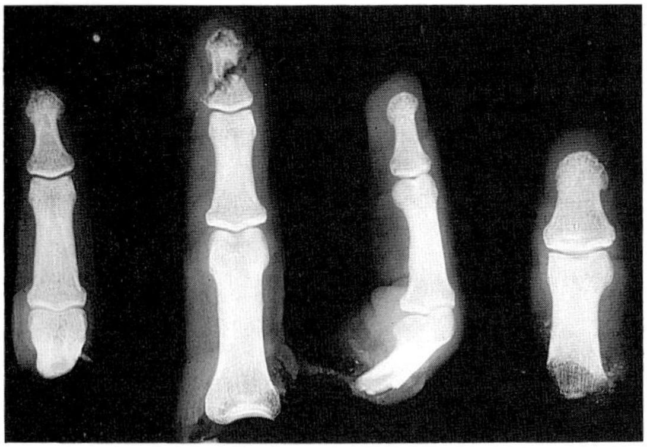

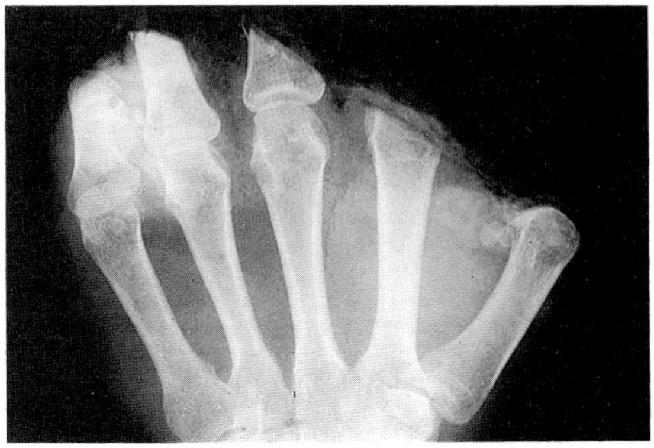

Figs 3.1 and 3.2 Lesions at several levels should be sought on the X-ray of the amputated parts, in order to choose the best method of internal fixation.

to include evaluation of the amount of skin loss, which may influence the decision to replant.

Assessment of the stump

It is important for the surgeon to ascertain the mechanism injury, because, to an apparently clean cut injury, avulsion damage may be added as a result of a patient's efforts to extract his hand from a machine. Furthermore, the degree of crush is also difficult to assess and is generally underestimated, and this worsens the prognosis.

It seems to us important to evaluate the arterial flow before applying clamps for anastomosis. Good blood flow should last at least one minute before any spasm occurs. (Fig. 3.3). Flow lasting only a few seconds indicates that a proximal lesion, such as extended intimal damage, is likely. In the case of poor blood flow, the artery should be dissected proximally for sufficient distance to find the cause of the problem. Such poor flow is especially significant when the patient has had an axillary block, as vasodilatation would be expected in such circumstances. Damaged arteries should be ruthlessly resected until good flow is obtained, the gap then being bridged with interposition vein grafts.

SURGICAL TECHNIQUES

The osteosynthesis

A number of techniques have been proposed for

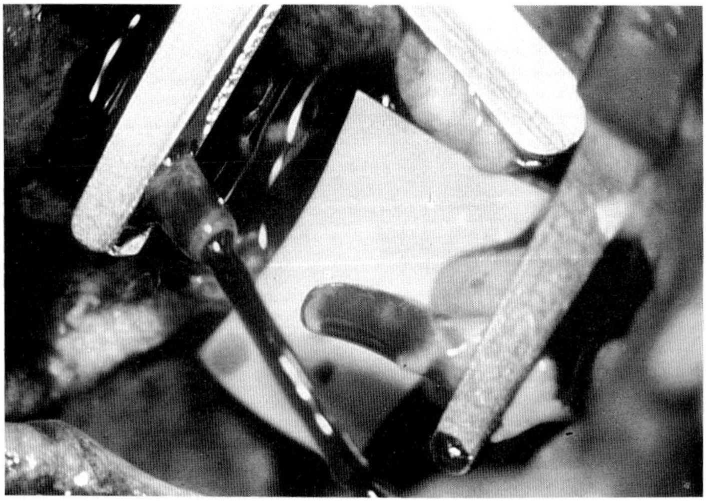

Fig. 3.3 The arterial flow is evaluated under the operating microscope. An unsatisfactory consistency of the arterial 'spurt test' should suggest proximal vessel damage.

osteosynthesis. For about ten years, along with Guy Foucher, we have been insisting upon the necessity of obtaining stable osteosynthesis, if possible using an intramedullary technique so that the surgeon is not handicapped during the rest of the operation; this is particularly to avoid damage to the neurovascular bundles by the use of Kirschner wires (K-wires), especially in adults. K-wires are responsible for infections (9.9% as against 4.5% for the intramedullary techniques) and they lead to rotational mal-unions in 4.1% as against 0.4% for the intramedullary techniques (Guy Foucher's statistical study).

We choose the cemented or non-cemented intramedullary techniques, such as the so-called 'bilboquet', or the blocked nail, or the cork screw when either the distal or proximal skeletal part is short and cannot provide sufficient anchorage for a conventional 'bilboquet' (Foucher et al 1977).

For a child, we use an axial K-wire, plus an oblique K-wire to prevent rotation.

We do not choose interosseous wire loop fixation in two planes, horizontal and vertical, because drilling four cortical holes seems to us to entail too much danger to the surrounding tissues and frequently leads to mal-union, either angulated or rotational.

An amputation through the PIP joint poses a difficult problem. When it is a clean amputation, with a very small defect at the PIP joint, it is possible to perform a PIP joint arthroplasty by volar plate interposition. This has allowed us to restore a useful range of motion, particularly in young children or teenagers; the results are not so good in the adult. For replantation, we have never taken the risk of using a Swanson's prosthesis to preserve joint function. When there is a contused wound of the joint with some tissue loss, an arthrodesis should be performed. This, of course, means that no functional movement will result, but when several digits are amputated, it is justified to proceed with such replantation to provide at least fundamental pinch grip. Arthrodesis should be in flexion ranging from 45–60° for the index or the long finger.

Flexor tendon repair

When the amputation is clean and sharp (as by a paper-cutter or a circular saw) it is preferable to repair both the sublimis and the profundus flexor tendons.

We repair the flexor tendons with an axial suture using a modification of Tsuge's method (Tsuge et al 1975). This suture technique is quick and strong, and is performed with an Ethicon PDS absorbable suture. In the case of the repair of the profundus tendon, the Tsuge's stitch is placed first, then two running sutures, one posterior and another anterior, are performed using a 6–0 suture. The same technique is chosen for the repair of the sublimis tendon, but close to the PIP joint we use only mattress sutures. The A2, A3 and A4 pulleys are partially resected, depending upon the position of the suture line.

Extensor tendon repair

If the ischaemia time is short, we would rather repair the extensor apparatus first with mattress sutures. This repair stabilises the finger in an intermediate semi-flexed position, and greatly improves the microsurgeon's access for nerve repair and arterial anastomosis.

Nerve repair

We prefer to repair the digital nerves prior to removing the arterial clamps, if time is not a critical factor. Indeed, we have noted poor results (two-point discrimination being greater than 12 mm) so far as the sensory recovery is concerned in several studies, if the nerve repairs are delayed until after clamp release because of worry about the duration of ischaemia time. This is because the resulting diffuse bleeding interferes with the proper alignment of the digital nerves.

We advocate the epiperineural suture technique. Contrary to the opinion of other authors (O'Brien 1977), we do not favour fascicular repair of the digital nerves. As these nerves are composed of approximately seven small fascicles, fascicular suture would require two 10–0 sutures for each fascicle, and in our opinion this accumulation of foreign material within the nerve would be greatly detrimental to axonal regeneration.

We do not use biological glue in the emergency situation for primary repair of nerves, because of the time needed to prepare it and because of tension. We reserve this technique for interfascicular nerve grafts.

ARTERIAL REPAIR

Arterial anastomosis

In the case of a sharp and clean arterial injury without any associated avulsion or crushing mechanism, an end-to-end anastomosis should be performed after resection of 1 mm of the arterial ends. Bone shortening allows anastomosis without tension.

For the beginner, it is advisable to use a double clamp which relieves tension and stabilises both arterial ends in the operating field. However, a double clamp is rather bulky and it is sometimes difficult to turn it in order to suture the posterior arterial wall.

With training, many surgeons use only a single clamp to perform such an anastomosis. Furthermore, it has been demonstrated that the turn over of a double clamp, thus twisting the artery, might cause intimal damage (Martin 1975). The placement of posterior sutures first eliminates the need to turn the clamp (Nathan 1976).

Whenever possible, two digital arteries should be repaired. All authors who have reported series of many patients agree that the maximum number of vessels should be repaired during digital replantation. This is equally true for arteries and for veins.

Interpositional vein grafts

When faced with an avulsed or a crushed amputated part, the appearance of the arterial ends might be misleading, and it is necessary to observe these arteries under the highest possible magnification of the operating microscope and to sharply incise them back to completely normal intima. The resulting arterial defects are reconstructed using interpositional vein grafts. These vein grafts are harvested from the volar aspect of the wrist, where vessels of varying diameters and lengths (up to 7 cm) may be found.

The vein graft should have a diameter close to that of the digital artery, remembering that a ratio of 1:2 should not be exceeded for haemodynamic reasons. A graft that is too short undergoes a reduction of calibre at its mid point that leads to thrombosis. On the other hand, a graft that is too long kinks, thus decreasing flow and also increasing the risk of thrombosis.

In so-called 'ring avulsion injury', which is an avulsion type of amputation caused by a ring, we suggest that only one vein graft should be performed. It should be done on the most avulsed side. Revascularisation of such a finger using two long vein grafts could lead to the development of a no-blood-flow area in tissues surrounding the PIP joint. Thus, it is important that the vascularisation of the skin envelope be established through the use of a distal arterial anastomosis at pulp level. To avoid too large a skin incision for the purpose of the vein graft, we use a mid-axial approach at the level of the DIP joint to perform the anastomosis between the vein graft and the distal digital artery; the graft is then threaded under the skin. The proximal anastomosis is performed just distal to the branching of the common digital artery at the level of the distal palmar crease. This technique is commonly used for replantation of an avulsed thumb (Figs 3.4, 3.5 and 3.6).

Neurovascular bundle transfer from another digit

Pho (Pho et al 1979) described the primary neurovascular bundle transfer from a healthy digit to revascularise an amputated digit and, in particular, an avulsed thumb. This procedure is reliable (Lobay & Moysa 1979) but we only use it as a last resort, to avoid the loss of arterial supply to a normal finger which might eventually be needed for a Littler's flap for sensory reconstruction of the thumb.

In the case of multiple digital injuries, we choose Tsai's technique (Tsai 1979), which uses a long vein graft with a 'bishop's staff' design to allow several end-to-side anastomoses for multiple revascularisations.

The re-established arterial circulation

At the time of tourniquet deflation or clamp

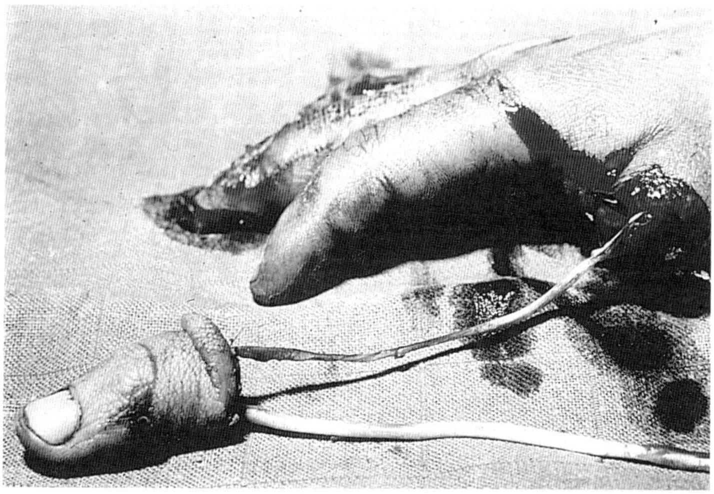

Fig. 3.4 A four-year-old child presenting with thumb avulsion. Tendons have been avulsed at the forearm level.

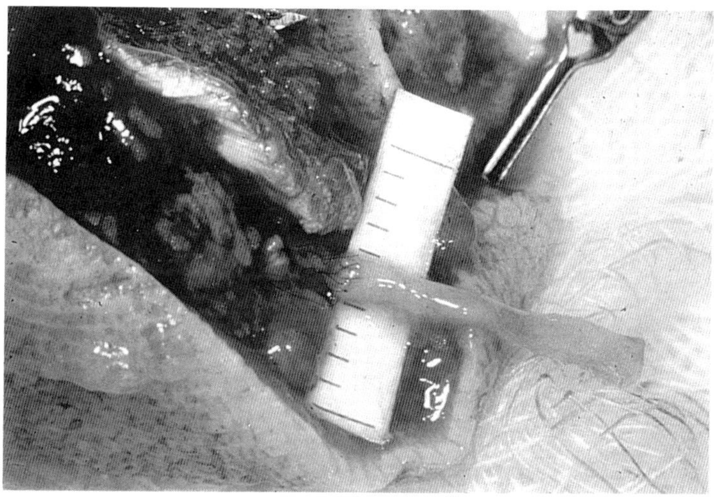

Fig. 3.5 Replantation of avulsed thumb. The distal anastomosis between the ulnar digital artery and the vein graft has been done first, before performing, in better conditions, the osteosynthesis.

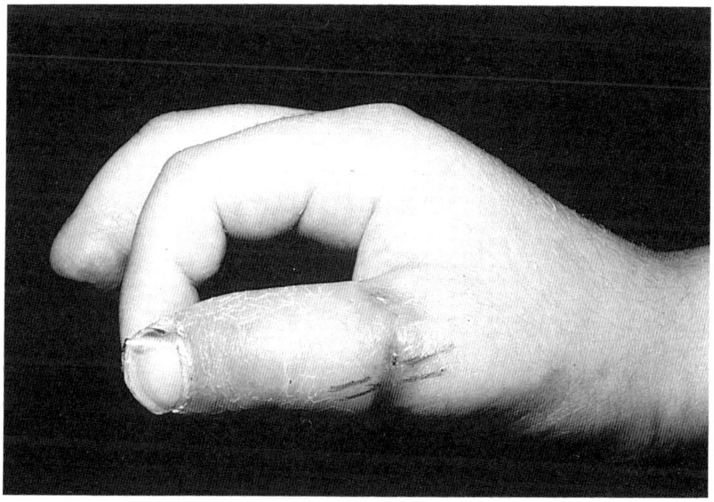

Fig. 3.6 Result three weeks after replantation of avulsed thumb. Later, tendon transfers were done to restore the extensor and flexor functions.

removal, we copiously irrigate the operative field with Buflomedil (Merle et al 1981) to reduce local vasospasm and to increase vasodilatation. If the arterial repairs do not leak and are patent, we quickly close the skin to let the arteries lie in their natural surrounding tissues.

VENOUS REPAIR

The rapid return of normal colour to the replanted digit is a good prognostic sign. A few seconds after restoration of arterial inflow, one observes spurting backflow from the severed veins. In our opinion, it is at that time that the best veins should be chosen, and dissected free over a length of several millimetres to allow placement of low pressure clamps. Direct end-to-end anastomosis is quite easy in the case of a clean and sharp amputation. While the optimal ratio of venous repairs to each arterial repair has never been clarified, we repair at least two veins to ensure adequate venous outflow and to limit postoperative oedema.

In the more difficult case of a dorsal skin defect with loss of venous tissue, two technical choices are available:

1. The more classical technique is to perform a vein graft, the length of which will depend upon the length of the defect. Long grafts may be required if the amputation is associated with some skin avulsion on the dorsum of the hand. Buncke (Buncke et al 1981) clearly demonstrated that such venous grafts are reliable after they have been covered with a split-thickness skin graft.

2. The second technique elegantly solves both the venous and skin problem. Foucher (Foucher et al 1980) developed the 'carrying-vein' flap concept. In the case of a reasonable chance of successful replantation when dealing with an amputation with long skin and vein defect, this author advocates the raising of a flag flap from a neighbouring healthy finger, bearing one or two veins divided at the PIP joint level. The two veins of this flap are anastomosed to the veins of the finger being replanted. This procedure allows skin closure and venous drainage at the same time. This technique can be useful for obtaining optimal venous return in stage 3 and 4 'ring avulsion' injuries; it is also well suited to thumb reconstruction, thanks to the index finger kite flap for dorsal defects at metacarpo-phalangeal joint or interphalangeal joint level. (Foucher & Braun 1979, Foucher et al 1980 & 1977, Foucher & Sibilly 1979, Foucher et al 1981 & 1978) (Figs 3.7 to 3.10).

SKIN COVERAGE

The cut surface of the amputated finger always bleeds, in spite of a meticulous haemostasis. This is secondary to the sympathectomy which has been obtained by the total amputation of the digit. Thus, the skin should be closed loosely, allowing drainage, to avoid haematoma formation which would, by mechanical compression, be a factor in the causation of vasospasm.

THE SPECIFIC PROBLEMS OF THUMB REPLANTATION

Whatever the state of the thumb, or the conditions of the transportation to the replantation center, its replantation should be attempted. Even if bone shortening of up to 5 mm or the use of multiple vein grafts are necessary, the indication for thumb replantation is maintained. If the digital nerves are avulsed, it will be possible later to perform nerve grafts and tendon transfers to restore the sensibility and motor functions of the thumb.

The ideal position of the patient on the operating table is prone, allowing the best access for the microsurgeon to repair the different structures. However, most replantations are performed under local regional anaesthesia with the patient necessarily supine; thus, to facilitate the procedure, we advocate, after debridement and the identification of every part to be repaired on the amputated thumb, the placement first of an intramedullary blocked nail, and then, if the thumb has been avulsed, the suture of an interpositional vein graft onto the artery of the part, before actually attaching the thumb to the hand. The tendon of the flexor pollicis longus, if it has been avulsed, is threaded through the digital canal using a silastic rod, and is then fixed to the transverse carpal ligament or to the palmaris longus tendon. It will later

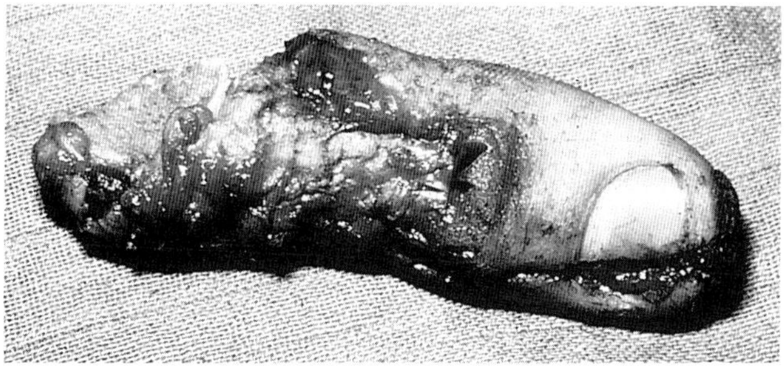

Fig. 3.7 Thumb amputation with dorsal skin defect.

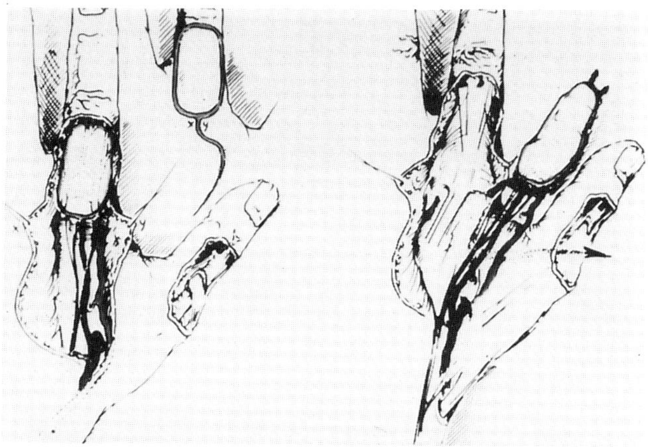

Fig. 3.8 A vein-carrying kite-flap (Foucher) allows restoration of venous return and provision of tension-free skin cover to the replanted thumb. (J W Littler's drawing).

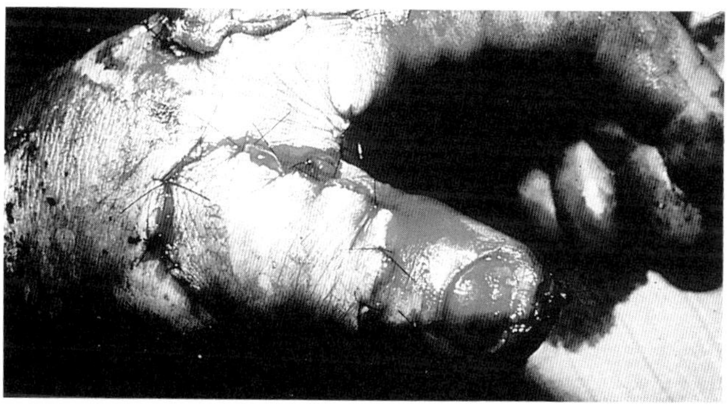

Fig. 3.9 Appearance of the thumb at the end of the replantation procedure.

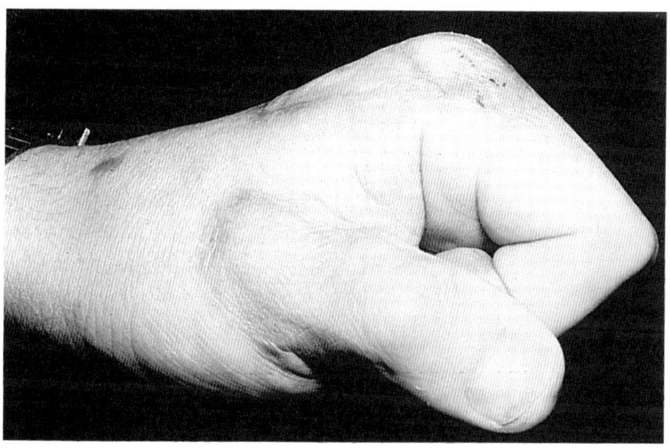

Fig. 3.10 Result six months after the thumb replantation.

be joined to a tendon transfer using the flexor digitorum sublimis of the ring finger.

So far as the extensor tendon is concerned, the same kind of procedure can be performed, and the tendon is fixed to the extensor retinaculum or the extensor carpi radialis brevis tendon. Later, its function can be restored using an extensor indicis proprius tendon transfer.

The arterial vein graft usually needs proximal anastomosis with the radial artery at the proximal intermetacarpal space. Sometimes, it is possible to use only a short graft, with proximal anastomosis to the principal artery of the thumb.

We avoid the transfer of a neurovascular bundle from the third or the fourth digit to revascularise an avulsed thumb as proposed by Pho (Pho et al 1979), so as to retain the possibility of performing a Littler's island flap transfer in case of poor sensory recovery (Littler 1953).

For venous repairs, we perform either vein grafts covered with a split thickness skin graft (Buncke et al 1981) or, more frequently, when dealing with a significant skin defect, we choose Foucher's kite flap according to the principle of a vein carrying flap, as described above.

DISTAL REPLANTATIONS

By distal, we mean amputations distal to the interphalangeal joint of the thumb, and distal to the proximal interphalangeal joint of the fingers.

Furthermore, a classification of these very distal amputations has been proposed which takes into account the possibility or otherwise of venous repair (Biemer & Duspiva 1977; Foucher et al 1981).

The replantation of distal parts of fingers is an excellent operation, because it guarantees a good functional result, even if there is little or no movement at the distal interphalangeal joint, thanks to a normal PIP joint. Furthermore, sensory recovery is rapid in view of the short distance to be covered by axonal regeneration. Finally, this kind of replantation is technically easy and quick.

The replantation of a distal phalanx needs only an osteosynthesis with K-wires, without any tendon repair. Most often, only one artery can be repaired, and it will be found at the mid-axis of the digit in view of the terminal distribution of the two digital arteries. The technical difficulties lie in its anastomosis, because the diameter of the artery will range only from 0.5 to 0.8 mm, and the surrounding tissues do not allow the use of a double clamp. (Figs 3.11, 3.12 and 3.13)

Any distal amputation located 2 mm proximal to the nail fold allows a vein whose diameter is suitable for microsurgical repair to be found. If venous outflow cannot be re-established surgically, its evacuation should be provided by incisions on the lateral aspects of the nail bed (Lendway 1973; Buncke et al 1981) or, if necessary, by the use of leeches.

It is accepted that five days are necessary for the natural re-establishment of some venous outflow. During this period, it is advisable to avoid any haemodynamic variation in the patient, by imposing bed rest, limiting manipulations of the replanted digit, and forbidding blood transfusions which might elevate the haematocrit too quickly and initiate sudden thrombosis.

Distal replantations are technically quite easy to perform, because they are seldom associated with cutaneous and tendinous problems; on the other hand, they require more precise postoperative monitoring. (Figs 3.14 to 3.17)

POSTOPERATIVE CARE

Monitoring

One has to be vigilant during the first five days following replantation; the complications of arterial or venous thrombosis are most often noted during this period. After the fifth postoperative day, venous neovascularisation is able to compensate for poor venous outflow. Arterial thrombosis is most often observed during the first day following replantation. Late thromboses have been most often induced by untimely blood transfusions.

Our usual means of monitoring of a replanted digit involve either comparative thermometric measurement (Baudet 1978, Silverman et al 1981, Stirrat et al 1978, Tricot et al 1979) or the use of laser-doppler. These methods allow the identification of the onset of arterial or venous thrombosis 15–20 min before the appearance of clinical signs. When there is the slightest doubt, the patient must

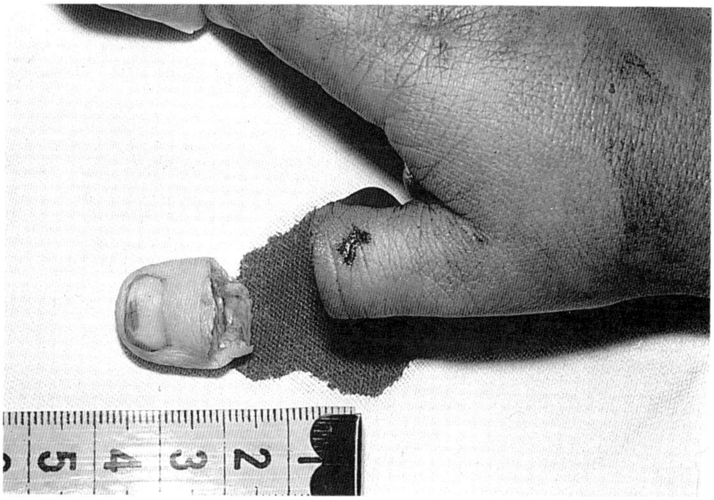

Fig. 3.11 Distal amputation of the thumb in an eighteen-month-old child.

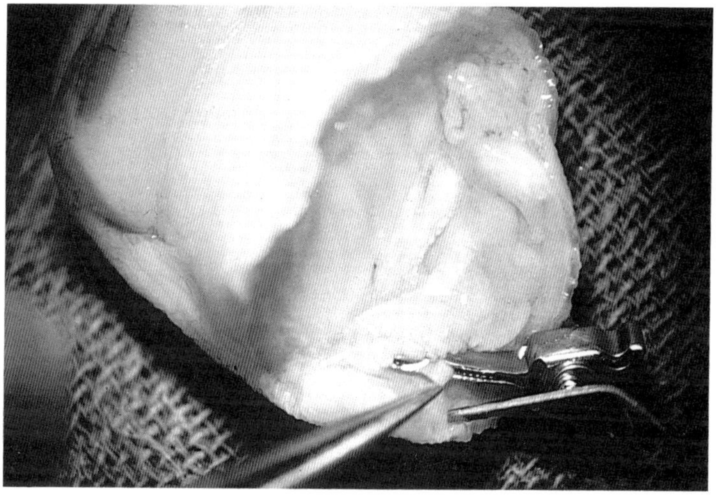

Fig. 3.12 The digital arteries have a diameter of 0.6 mm, and the arterial repair requires 11–0 suture size.

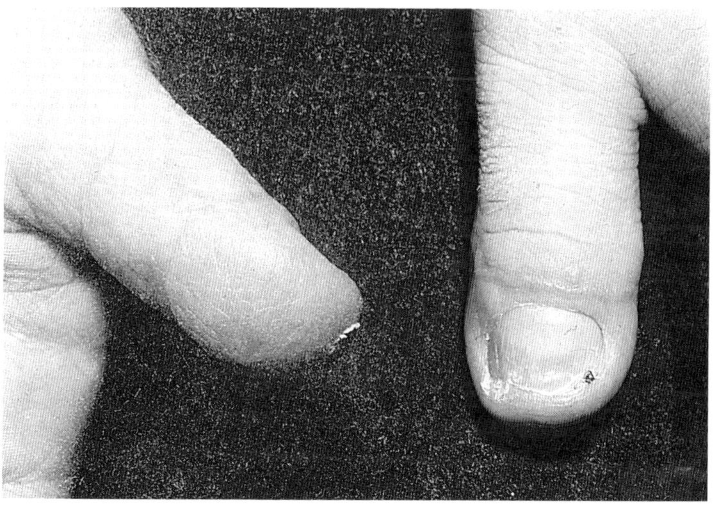

Fig. 3.13 Result of replantation after three months.

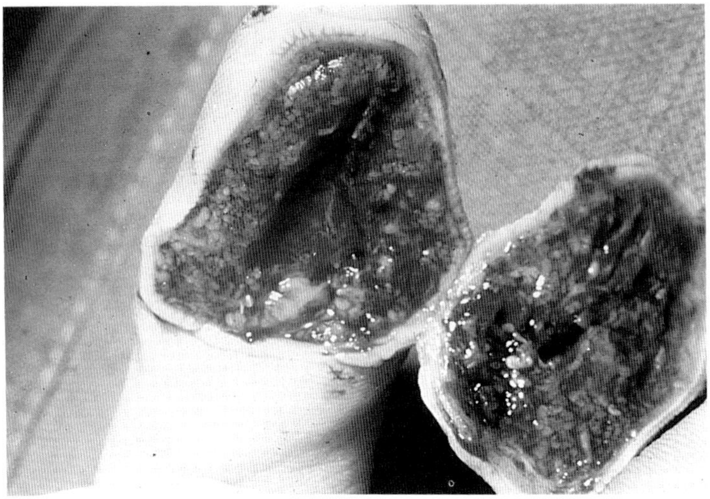

Fig. 3.14 Revascularisation of a thumb pulp flap.

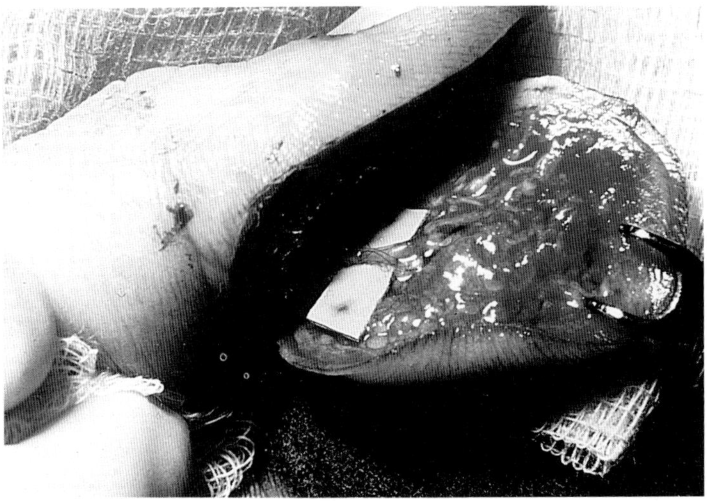

Fig. 3.15 The axial artery (0.5 mm) has been repaired using five 11–0 stitches.

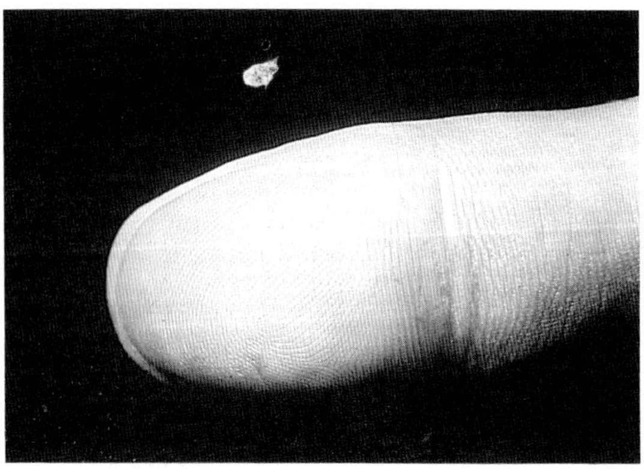

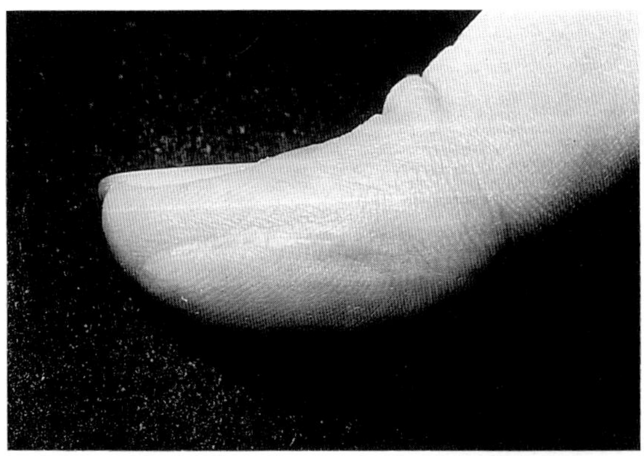

Fig. 3.16 and 3.17 Results three months after the procedure. The revascularisation has avoided any pulp atrophy, and has allowed a quick return of sensibility.

immediately be taken back to the operating room and new arterial and/or venous anastomoses performed. Too often, the decision to surgically check the anastomoses is taken after so much delay that vein grafts will be required instead of direct anastomoses, with a lower success rate.

When arterial thrombosis is the initial cause of the failure, one should consider that a crush or avulsion injury might have been responsible for the amputation. The use of vein grafts, with the proximal anastomoses in a healthy area, is the only technique able to ensure a successful replantation.

Postoperative aids

For our first digital replantations, we used a basic pharmacological regimen including low molecular weight dextran, vasodilators, inhibitors of platelet aggregation, etc. In the case of a non-smoking, non-obese, healthy patient, less than 40 years of age, we think that this is not useful; our experience has shown that such a protocol does not modify the results.

At present, we use only topical application of agents such as Buflomedil (Merle et al 1981) that are effective in offsetting local vasospasm induced by the clamps and the mobilisation of the neurovascular bundles. We reserve systemic Buflomedil administration, for 5 or 6 days only, for cases where there is significant sympathetic overactivity and/or a prolonged period of cool ischaemia.

We avoid haemodilution with high molecular weight products because, if stopped before the fifth postoperative day, a rebound effect is induced on blood viscosity, leading to an acute and irreversible thrombosis.

COMPLICATIONS

Early complications

Arterial and venous thrombosis

Arterial thrombosis is easily recognised when the surgeon is faced with a pale digit with sluggish capillary refill. The diagnosis is confirmed by the different methods of monitoring (Manke et al 1980), such as cutaneous temperature or laser-doppler discussed above. Rapid re-exploration should be the rule in order to limit additional ischaemia time.

Besides thrombosis at the anastomotic site, easily diagnosed and cured by limited resection, followed by a new direct anastomosis, a thrombosis can occur elsewhere at a site of intimal rupture and subadventitial dissection in the artery, well proximal or distal to the initial anastomosis. Its treatment consists of the re-establishment of continuity by the use of, sometimes long, vein grafts (5–7 cm), especially when the initial injury has been by avulsion.

For the thumb, when the proximal anastomosis of the vein graft at the level of the principal artery fails, the solution is to perform a longer bypass vein graft, to reach the radial artery in the intermetacarpal space.

Venous thrombosis may not be recognised for several hours. The observer can be fooled by the falsely reassuring appearance of a digit with a brisk capillary refill. A latero-dorsal incision close to the nail (Lendway 1973), or nail removal (Buncke et al 1981), decongests the digit for a few minutes. When there is the slightest doubt, it is better to re-operate on the venous repairs, because venous occlusion will soon lead to arterial thrombosis.

The abundance of the dorsal venous network allows us, in most cases, to perform a new direct suture, but any suture under tension should be avoided and a vein graft used.

In spite of some rare published cases, it is not appropriate to hope to save a whole replanted digit by using leeches or by nail removal; these techniques are only useful in case of distal replantations.

Postoperative oedema

Crushing injuries, a long ischaemia time, and errors during transportation, are cumulative factors responsible for significant postoperative oedema.

In order to avoid venous stasis, followed by thrombosis as a result of skin tension, it is necessary to remove some skin sutures, and then, if this is inadequate, dorso-lateral fasciotomies should be performed (Merle et al 1976).

Acute infection

Infection is still rare if the digit is well vascularised and if the repairs have been made with healthy tissues. Its cause is most often insufficient initial debridement and/or a non-stable osteosynthesis.

Acute infection can jeopardise the survival of the digit and, in any case, the functional result. Secondary operations are often delicate, and are successful only if it is possible to treat the cause of the sepsis; this is never easy, because of the tissue repairs that are exposed. It is often necessary to use cutaneous flaps to save those replantations that would otherwise produce poor functional results.

Late complications

Mal-union and non-union

Rotational mal-unions are those most frequently observed after replantation. They may result from either a positioning error during bone fixation — the fingers should all point towards the scaphoid when flexed — or an insufficient osteosynthesis with only a longitudinal K-wire.

The correction of these mal-unions should be done at least three months after the replantation, using a dorso-lateral approach (Bouchon et al 1984). The so-called 'bilboquet' (Foucher et al 1977b) osteosynthesis is the more secure method to ensure stability at the osteotomy, and to allow early motion when tenolysis and arthrolysis have also been performed at the same operation.

Non-unions are less frequent than mal-unions; they are due to an insufficient or bad osteosynthesis. Generally, the internal fixation has been done with two crossed K-wires which have maintained lack of apposition. Correction is done preferably through a dorso-lateral approach; the insertion of a cortical bone peg, taken from the ulna, will also realign the phalanx.

Internal fixation is performed with a mini-plate, screwed on the lateral side of the phalanx (Merle & Foucher 1986). This osteosynthesis is strong enough to allow the early mobilisation that is required when tenolysis of the extensor and flexor tendons, and arthrolysis of the PIP joint and sometimes of the MP joint have been performed during the same operation.

The treatment of mal-union and non-union is technically difficult and requires accurate knowledge of the details of the first operative procedure with regard to the nature and position of the neurovascular repairs. For difficult cases, and without such information, it is better to perform an arteriogram to evaluate the vascular state of the replanted digit. The surgical approach will preferably be on the side where thrombosis took place, or where no arterial repair was done.

No sensory recovery

A finger with no sensibility is a blind finger, useless and dangerous for a normal worker. It is therefore advisable to re-operate on the patient in order to restore at least protective sensibility to the replanted digit.

A direct approach to the primary nerve repair is dangerous, because it entails dissection near the arterial repair. We therefore prefer to perform nerve grafts, threading them beneath the skin.

For an avulsed thumb, repair using a long nerve graft is often a failure. The transfer of a tactile island flap, such as Littler's (Littler 1953) or Foucher's (Foucher et al 1978) ensures functional rescue.

Cold intolerance

Cold intolerance is a sequel to replantation frequently complained of by patients exposed to temperature variations. The problem often eases with the passage of time. Patients who had a total sympathectomy as a result of amputation, experience only a moderate response to therapy.

Tendon adhesions and joint stiffness

The functional results of proximal replantations are disappointing, because adhesion of the extensor and flexor tendons nearly always occurs.

It is advisable to propose tenolysis and arthrolysis 6 months after replantation. We advocate a dorso-lateral approach, which allows simultaneous access to the extensor and flexor apparatus. If the extensor apparatus tenolysis is relatively easy, on the other hand, the flexor tenolysis is more delicate, because it has to partially safeguard the A2 and A4 pulleys. If the flexor digitorum sublimis has been repaired and is restricting the flexor profundus function, then it should be resected. As PIP joint arthrolysis is most frequently for stiffness in flexion, it is necessary to release the volar plate at the proximal phalanx.

Postoperative motion has to be careful because of the length of the tenolysis, which results in devascularisation and may risk tendon rupture. The teno-arthrolysis exceptionally provides normal digital function, but most often leads to only a useful range of motion.

INDICATIONS

Digital replantations are not always successful and do not always result in good function.

The decision whether or not to replant a finger first requires an evaluation of the manual activities of the patient both at, and away from, work. For a patient whose job is, for example, wood-turning, the replantation of an index finger amputated proximally is dangerous, because the resulting finger, with limited mobility, will be susceptible to injury once again by machines.

With Foucher (Foucher et al 1978), we have proposed two successive scoring systems to clarify the indications for replantations. Each phalanx has a positive or negative score according to its location. We consider that if the patient has 10 points (see Fig. 3.18) an attempt to replant has to be made. Considering aesthetic and social factors, we give 4 more points to women, children, musicians, etc.

We would stress that the thumb remains an absolute indication, whatever the level of amputation, the mechanism of injury and the transportation conditions.

For proximal amputation of a single finger, we do not recommend replantation, particularly for a manual worker. On the other hand, two amputated rays indicates replantation of at least one of them. For the index or the long finger, we favour the long finger, to improve pinch and to widen the first web. The ring and little fingers attract a higher mark because they are fundamental to grip and provide stability to the handle of a tool.

When all five digits are amputated and technically replantable, we advocate the following order of replantation, considering the length of the operation and the risk of failure, which is higher for the last replanted. The thumb has priority, followed by the long finger, the ring and the little finger. The index finger can be excluded from the replantation if the risk of stiffness in association with the type of work would expose the patient to further trauma.

It is always advisable with multi-digit amputations, if the nature of the trauma to the thumb makes it impossible to replant, to attach the index finger to the thumb position. This will avoid the need for a secondary reconstruction by pollicis-

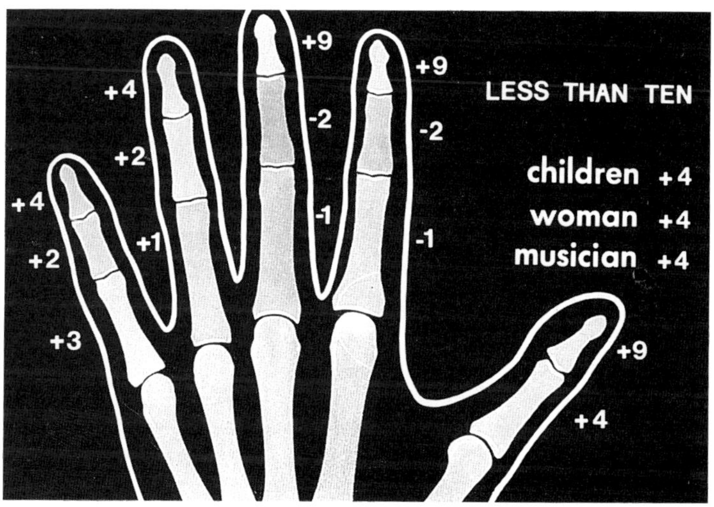

Fig. 3.18 Rating method used to evaluate the indications for replantation. A mark less than 10 is a contraindication. Thumb and distal amputations are over-evaluated, whereas an isolated proximal amputation of an index finger gets a negative mark. Four more points are always given to children, women and people with demanding manual jobs.

ation, osteo-plastic technique or a toe transfer, the results of which remain inferior to that of a successful replantation.

The more distal the amputation to the insertion of the flexor digitorum sublimis, the better the functional result of replantation will be. An intact PIP joint nearly always guarantees a useful result from digital replantation. With the proposed scorings, it should be noted that the digital extremities have higher marks, because the indications have to be according not only to the manual work of the patient but also to his needs at home, during his leisure time, etc. Many patients are, for example, musicians, or practise modelling, or electrical activities.

Replanting a distal phalanx is often an excellent operation.

Like Meyer (Meyer 1985) we consider that a doctrinaire attitude is not satisfactory, and that the surgeon should not feel trapped by rigid rules. Perfect understanding of the patient's lesions, and objective explanation to the patient concerning the likely results of the proposed replantations will lead to a good decisions.

THE RESULTS

A multicenter study performed in Shanghai, Zurich and Louisville (Wei et al 1981) showed a success rate ranging from 72.7 to 97.3%, according to the nature of the trauma. However, this high success rate includes every limb replantation.

The digital replantation series shows that the Asian continent has remarkable success. Thus, Tamai's results of 229 digits (including 91 partial amputations = 40%) showed 89.5% success (Tamai et al 1981), but mixing replantation and revascularisation enhances the results. In fact, in a statistical analysis from as early as 1984 of 125 replanted and revascularised thumbs (Merle et al 1984), we noticed that, when the amputation was total, the success rate was 59.7%, whereas when it was partial with total devascularisation, the success rate was 82.6%.

The success rate was reduced for certain types of lesions, particularly the ring avulsion injuries grade 3 and 4; we achieved 7% survival for grade 4, and 17% for grade 3. The statistical study performed by Dap of 90 cases of replantations and revascularisations of the thumb showed the importance of the influence of tobacco in Western patients (Dap 1982). A patient smoking more than 20 cigarettes per day had 20% less chance of success. The same is noted if the ischaemia time is over 6 hours when, in spite of good transportation conditions, the rate is 15% lower.

The worst lesions are those due to a crushing injury, whereas avulsion injuries have a success rate close to those of clean cuts, thanks to the systematic use of vein bypass grafts. The benefit of such replantations is unquestionably better, from the psychological, social and functional points of view, compared with that of a definitive amputation. A study by an insurance company (Dap 1989), of 40 accidents at work causing thumb amputation, demonstrated that replantation costs more than amputation, taking into account only the surgery and the time of working incapacity (6 months for an amputation; 8 months for a replantation); but long term, considering the permanent partial incapacity, we observe that for a totally amputated thumb, the incapacity can be 26% (average) whereas it goes down to 11% after replantation.

The saving for the French economy, for a replanted thumb in a 30-year-old worker, is over 10 000 U.S. dollars. This benefit is slightly lower if we consider the replantation of a finger at the proximal phalanx level, because it is often necessary to perform a flexor tenolysis within 4 or 5 months after replantation to get a useful range of motion (between +30° and +60° of active flexion).

CONCLUSIONS

Digital replantation should be performed by well-trained teams, because it is not only necessary to master vascular and nerve microsurgical problems, but also to obtain useful functional results through a full knowledge of osteosynthesis and of skin coverage.

The benefits for the patient, and for society, are obvious and justify such operations.

the dorsum of the index to the thumb. Plastic and Reconstructive Surgery 63: 344–349

Foucher G, Braun F, Merle M, Michon J 1980 Le 'doigt-banque' en traumatologie de la main. Annales de Chirurgie 34 (9): 693–698

Foucher G, Merle M, Michon J 1977a Intérêt de l'osteosynthèse dans la stabilisation des fractures du squelette metacarpo-phalangien. Annales de Chirurgie 31 (12): 1065–1969

Foucher G, Merle M, Michon J 1977b L'osteosynthèse Bilboquet. Annales de Chirurgie 31 (12): 1107–1108

Foucher G, Sibilly A 1979 La replantation et la revascularisation digitale. Pourquoi, quand et comment? A propos d'une serie de 42 cas. Journal of Medicine; Clinical, Experimental and Theoretical 10 (2): 69–73

Foucher G, Merle M, Braun J B 1981 Distal digital replantation is one of the best indications for microsurgery. International Journal of Microsurgery 3 (4): 263–270

Foucher G, Braun J B, Merle M, Sibilly A 1978 Le lambeau 'cerf-volant'. Annales de Chirurgie 32 (9): 593–596

Komatsu S, Tamai S 1968 Successful replantation of a completely cut-off thumb. Case report. Plastic and Reconstructive Surgery 42: 374–377

Lendway P G 1973 Replacement of the amputated digit. British Journal of Plastic Surgery 26: 398–401

Littler J W 1953 The neuro-vascular pedicle method of digital transposition for reconstruction of the thumb. Plastic and Reconstructive Surgery 12: 303–319

Lobay G W, Moysa G L 1979 Primary neuro-vascular bundle transfer in the management of avulsed thumbs. Journal of Hand Surgery 4 (1): 1–10

Manke D A, Summer D S, Van Beek A L, Lambeth A 1980 Hemodynamic studies of digital and extremity replants and revascularizations. Surgery 88 (3): 445–452

Martin L 1975 Apport du microscope électronique à balayage dans l'évaluation des traumatismes endotheliaux en microchirurgie vasculaire. Thèse Médicale, Nancy, 29 (11): 1019–1023

Merle M, Foucher G, Michon J 1976 Role de l'incision de décharge digito-palmaire dans la lutte contre l'oedemé post-traumatique. Annales de Chirurgie Plastique et Esthétique 21 (4): 263–266

Merle M, Foucher G 1986 Internal fixation for complex hand injuries. Technics in Orthopaedics 1: 14–17

Merle M, Della Santa D, Bayley Y, Chardonnal J, Foucher G, Benichoux R 1981 Buflomedil in vascular microsurgery. A study of the rate of blood flow in the rabbit femoral artery after replantation of the paw. International Journal of Microsurgery 3: 49–52

Merle M, Dap F, Foucher G, Bouchon Y, Michon J 1984 Réimplantation et revascularisation du pouce. Problèmes techniques et résultats. A propos de 125 cas. Chirurgie 110: 225–265

Merle M, Michon J, Foucher G 1976 Utilisation d'une cotation dans la réposition des doigts. Nouvelle Presse Médicale 36 (5): 2392

Meyer V E 1985 Upper extremity replantation. Churchill Livingstone, Edinburgh

Nathan P, Rose M C 1976 An alternative technique for microvascular suture. Plastic and Reconstructive Surgery 58: 635–637

O'Brien B, MacC 1977 Microvascular reconstructive surgery. Churchill Livingstone, Edinburgh

Pho R W H, Chacha P S, Yeo K Q 1979 Rerouting vessels and nerves from other digits in replanting an avulsed and degloved thumb. Plastic and Reconstructive Surgery 64 (3): 330–335

Silvermann D G, Cedrone F A, Hurford W E, Bering T G, Larossa D D 1981 Monitoring tissue alimentation of fluorescein with the perfusion fluoremeter: a new method to assess capillary blood flow. Surgery 90 (2): 409–416

Stirrat C R, Seaber A V, Urbaniak J R, Bright D S 1978 Temperature monitoring in digital replantation. Journal of Hand Surgery 3 (4): 342–347

Tamai S, Hori Y, Fukui A, Shimizu T 1981 Finger replantation. International Surgery 66 (1): 9–12

Tricot P, Bastien M, Choffat P, Merle M, Benichoux R 1979 Le triangle critique de surveillance des températures cutanées peripheriques au cours du choc ou après replantation de membre. Annales de Chirurgie 33 (9): 729–730

Tsai T M 1979 A complex reimplantation of digits: a case report. Journal of Hand Surgery 4 (2): 145–149

Tsuge K, Ikuta Y, Matsuishi Y 1975 Intratendinous tendon suture in the hand. A new technique. Hand 7: 250–255

Wei C Z, Meyer V E, Kleinert H E, Beasley R W 1981 Present indications and contra-indications for replantation as reflected by long term functional results. Orthopaedic Clinics of North America 12: 849–870

V. E. Meyer

4 Major limb replantation and revascularisation

GENERAL CONSIDERATION OF INDICATIONS

Upper limb amputations are serious compound injuries, the management of which demands not only microsurgical skill but also thorough competence in major traumatology, all aspects of hand surgery and a good knowledge of the pathophysiology of the post-ischaemia syndrome; the latter may be a source of life-threatening complications, a distinct difference to so-called minor (distal) replantations, where such severe problems do not exist.

The basic consideration of indications must embrace the general condition of the patient, his age, type of injury, level of injury, duration of tissue anoxia, occupation and psychological factors. Any decision as to whether or not to attempt to salvage an amputated or devascularised limb must be based on careful analysis of these parameters. Limb replantation and revascularisation surgery presents a heavy commitment for an institution. Due consideration must be given to all aspects of the organisation of a replantation center (Biemer 1988, Burton et al 1981, Meyer 1985a).

General condition of the patient

The general condition of the patient must be such that he presents an acceptable risk for undergoing the long and complex surgical procedure. Every patient must be carefully examined to detect concomitant injuries as well as pre-existing general health problems, for example cardio-pulmonary, vascular or metabolic disease. Also, severe mental handicap may possibly preclude an attempt at limb salvage. Any other serious or even life-threatening condition, for example traumatic shock, haemo-pneumothorax, intra-abdominal haemorrhage, cerebral injury, may either preclude replantation or must be appropriately treated before embarking on limb replantation or revascularisation. Haemorrhage must be under control, shock must be adequately treated, and in the case of rib fractures, a suction drainage of the pleural cavity should be established, before starting long-term anaesthesia, in order to eliminate the risk of pneumothorax under tension during the operation, etc. These concomitant injuries are much more frequent in proximal amputations than in distal ones, because of the usually much more violent nature of the accident in these cases. Therefore, an accurate history of the circumstances of the accident is most important, especially details of the mechanism of the injury, which may provide information about the type of contact surfaces, any exposure to abnormal temperature, chemical agents and the distribution of the forces involved.

Age

The age of the patient should be considered from a biological rather than a chronological point of view. In elderly individuals, distal forearm or hand replantations may be definitely worthwhile in well selected cases (Fig. 4.1 A–E). In practice, however, major limb replantation beyond the age of 50 should be a rare exception, because besides the potentially life-threatening risks discussed later, the functional results also become increasingly less favorable with age. The most obvious reasons for this are a higher frequency of joint stiffness, ten-

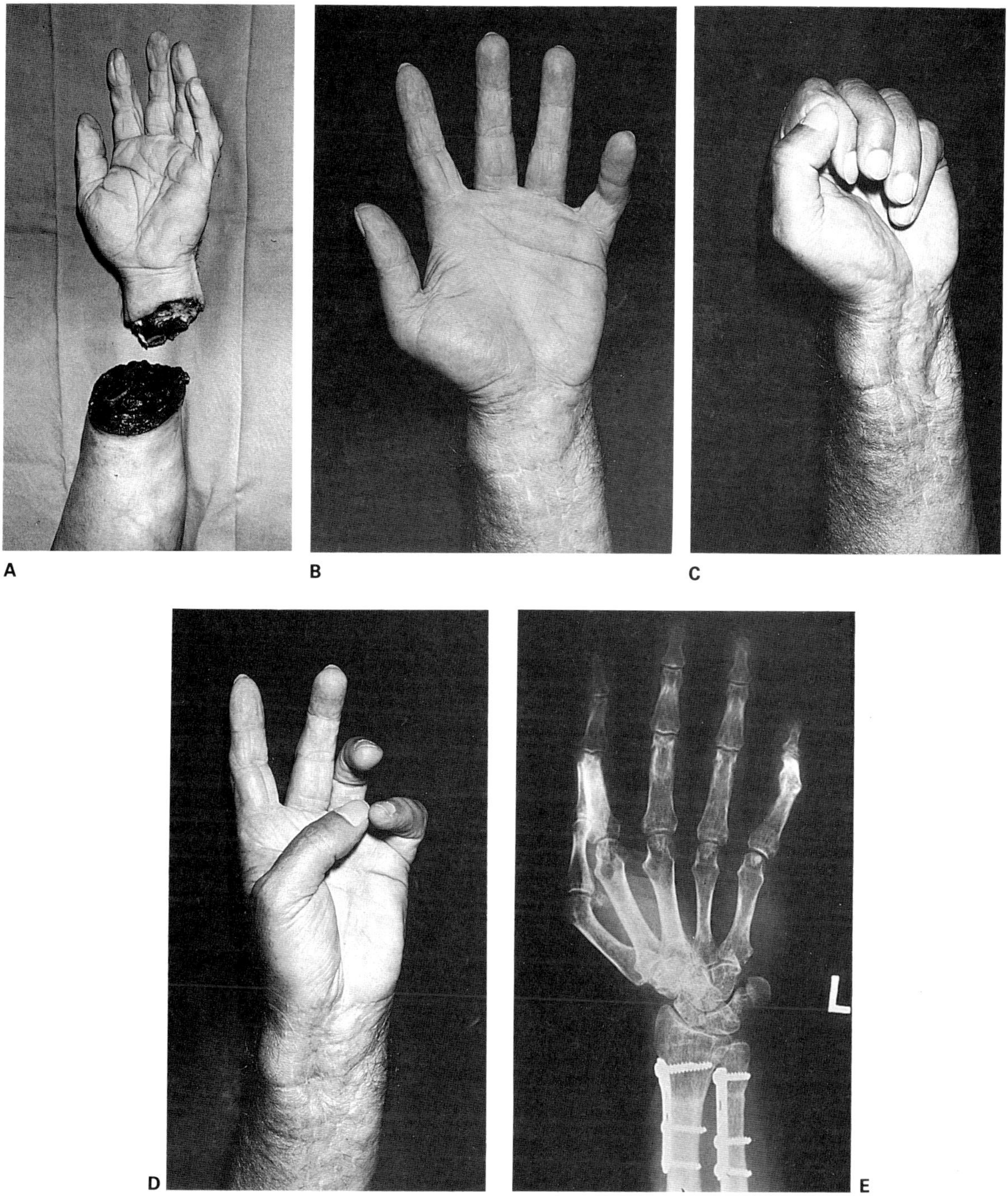

Fig. 4.1 **A.** Guillotine-like amputation in distal quarter of the forearm in a 62-year-old joiner. **B–D.** Condition 2 years after replantation with total primary repair. No secondary surgery has been performed in this case.
E. The X-ray taken 3 years after replantation shows perfect bone healing after rigid internal fixation by two AO-plates. This patient refused the removal of the metal plates because he was afraid of complications. This example shows that replantation of a hand may also be rewarding in well selected elderly patients. (**A** reprinted with permission from Meyer et al 1981. **B–D** reprinted with permission from Meyer V E 1983 In: Evarts C M (ed) Surgery of the musculoskeletal system, Vol. 1. Churchill Livingstone, New York.)

don adhesions, poorer nerve regeneration, little potential for sensory re-education and a high frequency of severe cold intolerance. In children, however, the indication for replantation and revascularisation is much less limited, as they have an amazing potential for nerve regeneration and sensory (self) re-education, and are, in general, free from such problems as joint stiffness and cold intolerance (see Ch. 5).

Type of injury

There are two important categories of injury to be distinguished:

1. Complete severance (i.e. amputation)
2. Incomplete severance with disruption of the main vascular system to the extent that the part distal to the injury would not survive without vascular reconstruction.

The surgical procedure for the first category is called *replantation*, the one for the second category is called *revascularisation for survival*. In fact, there are cases of incomplete severance in which the vascular damage is not so severe as to threaten the survival of the part distal to the injury. If, in these cases, vascular anastomoses are performed, they are done with the intention of improving the potential for functional recovery of the part; thus, this procedure is called *revascularisation for improvement* (Chen Zhong-Wei et al 1981, Meyer 1985a).

For later evaluation of functional results, the categories of revascularisations need further classification. This is a most difficult task, because there are so many possible combinations of severed and intact tissue structures. Biemer suggested a classification for cases of incomplete severance (so-called subtotal amputations) distal to the wrist which also could serve as a basis for cases with more proximal lesions (Biemer 1982, Burton 1981).

For cases with complete severance, the following classification into four categories of injuries has proved to be useful (Chen Zhong-Wei et al 1981, Meyer 1985a).

1. Guillotine-type amputation

Unless the amputated part has suffered significantly from anoxia, tissues will be normal except for those on the cut surface. Only minimal debridement will be necessary. The prognosis for survival is optimal. These injuries usually occur with high speed circular saws, metal plate, plastic and paper cutting machines, etc. (Fig. 4.2).

2. Crush amputation with local tissue damage

Some crush amputations have limited tissue damage proximal and distal to the level of amputation. More extensive debridement is required, with consequently more extensive shortening of the skeleton. In this way, the crush amputation is largely converted into a guillotine-type amputation, with correspondingly good prognosis for survival. These injuries may be caused by, for example, mechanical presses, with subsequent destruction of a segment of the extremity (Fig. 4.3).

3. Crush amputation with extensive diffuse tissue damage

A crush amputation with extensive diffuse tissue damage is usually the result of violent blunt trauma. The wounds are irregular, and the extensive tissue damage occasionally may even extend through the whole of the amputated part. Rotational forces may be involved, causing internal avulsive damage. Injuries of this type are mainly caused by gear drives, rollers, building and agricultural machinery, and sometimes by road traffic accidents. They require radical debridement and often it may be difficult to assess tissue vitality. Devitalised tissue, however, initiates an inflammatory reaction and — if it does not lead to infection — results in an increase of fibrotic tissue in the area which may interfere with function (Fig. 4.4).

4. Avulsion amputation

With avulsion amputation, the part is torn out rather than cut off or crushed. The result is that separation of the structures occurs at various levels, depending on the mechanical qualities of the different tissues. This type of amputation occasionally also involves diffuse crush injuries. In

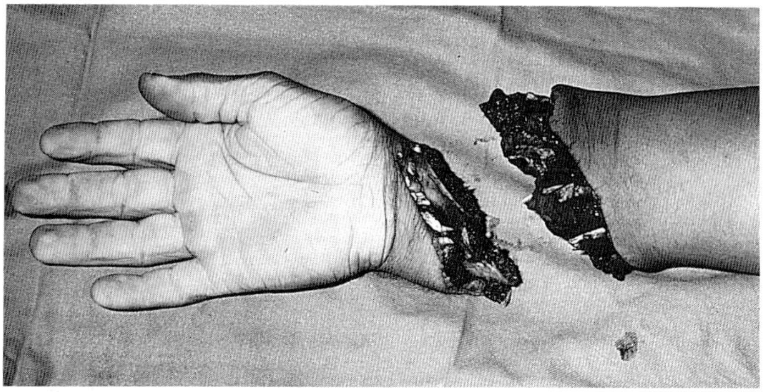

Fig. 4.2 Guillotine-type amputation by a plastic-cutting-machine. Labourer aged 21 years. (Reprinted with permission from Meyer 1985a.)

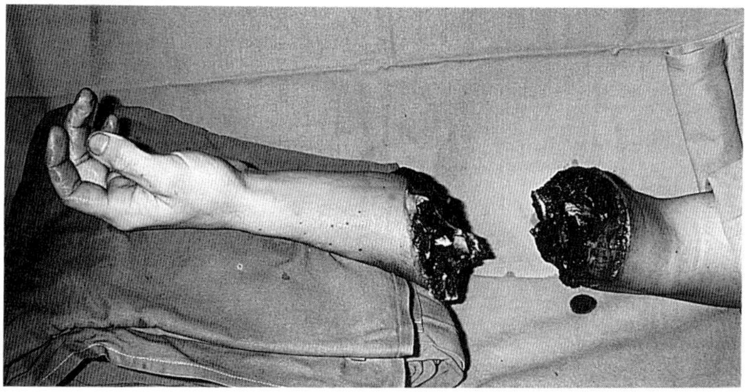

Fig. 4.3 Crush-amputation by a sheet-metal press. Locksmith, aged 20 years. (Reprinted with permission from Meyer 1985a.)

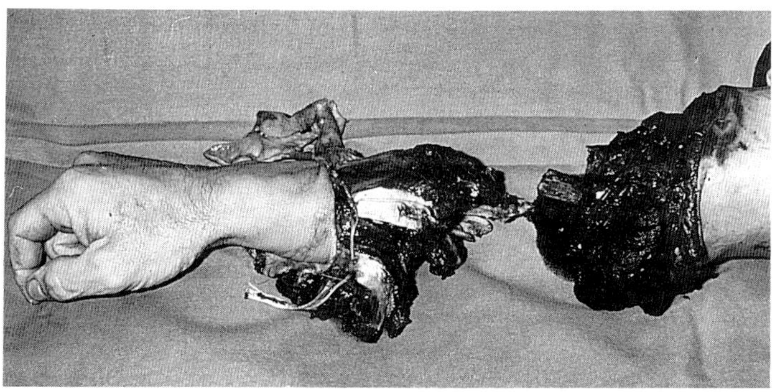

Fig. 4.4 Crush-amputation with extensive diffused tissue damage by a concrete mixer. Construction worker aged 31 years. (Reprinted with permission from Meyer 1985a.)

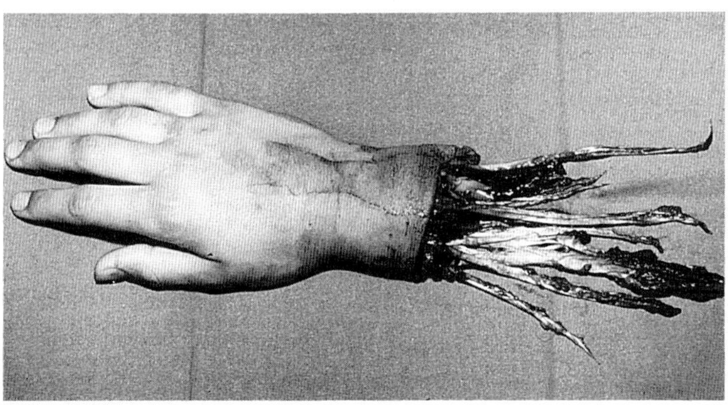

Fig. 4.5 Avulsion amputation in a mangle. Boy aged 11 years. (Reprinted with permission from Meyer 1985a.)

the vicinity of tendino-muscular junctures, the tendons are, as a rule, avulsed from their muscles. Vessels and nerves have sustained serious extensive traction damage.

These cases have the worst prognosis of all with respect to both survival and functional recovery. In most instances, extensive vascular grafts have to be interposed to re-establish circulation (Fig. 4.5). In fact, in avulsion amputations as shown in Figure 4.5, even the level of amputation is debatable. Looking at the amputated part, one could think of a hand amputation proximal but close to the wrist joint. However, with severance of nerves and tendon-muscle units at the level of the mid-forearm, the functional result to be anticipated will, at best, correspond to a proximal forearm replantation.

For cases with incomplete severance but disruption of the main vascular system (so-called subtotal amputation), in which there would be no survival without restoration of the vascular system, basically the same four categories of injuries may be applied. For later functional evaluation, however, all the structures preserved in continuity must be carefully protocolled. The enormous variety of possible types of such complex injuries makes it very difficult to establish a useful classification for comparable functional evaluation of final results. Of course, the part distal to the lesion must have a certain degree of physical integrity to justify an attempt at salvage.

Level of injury

The level of injury is a most critical parameter: the more proximal the injury is, the more conservative the attitude in establishing the indication for replantation. There are numerous reasons for this. In proximal amputations, there is an increasingly important muscle bulk in the anoxic or ischaemic part. Muscle is, above all the other tissues, the most susceptible to anoxic damage, which may give rise to serious complications in the later course.

The mechanism of injury is often extremely violent and thus results not only in an unfavourable type of injury, but also in important concomitant injuries which may take first priority for treatment.

In proximal amputations, the distance over which nerves must regenerate is correspondingly long and the chances for a more or less selective motor-sensory nerve repair are less favorable. Therefore, the functional results to be anticipated in each individual situation must be carefully balanced against the possible general risks for the patient which also are significantly determined by the level of injury.

There may be cases, however, where replantation or revascularisation for survival may be indicated despite the fact that the injuries sustained are such that functional recovery in the replanted or revascularised part is not likely to be great. For example, in the case of an amputation at the level of the upper arm, replantation may be indicated in order to regain valuable function in the elbow joint and make the forearm and hand a useful lever arm, even though significant prehensile recovery of the hand will not be achieved (Fig. 4.6 A–D). Sometimes, proximal replantations may also be indicated in order to improve later prosthetic fitting. An example of this would be disarticulation at the shoulder, including the entire scapula, where replantation may be indicated to maintain the arch of the shoulder, with an amputation possibly performed at the upper arm level at a later date (Piza et al 1977).

The level of amputation or incomplete severance is one of the most important determining factors with regard to the final functional result to be anticipated. A study at three replantation centers from three continents, using the same system of evaluation, has shown, for example, that a useful functional result of replantation at the shoulder level is the exception rather than the rule. In arm replantations, good results are achieved in only one-third of cases, whereas in the proximal forearm, 40% have good or excellent results; in the distal forearm and wrist (including carpus), good and excellent results are achieved in 80% of cases (Meyer 1985b, Chen Zhong-Wei et al 1981) (see Table 4.1).

The above analysis includes only cases of complete severance (amputation) and no revascularisation cases. If major nerves remain intact while other structures are severed, excellent results can also be achieved at proximal levels, such as in the arm (Fig. 4.7 A–H). Thus, the indications for

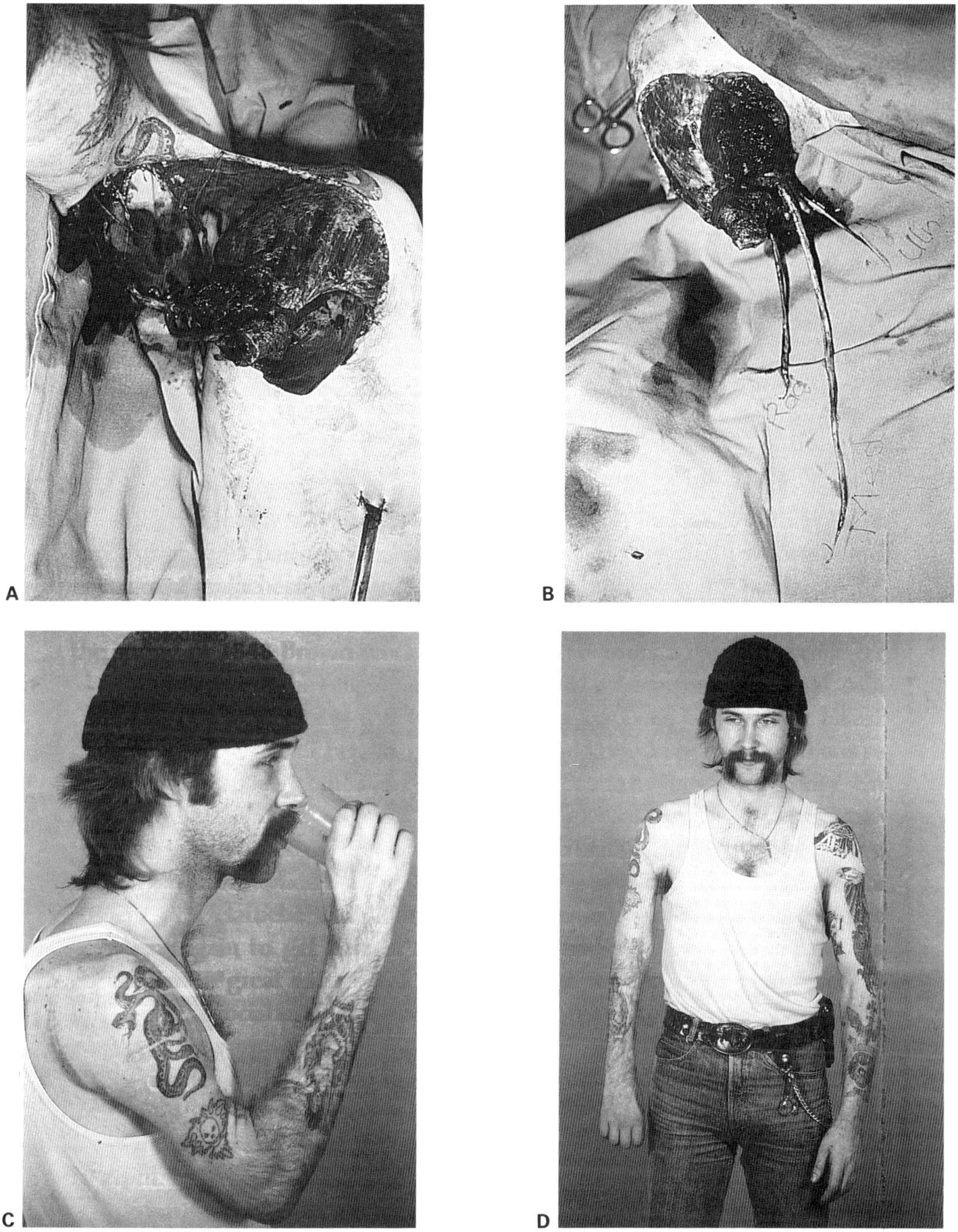

Fig. 4.6 **A.** Avulsion amputation of the right dominant arm in a 30-year-old labourer by a motorcycle accident. The only tissue structure in continuity is a heavily contused devitalised skin bridge which was excised during debridement. **B.** Proximal stump after debridement showing the avulsed radial, median and ulnar nerve. As significant concomitant injuries, this patient also sustained multiple rib fractures with haemothorax and lung contusions. Skeletal shortening in this case was 7.5 cm, and rigid internal fixation was achieved by an 8-hole AO dynamic compression-plate. All nerve stumps could be directly sutured after wide excision of the damaged segments. Total time of anoxia in this case was 9 hours, 2 hours at about 20°C and 7 hours at about 4–8°C. During the debridement, at least 50% of the upper arm musculature has been excised. After restoration of circulation, it took about 6 hours before the very pronounced muscle-rigor disappeared. The postoperative course was uneventful. **C** and **D.** Result two years after the accident: the patient has normal range of shoulder motion and a good function of the elbow joint, which makes the forearm a most useful lever arm. The prehensile capacity of the hand is marginal and not of relevant significance. However, sensibility in the hand is sufficiently protective.

Table 4.1 Functional result of major limb replantation. Cooperative study: Shanghai, Louisville, Zurich. (Chen Zhong-Wei et al 1981)

Level of amputation	*No. of cases*	*Grade I + II (%)*	*Grade III (%)*	*Grade IV (%)*
Shoulder	3	–	33.3	66.6
Arm	26	35	65	–
Proximal forearm	20	40	35	25
Distal forearm	48	79	21	–
Wrist (carpus)	30	83	17	–
Palm	54	60	33	7
Total	181	61	33	6

revascularisation do not parallel those for replantation. It is the specific nature, not the volume, of intact tissue bridges which is the most important factor. In revascularisation cases, there is often no distinct level of injury; tissue damage may be extremely extensive and, even by using long vascular grafts, it may occasionally not be possible to restore adequate circulation in the distal part. In such cases, the use of a temporary silicone-tube bypass has proved useful for evaluation (Fig. 4.8 A–D).

In major limb replantation and revascularisation, multi-level injuries are not a contraindication for replantation and revascularisation (Fig. 4.9).

Concomitant traction injuries of the brachial plexus may sometimes be difficult, or even impossible, to assess in very proximal amputation injuries. Evidence of severe traction injury of the brachial plexus should, however, preclude replantation of an arm, unless replantation would significantly contribute to the quality of later prosthetic fitting.

Duration of tissue anoxia — post-ischaemia syndrome

Anoxia causes progressive tissue damage leading finally to cellular necrosis. It is therefore necessary to restore circulation before significant irreversible damage has occurred. In replantation or revas-

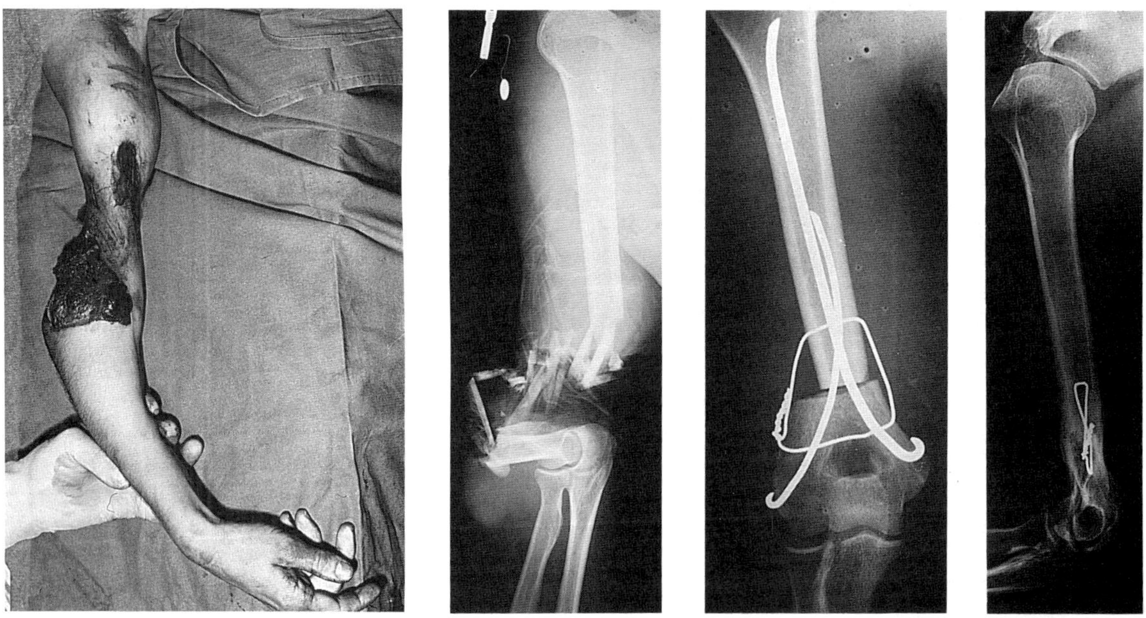

A B C D

Fig. 4.7 **A.** Incomplete severance of the upper arm in a 27-year-old woman who tried to throw herself in front of a train in a mentally depressed state. Her right dominant arm was the only part of the body which was injured. After debridement, the only structures in continuity were the median and ulnar nerves. **B.** Skeletal shortening in this case was 9 cm. **C.** Internal fixation was achieved by two rush-pins additionally secured by intra-osseous wiring. **D.** X-ray film taken at two years. Removal of intra-osseous wires is not needed, provided the curl is buried well.

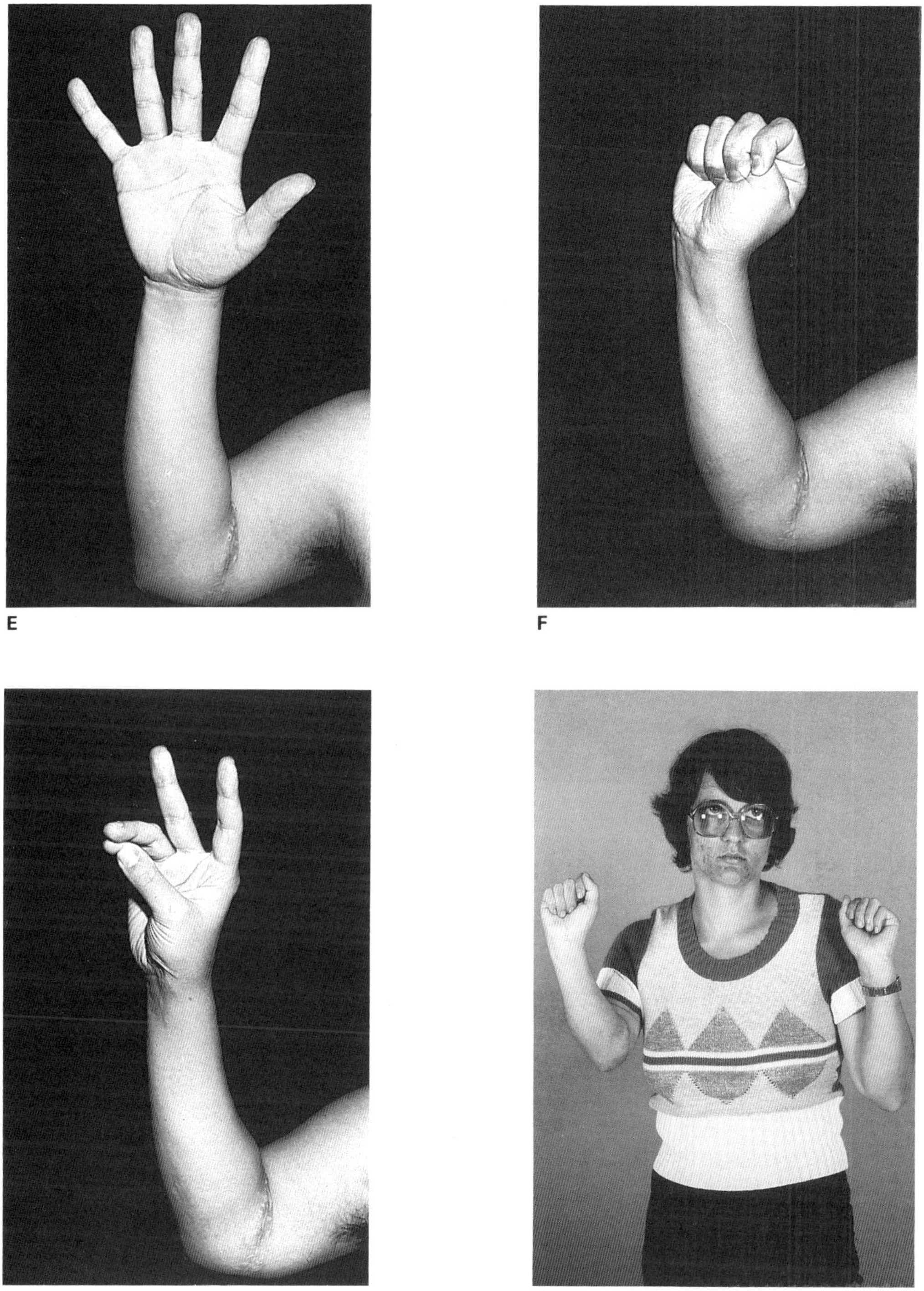

Fig. 4.7 (cont) E–H. Functional result at two years after total primary repair. There is normal hand function, as median and ulnar nerves have not been damaged and recovery of the sutured radial nerve was excellent. The clearly visible shortening of the upper arm does not significantly impair the overall function of this upper extremity. (**B, C** and **D** reprinted with permission from Meyer 1985a.)

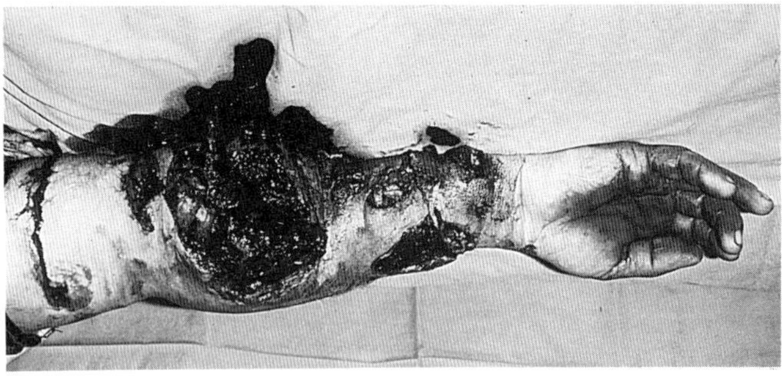

A

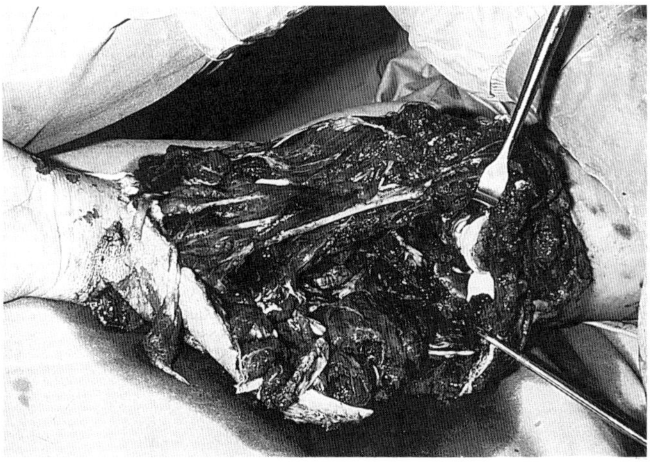

B

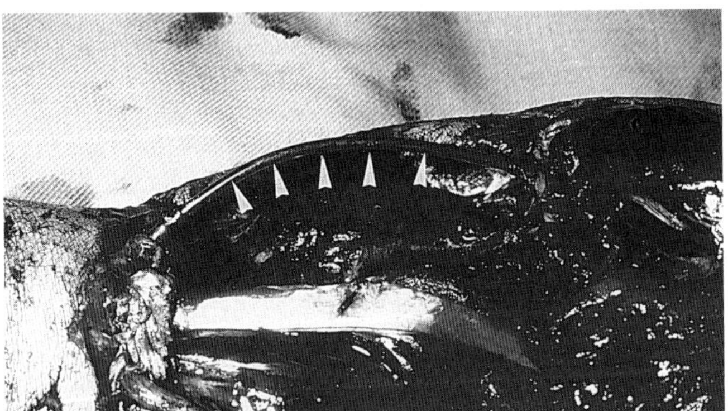

C

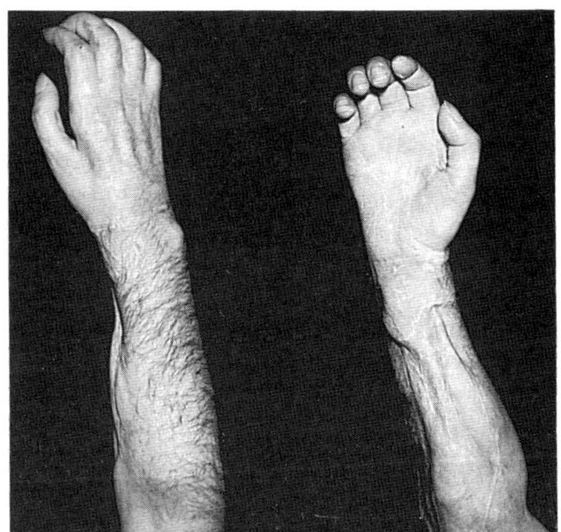

D

Fig. 4.8 **A.** Extensive blast-injury to the forearm and hand, with total ischaemia of the hand. **B.** Close-up view of the extensive muscle damage. **C.** Silicone bypass of radial artery (arrow). With this type of bypass, it is possible to establish very quickly whether or not vascular reconstruction will restore adequate blood supply to the hand; it also helps in the distinction between vital and devitalised tissue areas. **D.** Condition three years after the accident. There is no prehensile function of the hand and recovery of sensibility is very poor; however, the forearm and hand are very useful as a lever arm due to normal function of the elbow joint. (**A** and **C** reprinted with permission, from Meyer 1985a.)

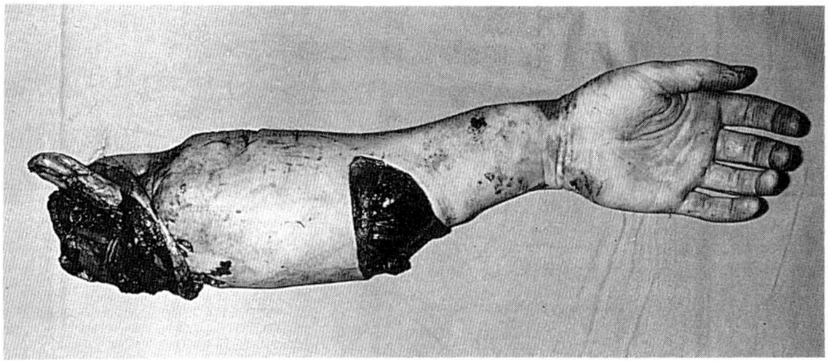

Fig. 4.9 Amputation proximal to the elbow joint with extensive crush and additional severance of the ulnar neurovascular bundle at the forearm level. In principle, such a two-level injury is not per se a contraindication to replantation; in this case, however, the patient died from traumatic cerebral haemorrhage.

cularisation of anoxic parts with a major muscle mass, early and late complications of the *post-ischaemia syndrome* remain a significant threat, no matter how sophisticated the technical infrastructure of a replantation center may be. Therefore this type of surgery cannot be considered as a simple routine procedure. Post-ischaemia syndrome is relatively new terminology and stands also for expressions such as tourniquet-crush-compression, and myonephropathic-metabolic-syndrome (Berger et al 1980, Brunelli 1981, Chen Zhong-Wei et al 1981, Doi et al 1983, Eriksson et al 1974, Malcom 1988, Matsuda et al 1978, McNeill & Wilson 1970, Steinau 1988).

Clinical and experimental data clearly demonstrate that the post-ischaemia (reperfusion) syndrome has the potential to lead to multiple organ failure and possibly death. Even during the replantation procedure, acute complications may occur. In one forearm replantation (shown in Fig. 4.3) we observed a rise of the blood potassium level up to 7 mEq/l after declamping, a value which may induce severe cardiac arrhythmias. Since that observation, we wash out the reattached part with arterial blood (1–2 units of conserved blood) before declamping the venous anastomosis. Steinau recently published a very extensive study based on his experimental work on post-ischaemia syndrome (Steinau 1988). Table 4.2 and Figure 4.10 have been taken from this remarkable work. These show the pathological conditions associated with post-ischaemia shock syndrome and post-ischaemia syndrome in major limb replantation. Any surgeon taking responsibility for such patients should have a good knowledge of this pathophysiology (Chase 1970).

There is no doubt that hypothermia effectively

Table 4.2 Major limb replantation: pathological conditions associated with post-ischaemia shock syndrome (Steinau 1988)

Local myopathy and capillaropathy	⟷	*Multiple organ failure (MOF)*
Acidosis		Systemic acidosis
Hyperosmolality		Volume deficiency
Oxygen free radicals?		Hyperkalaemia
Lysosomal proteolytic enzymes		Haemoconcentration
Histamine-like mediators		Coagulation dysfunction (microembolisation)
Coagulation dysfunction		
Compartment syndrome		Bacterial toxaemia?

increases the tolerance of tissues to anoxia. Every effort should therefore be made to cool the anoxic part as rapidly as possible to about 4°C. Hypothermia should be maintained until the main vascular system has been restored. At present, this is the only measure we use in clinical practice to increase tissue tolerance to anoxia. However, one should keep in mind that by perfusion with cooled physiological solution hypothermia is most rapidly initiated; also, recent experimental studies have shown that the use of special perfusates (perfusion solutions), such as oxygenated stroma-free haemoglobin solution, can effectively decrease anoxic tissue damage (Steinau 1988, Steinau et al 1980). Progress in this field needs careful attention because it will increase the safety of the patients in replantation and revascularisation procedures. Tissue protection in severed limbs is also a major issue in the futuristic perspective of allogenic limb transplantation.

In today's practice, any normothermic major anoxic muscle mass deprived of circulation for

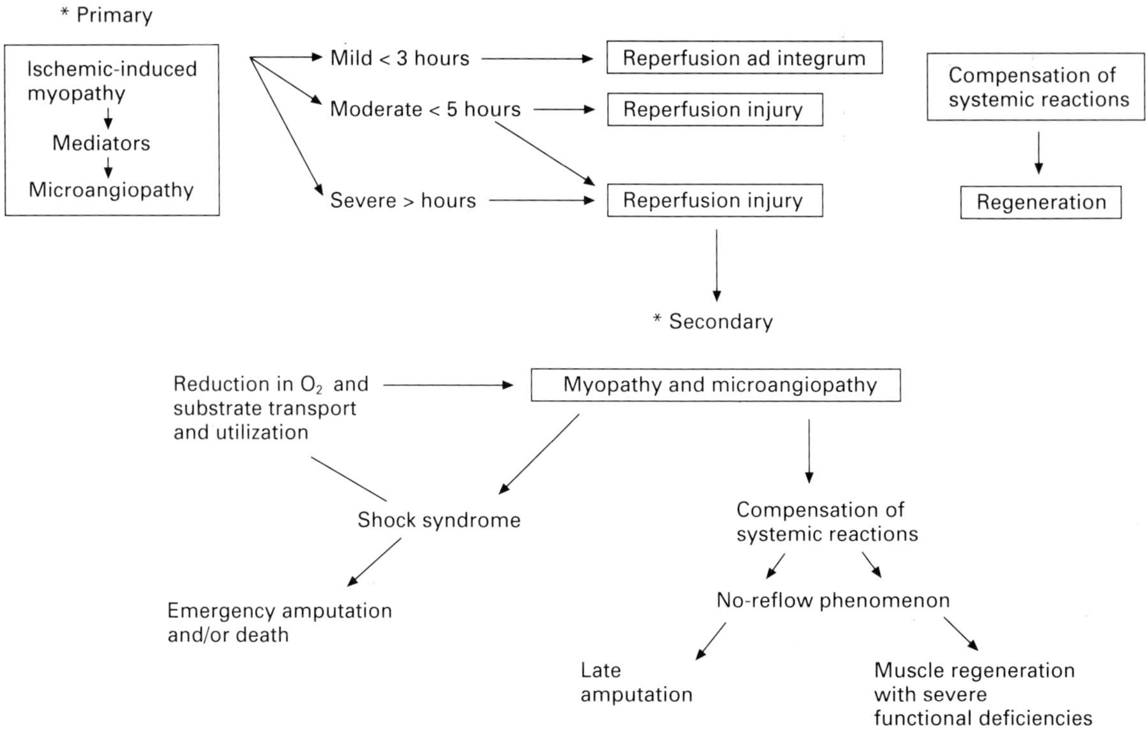

Fig. 4.10 Post-ischaemia syndrome in major limb replantation. Time-related pathophysiology as proposed by Steinau (Steinau 1988).

more than 4 hours must be suspect, and suspicion should geometrically progress in time (Brown 1981). This raises the question of what constitutes significant muscle bulk in major limb replantation surgery. The amount of muscle mass which may induce a severe post-ischaemia syndrome with multiple organ complications (renal failure, adult respiratory distress syndrome (ARDS), severe clotting disorders) is not exactly known. Of course, it is not only the muscle mass itself but also the extent of the anoxic damage which is a determining factor.

The intrinsic musculature of a whole hand, while being quantitatively impressive on cross-section (Fig. 4.11), and of critical functional importance, is unlikely to induce acutely life-threatening post-ischaemia syndrome. However, it may well become the origin for dangerous septicaemia if infection arises in severely damaged intrinsic muscles. In contrast, the volume of the musculature of a whole forearm or arm may well induce immediate dangerous complications, even during the replantation procedure, by the influx of high potassium content and toxic metabolites into the systemic circulation after declamping, as previously mentioned (Fig. 4.12).

Literature about these dangerous and sometimes even fatal complications is relatively scanty (Chen Zhong-Wei et al 1981, Eger et al 1974, Ferreira et al 1978, Hales & Pullen 1982, Jaeger et al 1981, Matsuda et al 1978, May & Gallico 1980, McNeill & Wilson 1970, Meyer 1985a, Russell et al 1984).

Psychological factors

The fact that circulation can be restored in an amputated or incompletely severed limb, and that by so doing survival of the part can be achieved, cannot be the sole criterion in deciding on a replantation procedure (Meyer 1979). Replantation should be considered only if in the individual situation a reasonable functional result may be expected. In the individual case, function does not necessarily mean prehensile capacity, but in

A

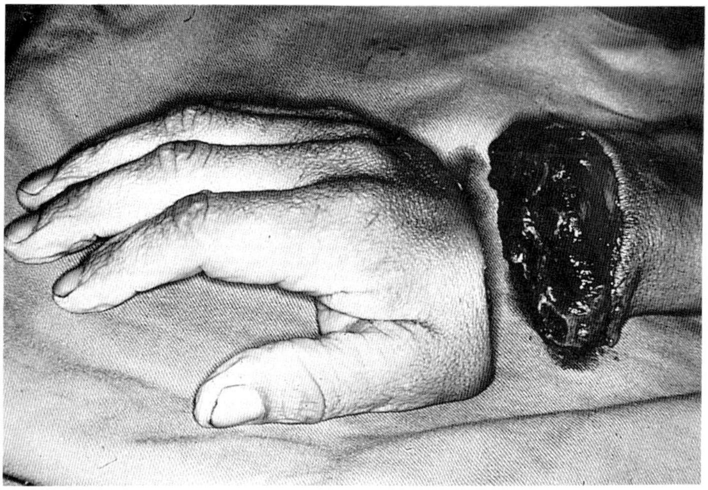

B

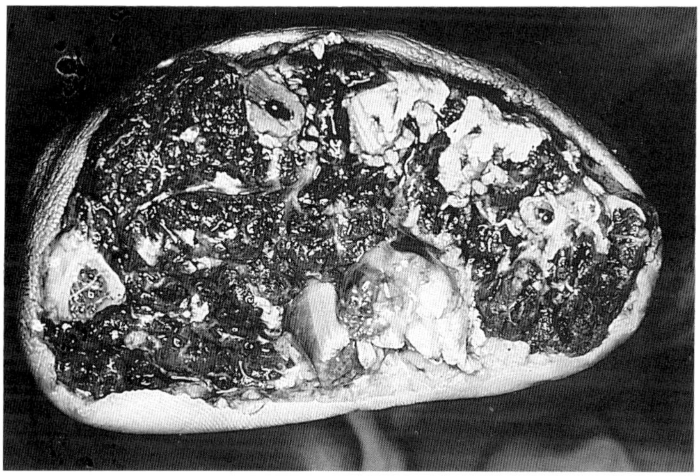

Fig. 4.11 **A.** Guillotine-type amputation by a woodshaper-cutter in a carpenter aged 28 years. **B.** Cross-section of the distal part shows the impressive muscle mass of the intrinsic musculature in a hand. (Reprinted with permission from Meyer V E 1981 Zum Problem der Kontraktur der kleinen Handmuskeln nach Mittelhandreplantation. Handchirurgie 13, 103–106.)

various degrees embraces also the aesthetic outcome and restoration of integrity of the body image. The concept of 'function' must relate to the patient's performance as a whole and not merely to prehensile capacity of the replanted part.

The psychological response to the injury, the integrity of body image and anxiety relating to possible disfigurement differ greatly between people from different cultures and ethnic groups, but also among individuals from the same cultural and ethnic group. Thus, the patient's emotional needs must also be considered and balanced against the functional (prehensile) requirements. In this delicate decision-making process, the patient should play an active role if possible; but often at this critical time he is under the influence of the mental shock sustained, and possibly even in haemorrhagic shock. Involving family members may be appropriate for getting helpful background information. In such severe cases of major limb loss, the most experienced surgeon of the replantation team should personally give the patient and his family detailed information and explanations about replantation (revascularisation) and all possible alternatives. He is the one who must take the final decision (Brown 1981, Meyer 1985a).

SURGICAL TECHNIQUE AND STRATEGY

Based on the considerable experience now accumulated, it has become possible to standardise

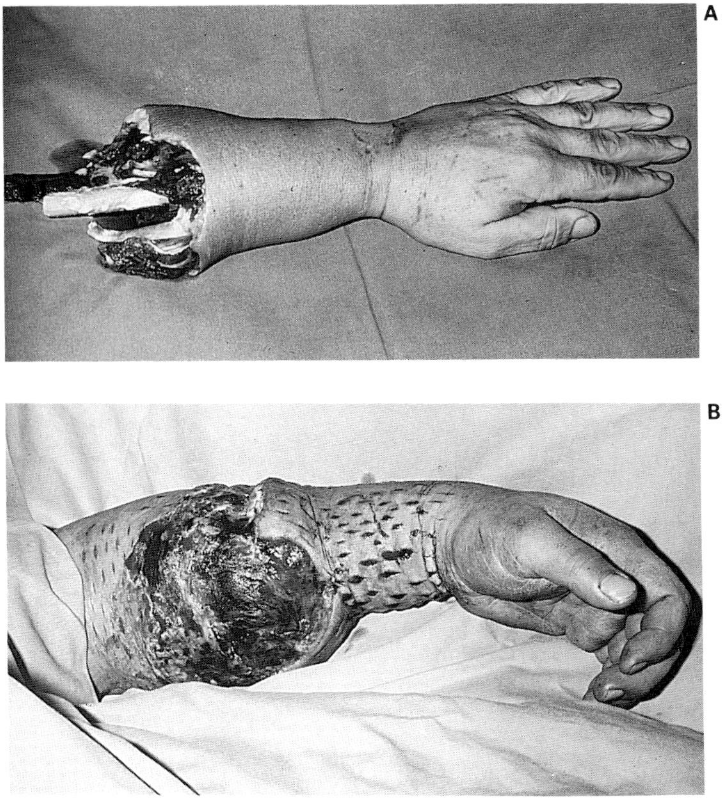

Fig. 4.12 **A.** Avulsion amputation of the proximal forearm by a conveyer belt in a 43-year-old farmer. **B.** Nine-days after replantation: extensive infection of the musculature with septicaemia and adult respiratory distress syndrome (ARDS). At this time, the forearm was amputated, despite the fact that there was excellent circulation in the hand, as this was the only measure able to control this life-threatening complication.

much of the surgical strategy. Nevertheless, it is necessary to approach each individual case without stereotyped preconceptions. Depending on the individual situation, different cases may require a different approach, if the best possible result is to be achieved. This is particularly true for revascularisation cases, where the spectrum of possible types and extensions of tissue injuries is immense. Therefore, many revascularisation cases are even more demanding in terms of surgical skills and experience than replantations 'in sensu stricto'.

External cleaning, disinfection and debridement

Before debridement is started, the skin of both the amputated part and the stump must be thoroughly cleaned mechanically without causing further damage to the tissues in the wound area. It has been found most effective to use sterile rubber brushes and physiological saline or Ringer's solution for this purpose. Of course, the fingernails are cut short. We do not use any soap and/or other disinfectant solutions at the stage of mechanical cleaning, as these may be toxic to tissues in the wound area. The wound areas themselves are thoroughly irrigated with physiological saline. After this, the skin is disinfected in the usual way, taking care to prevent the disinfectant from coming into contact with the wound area. We prefer uncoloured disinfectant solutions; assessment of later capillary refill in the skin will thus be optimal. The first principle in the treatment of injuries of extremities is to achieve uncomplicated primary wound healing. This applies no less in replantation surgery. Therefore, it is critically important that foreign bodies, and all tissue that is not viable or not well vascularised, be removed. The goal of primary wound healing will be jeopardised if foreign bodies, devitalised tissue or haematoma — which is in fact dead tissue — remain on either surface. Debridement comprises the economical, but at the same time sufficiently extensive, excision of clearly devitalised tissues and removal of foreign bodies in conjunction with thorough irrigation with Ringer's solution. In replantation and revascularisation surgery, every single step of the operation influences the ultimate success or failure of the operation as a whole. Nothing, therefore, in this type of surgery, including debridement, can be left to an inexperienced colleague. Total engagement of a competent surgical team is required from the beginning to the end, i.e. until dressing is complete.

In replantation surgery, wound surfaces are often exposed far longer than in any other type of surgery, so it is necessary to protect the patient by giving an effective shield of a broad-spectrum antibiotic before the operation starts. Antibiotic cover is in fact initiated as a part of the anaesthesia preparation, as also, of course, are preventive measures against tetanus.

Meticulous debridement may require several hours of work; preparation of the amputated part should therefore start as soon as possible, and certainly be on the way while the patient is being prepared for anaesthesia. Occasionally, the definite plan of treatment can only be formulated during debridement of the part and, later, of the stump. In the course of debridement, all anatomical structures that will be involved in later microsurgical reconstruction are identified and tagged with fine sutures. Cut vessels that are not anastomosed are ligated or coagulated in both the proximal and the distal part. A pair of magnifying spectacles giving × 2 or × 3 magnification will normally be adequate for this work. In cases of diffuse muscle damage and of contamination (especially farm injuries), we have found the use of gentamycin pellets an effective adjunct to prevent infection (Fig. 4.27C).

It is of utmost importance that the time of anoxia be reduced as much as possible; thus, two surgical teams are required at the debridement stage, one working on the stump and the other on the amputated part.

Continued cooling during the operation

At present, cooling is the only practicable method to effectively increase the tolerance of tissues to anoxia. Therefore, it must be as continuous as possible until circulation is restored to the anoxic part. The optimal temperature is 4°C. If there is any delay in starting the replantation because treatment of first priority is still under way (e.g. for shock), the debrided part is best transferred to a cooling pack (as described for transport) until replantation can be started. Amputated parts of any kind should never be thrown away before the operation is finished, even if initially considered unsuitable for replantation. They may prove a valuable source of tissues that may be required in the course of the operation. Once skeletal stabilisation has been achieved, the anoxic part should be cooled again by using frozen Ringer's solution packed in plastic bags. Care must be taken, however, that the anoxic part does not suffer from frost damage; the latter is best avoided by interposing thick layers of gauze compresses (Fig. 4.13).

In cases of incomplete severance which need revascularisation for survival, the same cooling method can be applied until the operation is started. Of course, cases of revascularisation for improvement need no cooling at all.

Extent and sequence of repair

Since we began our replantation work in 1974, we have striven for complete primary repair whenever possible. Over the years, this concept of total primary repair has proven its value. Firstly, secondary operations may be very demanding technically, and secondly they carry a considerable risk to the reconstructed vascular system.

A further factor of importance is that an intensive hand therapy program must be started as early as possible, in order to achieve the best possible result. Secondary reconstructions will cause serious interruptions and delays in these important efforts. Therefore, if at all possible, complete primary repair of all important structures should be the aim. On the other hand, the endeavour should never interfere with that of achieving primary wound healing. Where severed nerves can only be repaired with nerve grafts, primary nerve grafting is certainly indicated, providing that the nerve grafts can be harvested from non-replantable parts; alternatively, a nerve of minor importance from the replanted part itself, for example the superficial branch of the radial nerve, can be used. Primary use of nerves from uninjured areas (for

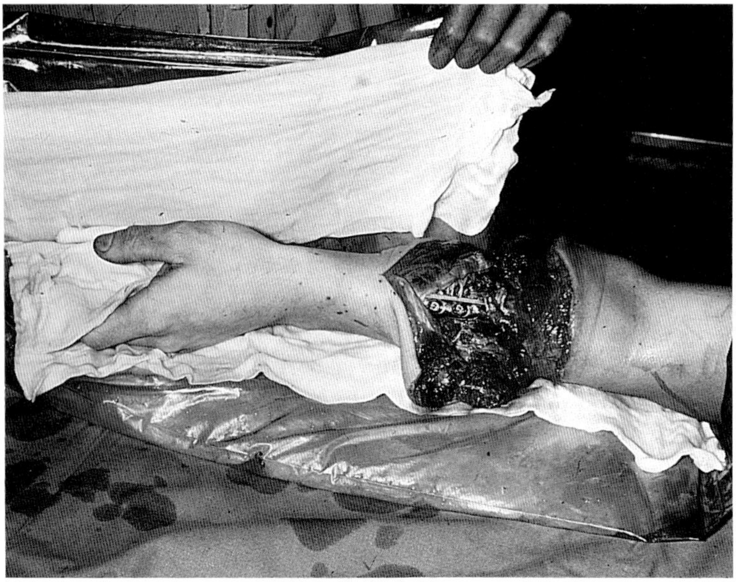

Fig. 4.13 Hypothermia is re-established immediately after skeletal fixation and maintained until circulation has been restored. This is best done by using packets of sterile frozen physiological solution. Freezing of the anoxic part is avoided by interposition of thick layers of gauze compresses. (Reprinted with permission from Meyer et al 1981).

example sural nerve) for this purpose is not justifiable as a rule, as these grafts will be lost if the replantation/revascularisation does not succeed.

The sequence of repair is largely determined by: the anatomical conditions pertaining to different levels of the injury; the need to restore circulation as rapidly as possible; and by the fact that optimum vascular repair is in general only possible after skeletal stability has been achieved. With few exceptions, then, skeletal stabilisation will be the first step. Apart from this, the sequence of repair depends on the individual situation in each case. As a rule, reconstruction should start with the deep structures and proceed toward the surface.

In the forearm, skeletal stabilisation is followed by efforts to repair the interosseous membrane and the major muscle septa, in so far as this does not interfere with subsequent neurovascular repair. This will make it easier to group the muscles in the anoxic part, which at this time does not yet show oedematous swelling. Muscles with poor potential for useful functional re-innervation are best excised. This gives immediate decompression, which facilitates the subsequent wound closure and minimises the final amount of fibrotic tissue in the area. In cases with large muscle bulk in the anoxic part, at least one large vein must be anastomosed before declamping the restored main arterial system to minimise the otherwise considerable blood loss once circulation is restored. This procedure needs to be strictly adhered to, particularly as successfully anastomosed vessels should not, on principle, be clamped in the further course of the operation once circulation has been restored, nor of course should the pneumatic tourniquet be reinflated.

As already mentioned, amputated parts containing relatively large muscle masses must be thoroughly irrigated with arterial blood (at least 1 unit of conserved blood), particularly if anoxia has been prolonged before the clamps on the anastomosed veins are removed. This is to keep the passage of toxic metabolites from the anoxic parts into the patient's blood stream as low as possible.

Especially in cases of prolonged tissue anoxia, the use of temporary vascular shunts may re-establish tissue perfusion and effective oxygenation very rapidly. This method also helps to determine whether or not vascular reconstruction will restore adequate blood supply to the anoxic part. It also allows identification of vital structures, thorough debridement and skeletal fixation prior to definite arterial repair. Thus, temporary arterial shunting is of particular benefit in difficult major limb replantations/revascularisations, such as avulsion, crush or blast injuries (Fig. 4.8 A–C) (Meyer 1985a, Nunley et al 1981). However, we do not consider vascular shunting as a routine method in major limb replantation/revascularisation, but as a useful adjunct in special situations.

Skeletal management

Skeletal shortening

Skeletal shortening is a most important principle in replantation surgery; it is performed in order to create the best possible conditions for subsequent soft tissue reconstruction. Only in rare exceptions is osteotomy to shorten bones not indicated. One such exception might be the highly unusual case of avulsion amputation by disarticulation with only minimal or no damage to the articular surfaces. In this type of case, eventually, joints can be restored by reconstructing the ligaments and capsule, and useful function may be regained. In such a case, however, it might be appropriate to consider skeletal shortening distal and/or proximal to the disarticulation site in the interest of the best possible soft tissue management.

Every amputation injury leads to more or less extensive segmental destruction of soft tissues. The extent of bone shortening should ideally be such as to allow nerves to be sutured without tension, blood vessels, muscles and tendons at near-normal tension, and the skin with minimum tension. Tendon-muscle units need to be shortened to about the same extent as the bones.

With osteotomy, care must be taken to see that as much of the periosteum as possible is retained. It is best to push the periosteum back in the proximal and distal direction prior to the osteotomy, like a cuff, afterwards pulling it back over the osteotomy site. This will promote rapid and reliable bone union.

Forearm and upper arm amputations usually involve extensive soft tissue damage. Osteotomy must therefore be particularly radical. No compromise is possible (Fig. 4.7 A–H). Insufficient shortening of the skeleton leads to soft tissue necrosis with all that this entails (infection, septicaemia, etc.), so that not only the reattached or revascularised part, but the patient's life, is put at risk. If the part survives, expensive secondary procedures will be necessary to restore soft tissue coverage and to treat possible pseudo-arthrosis, all of which will greatly increase morbidity (Fig. 4.23). Even if the revascularised part survives, deep infection will always have a serious effect on the final functional result. Inadequate bone shortening in replantations proximal to the wrist joint is one of the commonest faults in replantation surgery. The importance of sufficient skeletal shortening cannot be overemphasised.

Bone fixation

Another basic principle in skeletal management is accurate restoration of skeletal axes, securing them by rapid bone fixation. Primary stability for unresisted active movement has the great advantage that the time period of immobilisation depends only on soft tissue healing. The result is that the critically important hand therapy program can be started earlier in these cases, and can be more intensive and effective, as there is no need to wait for bone union. The method of bone fixation used must, in every case, be in optimum accord with the given biological situation. The soft tissue status, being primarily determined by the type of injury and the level of amputation, needs to be particularly taken into account. In general, we strive for rigid internal fixation. In some cases, however, the use of an external fixateur may be indicated, especially if the extent of soft tissue damage is difficult to assess primarily, a situation in which we are reluctant to implant foreign material.

For rigid internal fixation different methods may be applied. If the level of injury is not critical with regard to the skeletal situation and the surrounding soft tissues, bone plates offer the distinct advantage of a most reliable primary stability which is otherwise difficult or impossible to achieve. This is true, in particular, in the area of the diaphysis, where bone union is known to take a long time. In these cases, we prefer the so-called dynamic compression plates (Fig. 4.14 A–C). In areas which are close to joints, however, the plates may function rather as pure neutralisation plates or, if possible, as tension band plates. The use of bone plates does, however, call for a relatively wide-ranging dissection of soft tissues. With upper arm amputations close to the elbow joint, where two plates would be required to give reliable stabilisation of the condyles, we do prefer the

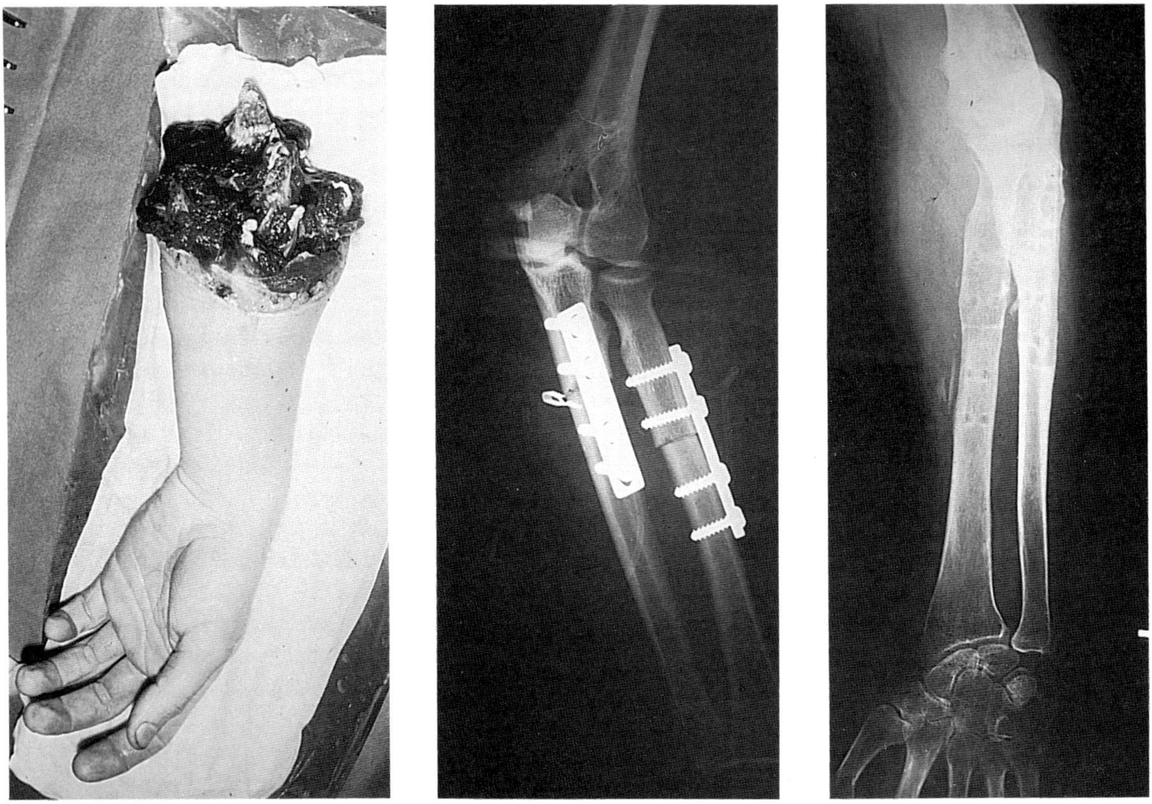

A B C

Fig. 4.14 **A.** Proximal forearm amputation with local crush. **B.** Rigid internal fixation with DC (dynamic compression) plates on radius and ulna. **C.** Condition 18 months after accident following removal of the plates. (Reprinted with permission from Meyer 1985a.)

much less traumatic Rush-pin fixation, which we complement with additional stabilisation using intra-osseous wiring (Fig. 4.7 A–H). Intra-osseous wiring has also proved effective in extremely distal, close-to-the-wrist joint amputations in the forearm, where the distal fragment is too small to securely anchor the screws of a plate (Fig. 4.15 A–D).

When amputation has been through a joint there are three basic options for skeletal stabilisation. In the rare case where the articular surfaces remain intact, the joint can eventually be restored as previously mentioned. We do not have particular experience with such cases at the level of the wrist and elbow joints; however, we have done this in a case of disarticulation avulsion amputation of all fingers through the MP joint and these joints have functioned well for more than 10 years. Joints with a major functional role should, whenever possible, be restored using Kirschner wires, intra-osseous wiring and screws. In the majority of cases, however, joints that have suffered transarticular amputation cannot be reconstructed. Fixation must be achieved either by primary arthrodesis or by arthroplasty. Both methods will almost always permit adequate bone shortening. A primary arthroplasty for the wrist or elbow joint of one or another form may be a rare exception if this is indicated at all in this type of surgery. However, we would not absolutely preclude this possibility, especially for the elbow joint, where arthrodesis represents a major handicap.

Repair of musculotendinous units

For an optimal functional result, primary repair of musculotendinous units must be the aim. If this is not achieved, contracture will rapidly lead to irre-

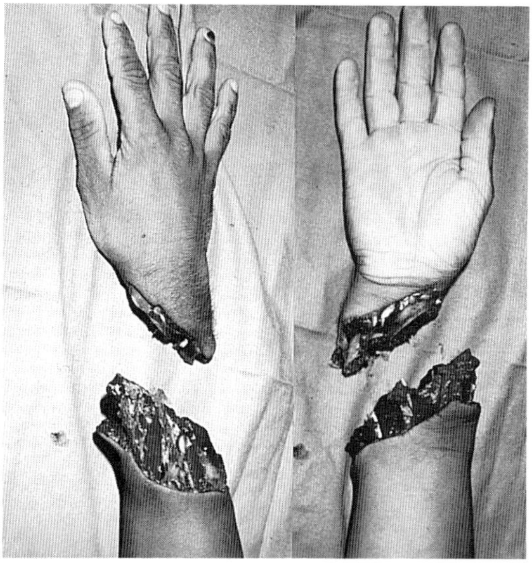

A

Fig. 4.15 A. Guillotine-type amputation in a 21-year-old labourer by a plastic-cutting machine. **B.** By using intra-osseous wiring at the radius in conjunction with a Kirschner wire, this joint could be preserved. The ulna was fixed by a $\frac{1}{3}$ tubular plate. **C.** X-ray taken at $1\frac{1}{2}$ years after the accident after removal of both the plate and Kirschner wire, as well as of the curl of the intra-osseous wire. **D.** The functional result is documented $3\frac{1}{2}$ years after reattachment with total primary repair. There was no secondary surgery except for removal of the metal implants. Mainly due to the remarkable re-innervation of the intrinsic muscles, and the most favourable level of amputation, which is proximal but close to the wrist joint, this patient has achieved an excellent result. Initial skeletal shortening in this case of a clean-cut amputation was 2.5 cm. The two-point discrimination in the median nerve distribution is 6 mm, and in the ulnar nerve distribution 8 mm. There is only very moderate cold intolerance. (Reprinted with permission from Meyer 1985a.)

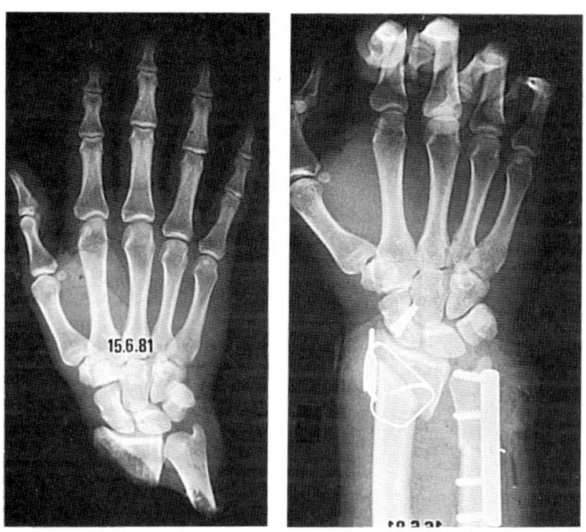

B

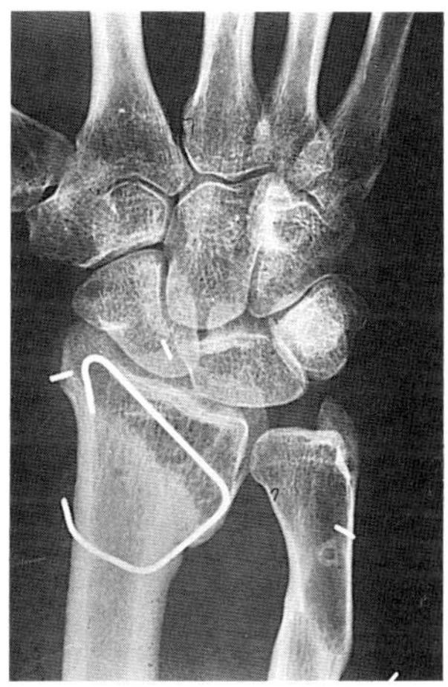

C

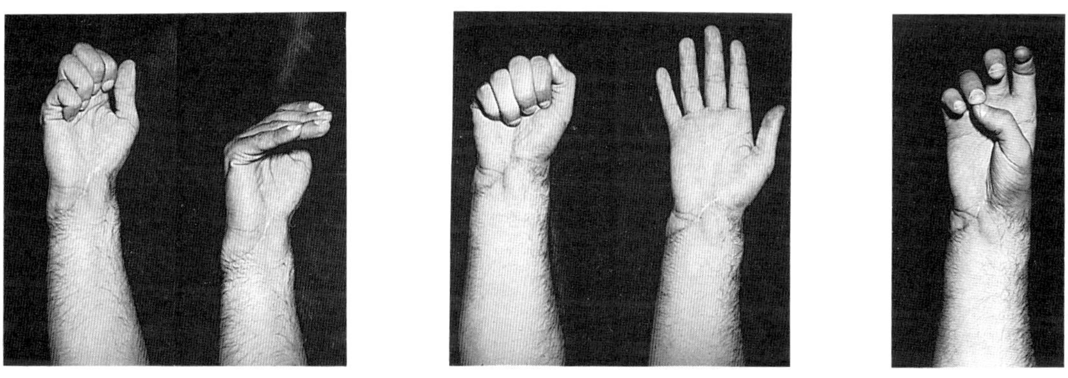

D

versible shortening of the muscle. In the arm and forearm, it is preferable to carry out muscle repair immediately after skeletal fixation, with due regard to subsequent neurovascular repair. This makes it possible to prepare optimum conditions for neurovascular repair, and the re-established muscle tension will help to prevent later oedema. As already mentioned, only the most important musculotendinous units are repaired; muscles not repaired are, on occasion, better excised, especially when useful re-innervation is unlikely, or when the muscle is severely damaged by anoxia and/or crush. This achieves effective immediate decompression, and ultimately reduces the volume of fibrotic tissue in the area (Brunelli et al 1988, Meyer et al 1981). Basically, there are three types of musculotendinous repair: 1) tendon-to-tendon, 2) tendon-to-muscle and 3) muscle-to-muscle coaptation.

Tendon-to-tendon repair is done using the well-known methods of modern hand surgery. Tendon-to-muscle coaptation is required especially with avulsion amputations, and requires implantation of the tendon in the muscle (Fig. 4.16). This is achieved by careful dissection and longitudinal division of the muscle. The tendon can only be fixed with loose mattress sutures. If the sutures are too tight, ischaemia will lead to fibrosis of the muscle. Muscle-to-muscle coaptation is also achieved with loose mattress sutures; whenever possible these are anchored in the muscle septa. Except in cases where tendon-muscle transpositions are performed as a part of the primary procedure — and this is done quite often — it will be necessary to shorten the musculotendinous unit almost to the same extent as the bone, to ensure normal tension when the repairs are complete. Normal tension has been achieved if the hand and finger joints are in normal resting attitude after the operation.

Vascular repair

Experience has shown that it is a definite advantage to use microsurgical techniques also for the anastomosis of larger vessels in the arm and forearm (Meyer 1979).

A

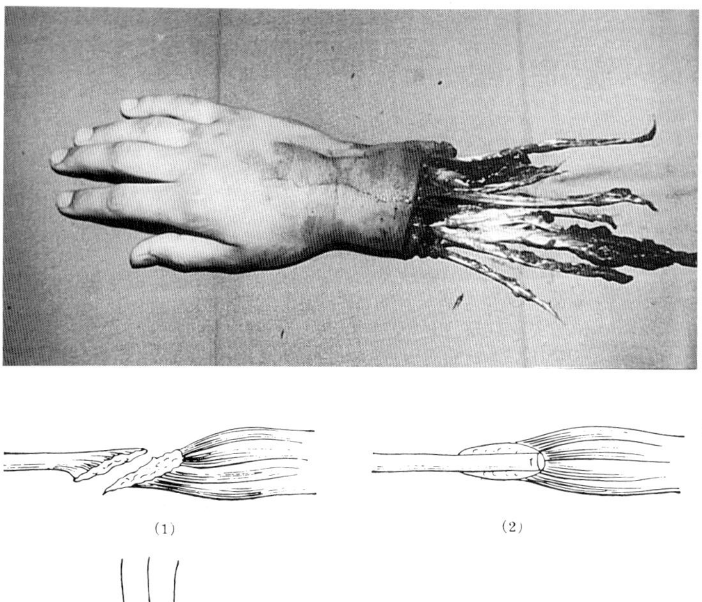

B

Fig. 4.16 To restore tendon and muscle units in avulsion amputations (**A**), the torn tendons need to be implanted in the muscle belly. **B**. The diagrams (1–4) show the individual stages of implantation as described by Chen Zhong-Wei. (Reprinted with permission from Meyer 1985a.)

Successful re-establishment of circulation is the prime condition for survival of the part distal to the injury, just as optimum nerve repair is a major factor for restoring optimum function. The aim of vascular reconstruction must be to achieve the best possible arterial blood supply for the anoxic or ischaemic part in conjunction with minimum inhibition of venous return. The theory that there is an advantage in anastomosing only a minimum number of veins, to reduce the risk of postoperative venous thrombosis by having maximum flow through the repaired veins, is not supported by clinical experience. The principle, therefore, is to anastomose as many veins as possible. Even then, only a small number of the venous return channels, in amputation cases (as compared to normal) will be restored. The result is that, despite the most extensive venous repair possible, the rate of flow is still abnormally high across each venous juncture. Thus, in replantation and also in serious revascularisation cases there will always result, postoperatively, a situation of relative venous congestion which may of course be of transient nature. This relative inhibition of the venous return, and a temporary complete stoppage of lymph circulation, are additional important factors in the development of postoperative oedema. If deliberate reduction in the number of possible venous anastomoses causes a further unnecessary restriction of the venous return, postoperative oedema must, as a result, be even more severe. One of the main aims with all surgery of the extremities, however, is to keep oedema to the minimum, and to counteract any existing oedema by initiating an intensive exercise program as soon as possible. Persistent oedema will cause a cellular reaction with subsequent collagen formation, which will impair tissue gliding and cause stiffness of joints.

It takes up to eight days for lymph vessels distal to the injury to establish new connections with proximal lymphatic channels (Piza-Katzer et al 1987). In major upper limb replantation, it has been proven that even main lymphatic collectors will reconnect spontaneously (Vogt et al 1970).

Arteries should also be repaired to the fullest possible extent. In the forearm, continuity of the radial and ulnar arteries should be re-established wherever feasible. Of course, the final result will depend not only on the number of vessels repaired, but even more so on the technical quality of anastomoses.

Unlike the case of nerves, normal tension should be aimed at in vessel repair. But it is important to realise that vascular anastomoses under increased tension have a much poorer prognosis than anastomoses with normal, or only minimal, tension. As already stated, at least one large vein needs to be anastomosed before the repaired arterial system is declamped. This reduces blood loss which otherwise may be considerable and difficult to control without putting back the arterial clamps. Again, the anoxic part should be flushed with at least one unit of conserved blood before removing the clamps on already anastomosed veins, to reduce the amount of toxic metabolite which will get into the patient's circulatory system. A very common fault, apart from excessive tension at the anastomoses, is inadequate debridement of damaged vessels. No compromise is possible in this matter; it is better to use an interposition graft rather than to anastomose with increased tension. The patency rate of an autologous vein graft with two technically perfect anastomoses will be very much better than that through a simple anastomosis that is under increased tension (Brown 1981, Fujikawa & O'Brien 1975).

The failure of vascular anastomosis is almost always a consequence of inadequate judgment of the overall situation, insufficient debridement and poor anastomotic technique. Subsequent anticoagulant medication will not prevent the consequences of such errors. These points, therefore, need due consideration (Hayhurst & O'Brien 1975).

As mentioned above, the principles of microvascular techniques (described in greter detail in Ch. 2) are also advantageously applied to the larger vessels of the arm and forearm. First of all, it is necessary to cut away all thrombosed and damaged parts of the vessel until normal tissue is left (Fig. 4.17 A). The loosely attached, easily mobile tissue layers of the adventitia are then cut back in a cuff-like manner (Fig. 4.17 B). This prevents entrapment of adventitia tissue in the lumen of the anastomosis, which may otherwise give rise to thrombosis (Fig. 4.17 C). Before the suture is commenced, the vessel stumps are dilated with a pair of forceps. This mechanical dilatation will not only eventually eliminate pre-existing spasm of the vessel stumps, but also paralyse to some extent the smooth musculature of the vessel wall for some time, and thus counteract the tendency to spasm in the area of the anastomosis (Fig. 4.17 D). For all forceps manipulation of the vessels, we use the so-called vessel stretcher forceps of Acland, which have particularly fine rounded and polished tips (S & T Marketing Ltd, CH-8211 Neuhausen-Rheinfall, Switzerland). These forceps are not only suitable vessel stretchers, but also serve as an excellent counterpressure instrument and as knotting forceps when suturing (Fig. 4.17 E). The finest possible suture material that will still give reliable juncture of the vessel in question is always used. In the arm and forearm, this is usually a 7–0 to 9–0 thread mounted on a flat-bodied, non-cutting needle. The suture must include all tissue layers of the vessel wall, and it should be at right-angles to the wall to achieve optimum adaptation. Oblique or tangential stitches will cause inversion of the wall and this must be avoided at all cost (Fig. 4.17 F).

As a rule, we do not use continuous sutures for vascular anastomoses in the extremities. Also, for the larger vessels in the arm and forearm we definitely prefer anastomoses with interrupted sutures. This offers the advantage that vascular stumps which may not have been fully dilated during anastomosis will be able to dilate fully at a later stage, which may even be as late as the day after the operation. A continuous suture will prevent this, with the result that maximum spontaneous dilatation will produce circular constrictions which will give rise to turbulences and related subsequent problems.

The first two sutures are placed at an angle of 120° as stay sutures. Slight pull on these sutures will cause the posterior wall to fall open, so that the anterior wall of the vessel can be sutured without danger of including parts of the posterior wall, exactly as in small vessel anastomoses (Fig. 4.17 G). The distance between the sutures should be such that the anastomosis may be expected to be leak-proof after removal of the vascular clamps (Fig. 4.17 H). Minor seepage from the suture holes or from between individual sutures is of no significance, and will usually cease within one or two minutes.

Double approximator clamps have proved particularly useful in vascular anastomoses when no efficient assistance is available. These double clamps need more space, however, so their use is somewhat limited according to the individual anatomical situation. For vascular surgery in the arm and forearm, we found Acland's vascular clamps (S & T Marketing Ltd) most useful, except of course in the proximal area of the arm and at the level of the axilla where the common vascular instruments are used.

Vascular end-to-end anastomosis using sutures is time-consuming and often technically difficult. For years, therefore, new proposals have been made for quicker and simpler alternatives (Meyer et al 1980, Nakayama et al 1962, Oestrup 1976, Nylander et al 1989). However, at this time, none of these alternatives has replaced the old classical technique for general use. Nevertheless, the ongoing process of developing new vascular techniques deserves due consideration.

In our experience, vascular interposition grafts are often needed, especially in severe revascularisation cases; for this, we always prefer autologous veins. This makes it possible for the dissection of the graft to be done by a separate team, and thus the work at the upper limb need not be interrupted. Usually, we take a segment of the greater or lesser saphenous vein. All side branches of the vein segment must be carefully ligated as closely as possible to the wall of the vein to avoid blind sacs liable to produce turbulence in the graft. The vein is then washed out with heparin-Ringer's solution; in doing this, the vein segment can be distended by intraluminal fluid dilatation, which also helps in detecting leakages and constricting fibrous tissue strands. A suture at the distal or proximal end will serve as a marker to facilitate directional orientation with regard to existing valves. Vein grafts increase in both diameter and length when submitted to arterial pressure. Therefore, its original diameter needs to be slightly less than that of the artery, and its length slightly shorter than the defect.

Many of the previously described mechanisms of injury, such as crush, traction and explosion injuries, may lead to partial lesion of the vessel wall. Circular disruption of the intima with subsequent intussusception of the intima distally is the most classical form with blunt injuries (Fig. 4.18 A–B).

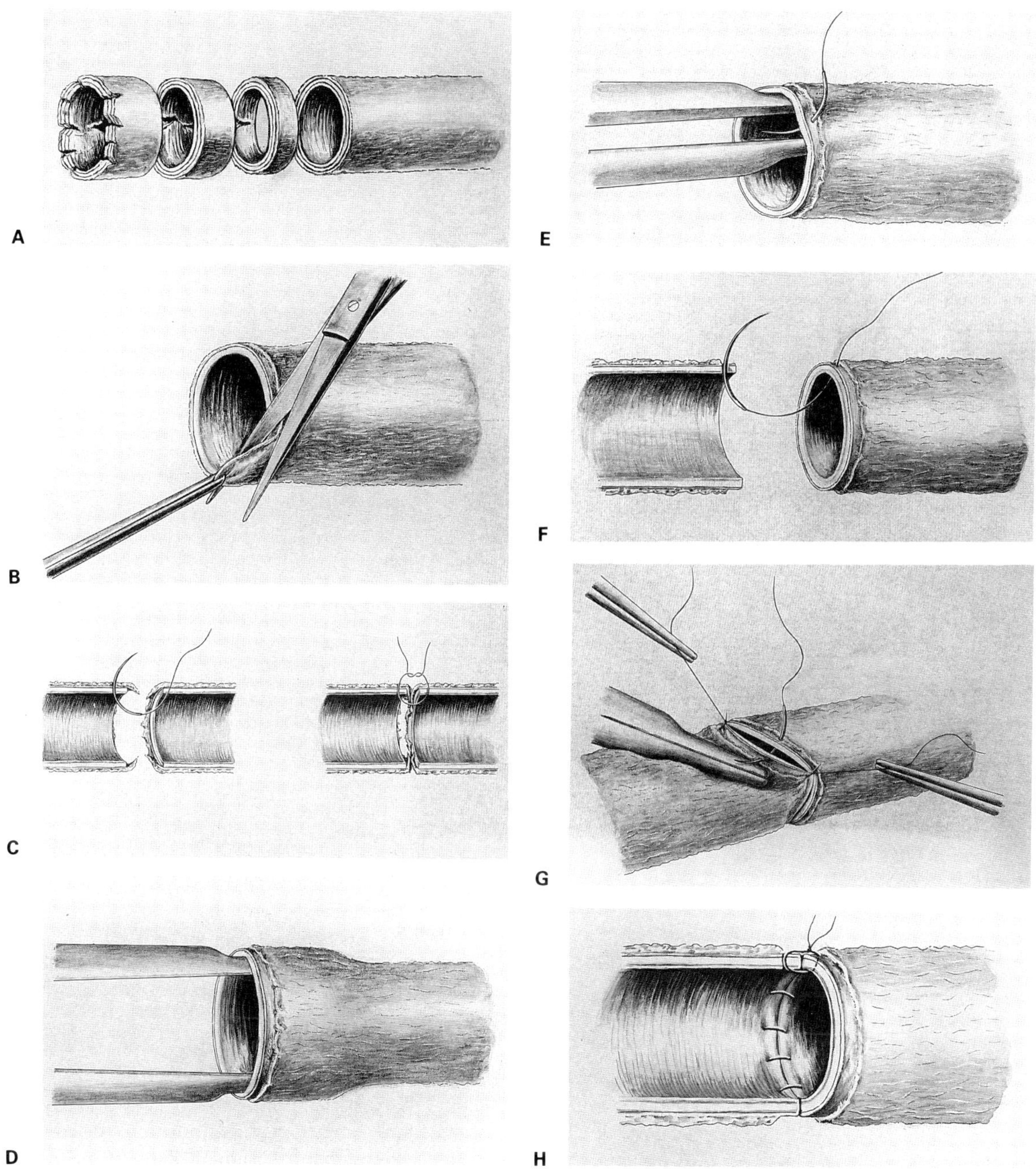

Fig. 4.17 **A.** Damaged part of vessels must be cut back until only normal tissue is left. This is an absolute precondition for successful microvascular anastomosis. **B.** Cuff-like resection of the loose, easily mobile tissue of the adventitia to prevent adventitia becoming entrapped in the subsequent suture. **C.** If the adventitia has not been sufficiently cut back, fronds of it are easily trapped in the lumen of the vessel and may well be a possible cause for subsequent thrombosis. **D.** Careful dilatation of the vessel ends. This makes suturing easier and prevents vascular spasm in the area of the anastomosis. **E.** Atraumatic vascular suturing requires the use of a counter-pressure instrument. The vessel-stretcher forceps shown here have proved most useful in our experience. **F.** For optimum adaptation, the suture should be at right angles to the vessel wall and pass through all three layers. **G.** Two guide-sutures placed at an angle of about 120° will cause the posterior wall to fall open. This largely avoids the risk of parts of the posterior wall being included in the suture of the anterior wall. **H.** The distance between individual sutures should be such that the resulting anastomosis may be expected to be leak-free. Individual sutures must not be pulled too tight. They should always remain visible as a loop having at least the thickness of the vascular wall. (Reprinted with permission from Meyer 1985a.)

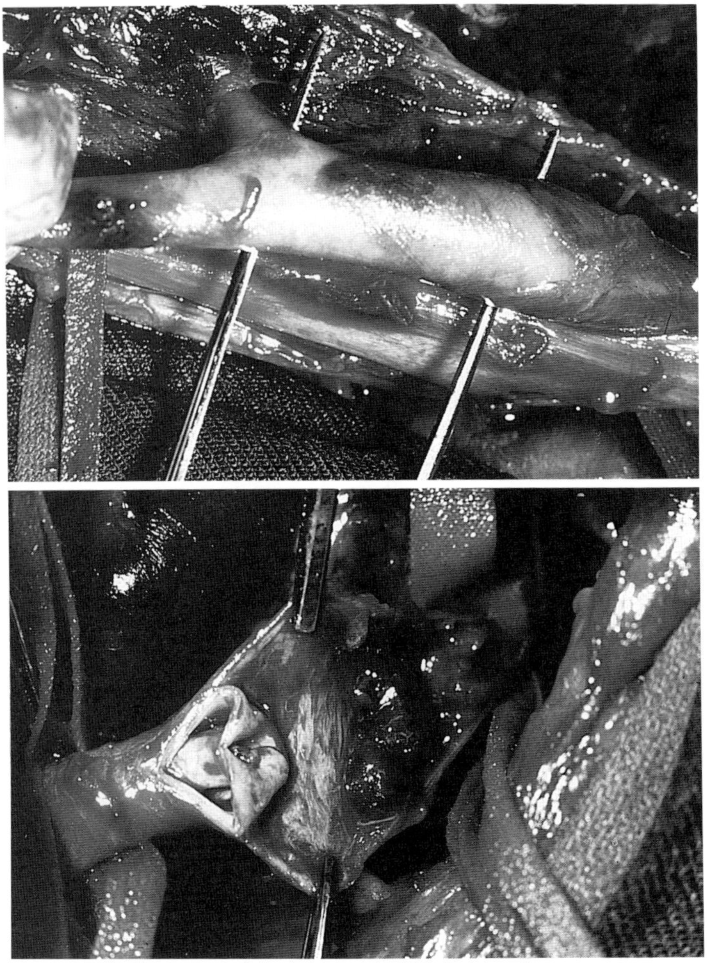

A

B

Fig. 4.18 **A.** Blunt trauma to an axillary artery. On surgical exposure, the site of the lesion is easily located by the haematoma within the vessel wall, in which area palpation of the vessel shows a circumscript hardening (segment between the tips of the forceps). **B.** Conspicous intussusception of the inner layers of the arterial wall after arteriotomy. In such a situation we perform resection of the damaged vascular segment and an autologous interposition graft if direct anastomosis is not possible. (Reprinted with permission from Meyer & Largiadèr 1989.)

In larger arteries, this was formally treated by longitudinal arteriotomy, refixation of the intima by a few sutures, and closures with or without vein patch angioplasty. We found, however, that excision of all damaged-vessel wall and reconstitution of continuity by direct end-to-end anastomosis or insertion of a vein graft gave superior results, even if a vein graft had to be doubled to accurately match a larger vessel diameter (Fig. 4.19) (Meyer & Largiadèr 1989). If ever the extent of vascular injury is not clear from the clinical findings, we make liberal use of arteriography before or, if necessary, even during the operation. This may be extremely helpful, particularly in multi-level injuries.

Trauma-related spasm is, with rare exceptions, of segmental nature. Usually, the spastic segment is located in the area of the main injury. Compression from outside may imitate vascular spasm, as for example in compartment syndromes. Younger individuals are most prone to develop spasm, and spasm may even have a similar appearance to thrombosis on the arteriogram, especially if this is not of high quality. In doubtful situations, it is advisable to leave the catheter in place for administration of spasmolytic drugs, such as lignocaine, in combination with warming up the extremity and a second arteriogram at a later stage. This refers especially to cases of incomplete severance.

Because clinical diagnosis of compartment syndrome is not possible in most of these severe injuries, especially if there is considerable concomitant nerve damage, we regularly perform

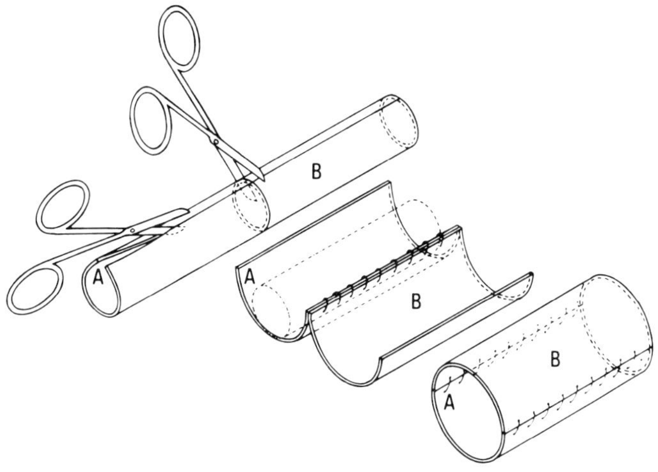

Fig. 4.19 For bridging a gap in a large proximal artery, a graft of the greater saphenous vein may occasionally be too small in diameter. The illustration shows the technique we use to double the diameter by two segments of the greater saphenous vein. Both segments (A and B) are split longitudinally and then united by running sutures. (Reprinted with permission from Meyer & Largiadér 1989.)

fasciotomies as a part of the primary procedure in all major replants and cases of revascularisation for survival.

Nerve repair

The final function of a replanted extremity is in large part determined by the quality of nerve repair and resulting nerve regeneration. This is one of the main reasons why the clear distinction between replantation and revascularisation cases must be made. Whereas in replantation, by definition, all the structures including the nerves are divided, in revascularisation cases it may well be possible that one, several or even all major nerves remain intact. This makes any classification of revascularisation cases both difficult and questionable.

In contrast to complete severance, where the type of injury can be divided into a few categories, the possible combinations of tissue lesions in cases of incomplete severance of the upper limb are so numerous that any system of classification would probably have so many categories of lesions as to become impractical.

Unfortunately, in revascularisation cases, there are often severe nerve lesions in continuity, which tend to have a poor prognosis for useful recovery and may eventually call for secondary neurolysis or even nerve grafting.

Nerve repair in replantation surgery has some special aspects only with regard to deciding whether nerve repair is to be a primary or a secondary procedure. These have been discussed above, in the section on 'extent and sequence of repair'.

In contrast to other forms of nerve injury, suitable skeletal shortening will, in the case of replantation surgery, create uniquely favourable conditions for direct nerve repair without any tension. Even the normal tension due to the elasticity of the nerve can be fully eliminated and will not influence the scar formation at the coapted nerve stump surfaces. On the other hand, it is not advisable to insist on primary suture in every case. There are situations when secondary nerve repair is likely to give a better result. This is particularly true when nerves have been damaged over a long distance. In our experience, secondary nerve repair in this category of upper limb injuries always calls for the use of autologous nerve grafts.

The surgical technique and strategy used to repair severed nerves in replantation and revascularisation surgery does not differ in principle from that used in isolated or less complex injuries. The reader is therefore referred to Chapter 14, in which the state of the art is described in great detail (Jabaley 1984, Mackinnon & Dellon 1988, Meyer 1988, Millesi 1979, Sunderland 1978).

There are only two technical points which I would like to mention:

1. As mentioned already, adequate bone shortening creates a situation which enables an absolutely tension-free nerve juncture, in which case the use of a low-reactive tissue glue (Tissucol® (Immuno Ag)) to keep the nerve juncture aligned may be considered. This reduces, or sometimes

eliminates, the suture material needed (Egloff & Narakas 1983, Narakas 1988, Smahel et al 1987).

2. In this type of injury severed nerve ends need to be freshened in all cases. This must be done with great care and precision, in order to remove the least necessary amount of nerve tissue. Millesi has developed scissors for cutting small nerves and single fascicles (Millesi 1979). These have serrated blades which prevent the nerve from slipping as it is cut, without any additional holding device. We have found these scissors very useful for trimming small nerves, groups of fascicles and single fascicles. However, all scissors have the effect of crushing tissue, and should therefore be avoided whenever the diameter of the nerve permits cutting with a sharp blade. Using a blade, however, one has the problem of fixing the nerve while cutting. For this purpose, we have developed a series of simple nerve-holding forceps of different calibre (Fig. 4.20). These nerve holders permit atraumatic fixation of the nerve ends, and make it possible to achieve accurately clean-cut surfaces (Fig. 4.21 A–B) with a minimum loss of nerve substance; by this technique, slices of 1 mm or even less may be obtained (Fig. 4.22). They are very easy to handle, even in areas of difficult surgical exposure. In fact, they are equally useful for cutting other cylindrical structures which may require a clean-cut surface, such as tendons and vessels (Meyer et al 1980). A clean-cut surface of the nerve ends is important for accurate mirror-like identification of the corresponding fascicles or groups of fascicles on either surface.

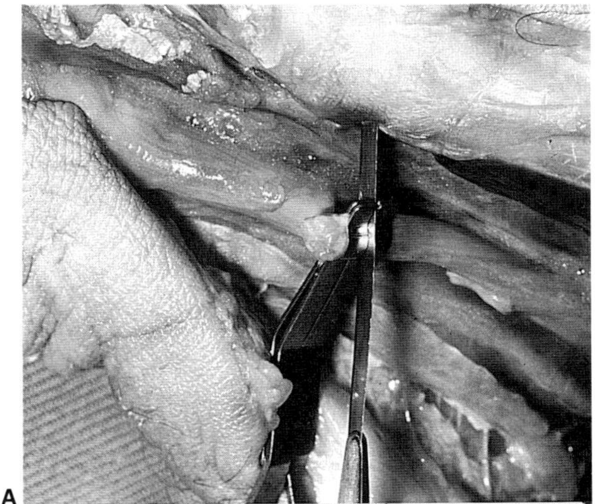

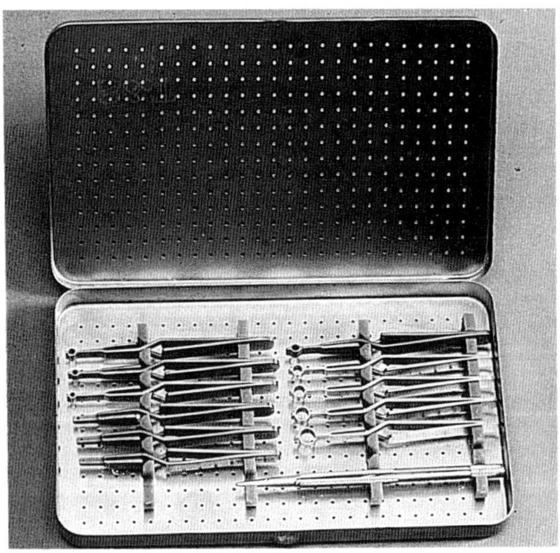

Fig. 4.20 A wide range of forceps of different calibres has been developed to adjust to the different diameters of cylindrical anatomical structures, including those other than nerves. Manufactured by S & T Marketing Ltd., CH 8212 Neuhausen am Rheinfall (Switzerland).

A

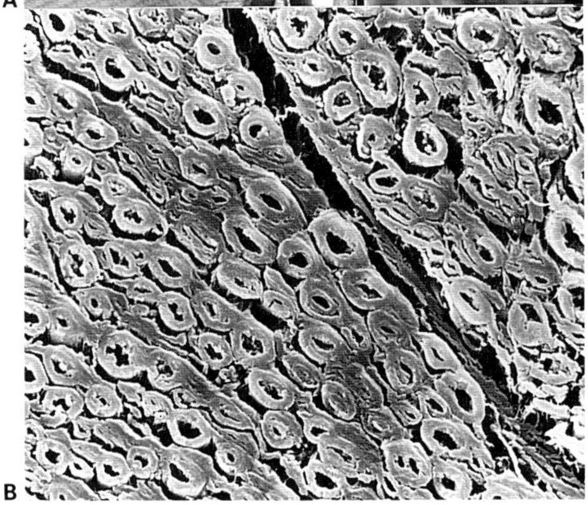

B

Fig. 4.21 **A.** The nerve stump is fixed by a special nerve-holding forceps of appropriate calibre which has a slot in its branches thin enough to pass a razor blade.
B. Scanning electron micrograph of a human sural nerve showing the clean-cut surface attained.

Wound closure and decompression

To keep inflammatory reaction at a minimum and to favour primary wound healing, only tissues that are clearly viable should be used for wound closure. Skin tension should be such that, on the one hand, the skin itself is not subject to ischaemia

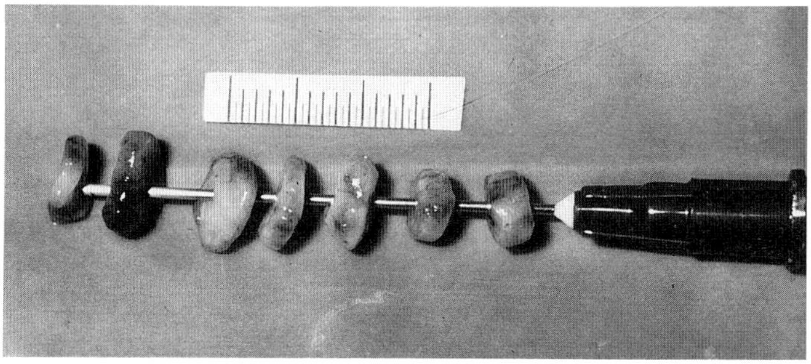

Fig. 4.22 With the special forceps shown in Figure 4.20 it is possible to get slices of about 1 mm thickness.

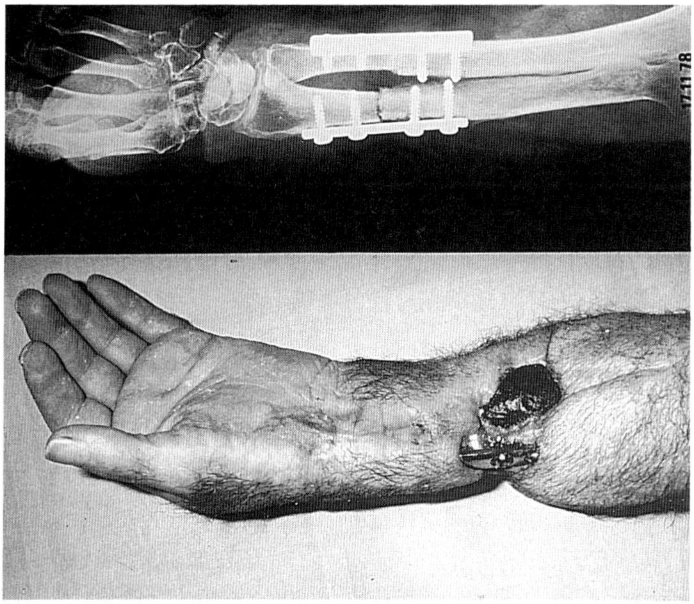

Fig. 4.23 Forearm replantation in a 45-year-old manual worker. Correct rigid skeletal fixation achieved with two dynamic compression plates after initial bone-shortening of 4 cm. Skeletal shortening, however, proved to be insufficient and resulted in undue tension for wound closure. Consequently, soft tissue necrosis with exposure of the plate on the radius, and non-union of bones occurred. A distant pedicle flap was needed to achieve healing, and the final functional result turned out to be poor. Moreover, the morbidity in this case was significantly increased with all socio-economic consequences. (Reprinted with permission from Meyer 1985a.)

and, on the other hand, any reconstructed vessels are not under undue pressure.

In all cases where bone shortening has been performed, uncomplicated wound healing depends largely on the extent to which the skeleton has been shortened with regard to the extent of the injury. At the level of the forearm, it is of little consequence to the patient whether the bone was shortened by 3 or by 5 cm but the extra 2 cm can be of vital importance where wound closure is concerned and, at times, even decide whether replantation will be successful or not. At the level of the upper arm, we found that even radical shortening by as much as 9 cm is of negligible functional consequence (Fig. 4.7 A–H).

There is a danger — not to be underestimated — that, due to fatigue after 8–14 hours at the operating table, surgeons may resort to unacceptable compromises when closing the wound. There is also a tendency to leave wound closure to younger, less experienced colleagues. If the edges of a wound become necrotic, it may be possible to keep infection limited by early excision of all necrotic tissue. The revascularised part may survive, but progress will often then be greatly delayed and expensive treatments become necessary. This is illustrated by the case shown in Fig. 4.23 where the bone had not been sufficiently shortened. Soft tissue necrosis with localised infection interfered with bone healing, and pseudo-arthrosis developed; moreover, there was extensive fibrosis of all soft tissues in the area, especially musculature. It finally became necessary to perform an abdominal flap procedure to restore soft tissue coverage, after which the pseudoarthrosis was treated with cancellous bone grafting. All this resulted in a delay of rehabilitation of more than one year. It is easy to imagine the enormous additional socio-economic impact of such a case, which could probably have been avoided by a more radical initial bone shortening.

In parts with large anoxic and/or ischaemic muscle bulk, it must be taken into account that, once circulation is restored, the muscle tissue may develop quite considerable oedematous swelling for a period of time; therefore, in every one of these cases, without exception, we perform primary decompression of all muscle compartments by fasciotomies. There are a number of methods to reduce undue tension at the skin sutures:

1. *Relief incisions and primary use of a split-thickness skin graft to cover the defect.* Experience has shown that vascular repairs, including interposition vein grafts, may be covered directly by split-thickness skin grafts without increasing the risk of thrombosis. However, we practise this method only in situations where, for whatever reason, no better soft tissue coverage can be provided.

2. *Staggered rows of stab wounds* (author's method). The use of staggered rows of stab wounds to allow for expansion of skin areas has been known for a long time (Lanz 1908). It has been successfully used for years with free skin graft (mesh graft). It appears that even the ancient Egyptians employed the principle of draining fluids from swollen extremities for decompression by making series of multiple skin incisions (Balsamo & Rapontico 1745). Apart from primary decompression by making multiple small skin incisions, these also provide immediate external lymph drainage, and this also helps to counteract postoperative swelling.

Staggered rows of stab wounds will assist considerably in the decompression of the skin and soft tissue envelope after revascularisation, particularly in cases with bone shortening, in which the relative excess length of the skin sleeve can be converted into an increase in diameter. With consistent application of this principle, in conjunction with primary fasciotomies, we have never had to perform a secondary operation for decompression in more than 12 years. Healing progresses normally and the scars that remain are not very noticeable, certainly much less so than the scars produced by a major relief incision and subsequent skin grafts (Figs 4.24 to 4.26).

In 1968, clinical proof was given that after replantation of an amputated arm even major lymphatics do reunite (Vogt et al 1970). At this time, we have seen only one major replant with persistent oedema.

3. *Pedicle or free flap procedures.* Occasionally, a skin flap is necessary to provide adequate soft tissue coverage. In our view, the groin flap either as a pedicle flap or as a free flap, is an excellent choice for many of these cases (Fig. 4.27 A–E and Fig. 4.28).

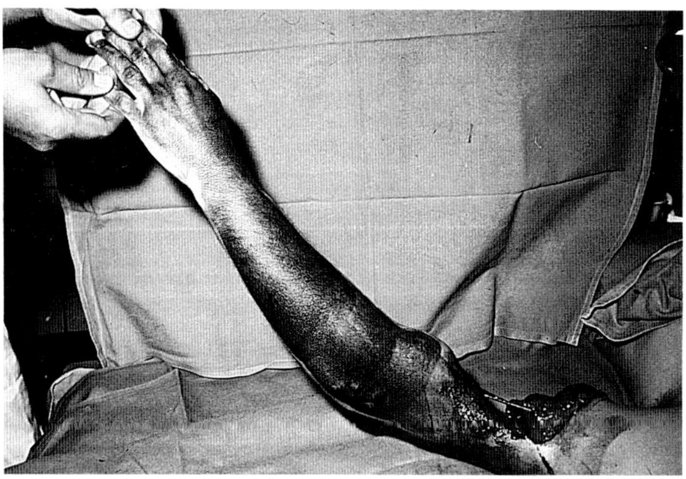

Fig. 4.24 Incomplete upper arm severance by colour application rollers (distance between rollers 2–5 cm) causing very severe diffused crush injury of the whole amputated part and fracture of the forearm. Printer aged 22 years. On admission to the hospital, the whole arm was stained with blue printing ink. The only structures in continuity were a badly crushed bridge of skin 3 cm in width and an extensively lacerated cephalic vein. Both were cut away during debridement. A temporary silicon bypass in the brachial artery showed that the hand could be effectively revascularised. (Reprinted with permission from Meyer 1985a.)

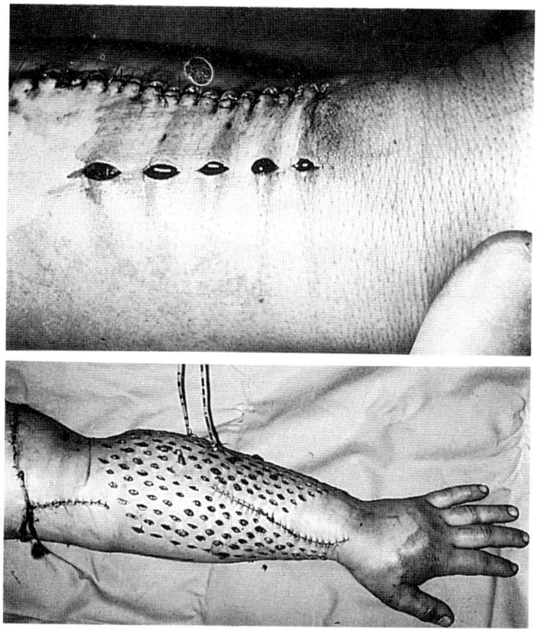

Fig. 4.25 Complete decompression of the skin and soft tissue envelope with primary subcutaneous fasciotomy resulted in sufficient release of tension to allow effective capillary circulation. (Reprinted with permission from Meyer 1985a.)

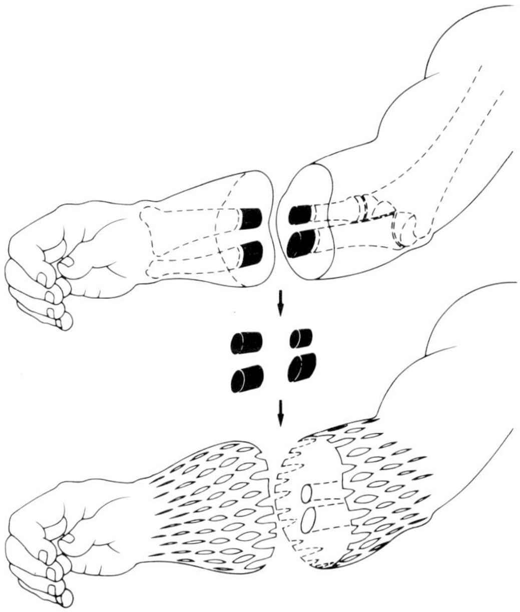

Fig. 4.26 This diagrammatic illustration shows how the relative redundancy of the skin sleeve obtained by skeletal shortening can be transformed in a significant increase of circumference. In combination with primary fasciotomies, this offers optimal condition for successful wound closure with sufficient soft tissue decompression and efficient early lymph drainage. In performing the multiple stab wounds in the skin, care must be taken to avoid injury to the superficial veins. (Reprinted with permission from Meyer 1985a.)

High grade haemostasis must always be the aim in replantation surgery. However, as tissue damage tends to be extensive, it can of course never be complete, and additional wound drainage will often be required. In major limb replantation, so-called 'easy-flow' drains, or on occasion also suction drainage, are used.

Dressings

The dressing is a major, and often critically important, part of the operation. It should not be left to anyone who is unaware of this fact. The following technique has proved to be effective. First of all, soft gauze compresses, moistened with Ringer's solution or physiological saline, are completely unfolded and loosely placed between individual digits; this will prevent skin maceration between the fingers. The gauze compresses, which run lengthwise, completely cover all wounds in the forearm and arm, including any drainage tubes if present. To complete the dressing, the first layer is then covered with a second layer of moist gauze compresses, again running lengthwise. Gauze or gauze dressings should never encircle the extremity, so as to avoid any circular constriction. This loose, sterile dressing is contour-bound and padded with a Dacron fibre felt bandage. Compared to normal cotton wool, Dacron padding has the advantage that it does not compact when moisture soaks through; thus it allows the air to circulate. As the compresses (moistened with electrolyte solution) dry out, considerable capillary suction is created in the area of the wounds and drainage tubes, providing for excellent drainage. At the same time, the contoured dressing achieves a certain stability of its own as it dries. The strong suction effect produced is also evident from the fact that blood seeping from the wounds becomes distributed all over the dressings, and no dried blood is left on the skin when the dressing is removed.

A plaster slab is used in all cases, at least to

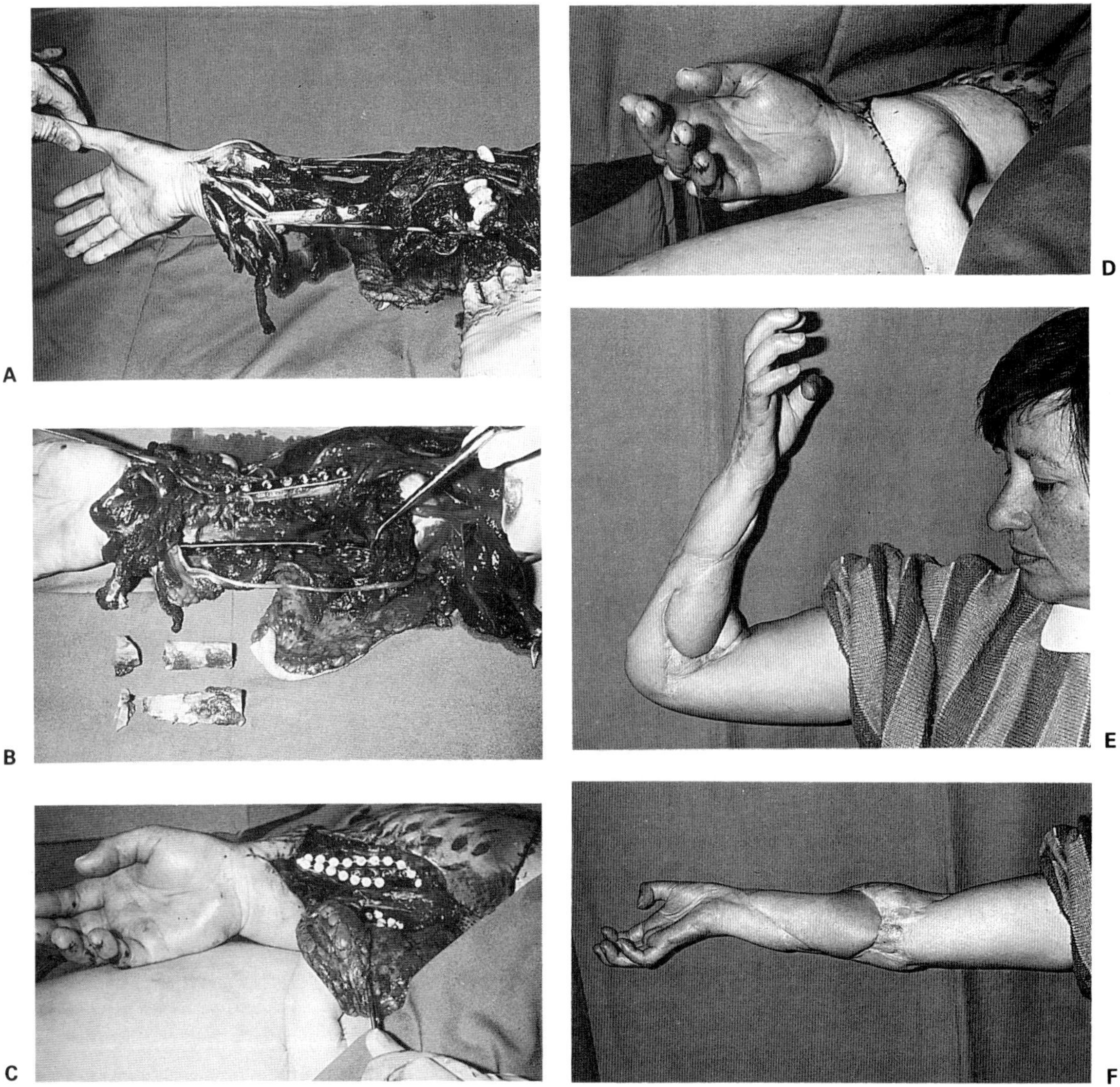

Fig. 4.27 **A.** Severe injury of the forearm in a 38-year-old woman by a mangle with complete stoppage of circulation in the hand. **B.** Condition after radical debridement and skeletal shortening of 6.5 cm. **C.** Application of gentamycin pellets in order to prevent infection in this forearm with extensive tissue damage. **D.** Wound closure in this case required extensive soft tissue replacement, which was provided in this case by a pedicle groin flap. **E.** Condition 3 years after the accident. There is protective sensibility in the hand but no really significant prehensile capacity. **F.** The advantage of this limb salvage is the preservation of body integrity and the usefulness of the forearm and the hand as a lever arm.

stabilise the wrist and finger joints. The hand is ideally immobilised in the so-called 'protective position' — the best way of avoiding joint stiffness due to immobilisation. In replantation, however, flexor and extensor units have been severed, and it is therefore necessary to accept the position spontaneously assumed by the hand (Beasley 1981).

The dressing put on in the operating theatre must not be removed for 8–12 days, unless there are special reasons for inspecting the wound, such as persistent fever or the need to remove drainage tubes. Postoperatively, the revascularised part is kept in an elevated position (10–20 cm higher than the right atrium) to assist venous return.

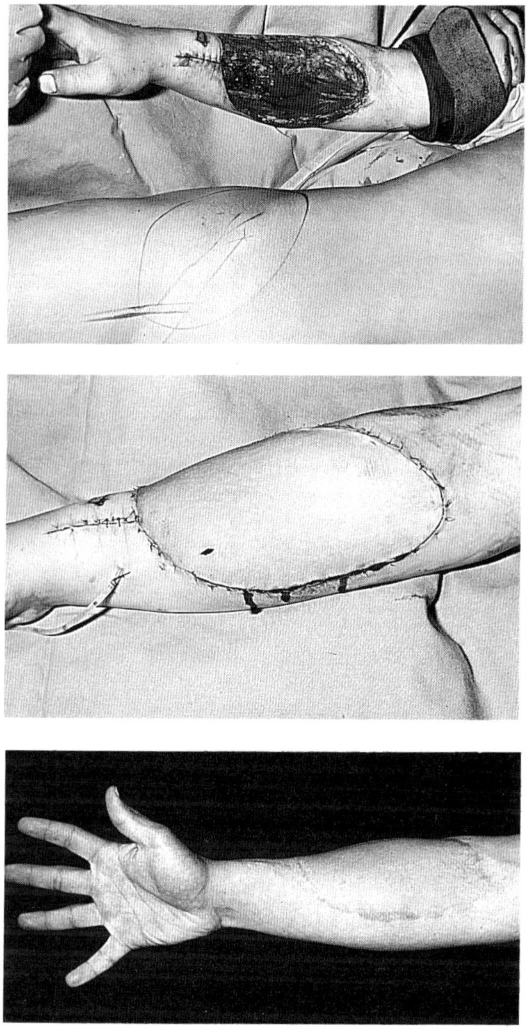

A

B

C

Fig. 4.28 **A.** Extensive bone and soft tissue defect in a forearm of a 14-year-old boy. Total primary repair of all divided structures, including restoration of a defect of the radius of 4 cm by a bridge-plate and cancellous bone grafting. **B.** Reconstruction of the soft tissue defect by means of a free microvascular groin flap. **C.** Condition 2 years after the accident with excellent function of the hand and a very satisfactory aesthetic result without any corrective secondary surgery in this case. (Reprinted with permission from Meyer V E 1988 The role of microsurgical techniques of treatment of upper limb amputation. In: Tubiana R (ed) The hand, Vol. III. W B Saunders Company, Philadelphia, p 951–971.)

POSTOPERATIVE MANAGEMENT

Surveillance

If the revascularised part contains a fairly large amount of musculature, renal and pulmonary function as well as serum electrolytes need to be watched carefully during the first days to ensure early detection and treatment of possible post-ischaemia syndrome.

Many of these patients suffered considerable blood loss at the time of the accident and during surgery. It is difficult for the anaesthetic team to assess the amount of blood lost during the operation, because of the generous use of wound irrigation during the operation. This makes it necessary to complete blood replacement postoperatively in almost all cases. Assuming that oxygen exchange and flow properties of blood in the microcirculation seem to be optimum at a PVC of 32–35%, we only transfuse sufficient blood postoperatively to get a stable reading at this level (Messmer 1973).

The circulation in the revascularised part is monitored every 30 minutes for the first 8 hours after the operation, then hourly for 48 hours and finally every 2–3 hours until the sixth postoperative day. It is during this period that postoperative vascular thromboses occur. Monitoring of the circulation is best based on the following clinical criteria: skin color, skin temperature, capillary filling and tissue turgor. As nursing staff change shifts frequently nowadays, it is often difficult to ensure good continuity of this fairly demanding surveillance. It has thus proved most effective to involve the patient in the monitoring process as soon as possible; after all, he has the greatest interest in making sure that the operation is a success. In major limb replantations, we see no need for any electronic monitoring device.

Medication

The best method of preventing postoperative thrombosis of vascular anastomoses is perfect surgical technique. Medication cannot prevent the consequences of bad technique with vessel anastomosis. Thus, in guillotine-type amputations, medication for the prevention of thrombosis in the revascularised part is not required. On the other hand, in extensive tissue crush and/or avulsion with the possibility of diffuse damage to the vascular system, which cannot be fully eliminated by extensive debridement, medication to prevent thrombosis is indicated. In these cases, we give 10 000 units of heparin by infusion and 3 × 300 mg doses of acetylsalicylic acid daily for one week. Due to life-threatening anaphylactic reactions, we have stopped using low-molecular-weight dextrans as an adjunct to improve the flow properties of the blood.

Exposure of the wound is extremely long in replantation and revascularisation surgery. Therefore we always give antibiotic cover, using a broad-spectrum antibiotic. This is started preoperatively when preparing the patient for anaesthesia. If the postoperative course is normal, we continue antibiotics only until the fifth postoperative day. Of course, tetanus prevention must not be forgotten, as in all cases of injury.

Local complications

The earliest local complication is thrombosis of vessel anastomoses. If this occurs, it is almost always within the first five days. The only case of thrombosis we have seen in replantations after the seventh postoperative day, was in a digital vein on day 16.

Arterial thrombosis

If arterial occlusion has occurred, the revascularised part looks pale, and turgor is clearly reduced, particularly in the terminal phalanges. Pressure on the nail is not followed by evident capillary refill in the nailbed. If no blood, or only a small quantity of very dark blood, flows from a stab wound in the digital pulp, arterial occlusion is even more likely. Of course, the pulse of the radial and/or ulnar artery at the wrist is absent. With all types of circulatory disorder, the first step must always be to remove the dressings and, if necessary, also some of the stitches. If this does not restore circulation, immediate revision of the anastomosis is indicated.

Venous thrombosis

If the venous return is impeded, the revascularised part appears cyanotic and tissue turgor is increased. Capillary refill after brief pressure is greatly accelerated. The pulse of the arteries at the wrist is still present. Following a stab incision in the digital pulp, dark venous blood will emerge first under pressure. With the venous pressure thus relieved, the finger may temporarily turn pink again. The first step is again to check the positioning of the extremity and the dressings. If this does not correct the situation, it will be necessary to remove the dressings and some of the skin sutures in the region of the venous anastomosis. If this proves unsuccessful, surgical revision must immediately be undertaken.

Necrosis

Apart from vascular thrombosis, necrosis of wound margins is the most common early complication. If this is merely superficial, and strictly limited, it will not necessarily lead to infection and may be ignored. Any more deep-seated necrosis will, however, require early debridement to prevent infection. If there is extensive infection of large muscle bulk, which occurs particularly in farming injuries, early amputation must be considered, even though circulation in the hand may be fully intact, in order to prevent or combat potential life-threatening septicaemia (Fig. 4.12 A–B).

Systemic complications

Systemic complications specifically related to revascularisation of a significant muscle bulk are: the post-ischaemia syndrome; septicaemia from infected necrotic soft tissue, particularly musculature; or a combination of both. The basic pathophysiology of post-ischaemia syndrome is summarised in the section on duration of tissue anoxia — post-ischaemia syndrome (p. 42).

We have ourselves observed one case of a forearm replantation after a farming accident, in which the patient developed a combination of post-ischaemia syndrome and subsequent severe septicaemia with adult respiratory distress syndrome (ARDS). On the ninth postoperative day, upper arm amputation had to be performed while circulation in the hand was still intact. A few days later, the patient recovered and respiratory assistance could be discontinued (Fig. 4.12 A B). In our series we have had no death and no complication from prolonged general anaesthesia.

PHYSICAL THERAPY

An intensive postoperative hand-therapy program is of critical importance for optimal functional results. Wherever the conditions of the wounds permit, all small joints not immobilised by the dressings are very gently taken through slight passive movements at the beginning of the second postoperative week. In the third postoperative week, graduated active exercises are done under the supervision of a hand therapist. After the third week, the patient is requested to carry out a daily program by himself, prescribed for him on an individual basis. With non-rigid bone fixation, this hand therapy programme can only be started when adequate skeletal stability has been achieved by bone healing. From the beginning, very special attention must be given to joints proximal to the injury, particularly the shoulder joint. Where long-term muscle denervation must be anticipated, early fitting of hand splints is indicated. These splints serve to keep the finger joints in the best possible position, particularly at night, and also serve to prevent, as far as possible, both the damaging effects of immobilisation due to shrinking of joint ligaments and capsules, and fixed malposition, for example adduction contracture of the thumb. Optimum postoperative physical therapy must be guided and controlled by the surgeon who took overall responsibility for the particular case. Active movement exercises are of prime importance; if the patient cannot be adequately motivated, optimum results will not be achieved. The issue, therefore, depends not only on good knowledge of functional anatomy and the technical skill of the hand therapist but also very much on psychological skill in dealing with the patient (Hunter et al 1990, Wynn Parry 1973).

ACKNOWLEDGEMENTS

The author expresses appreciation to the Foundation for Hand Research Inc., New York, N.Y., for the gracious suport in the production of all drawings for chapter 4.

REFERENCES

Balsamo, Rhapontico 1745 Medicina Aegyptiorum Gerardum Potvliet. Institute for History of Medicine, Vienna
Beasley R W 1981 Hand injuries. W B Saunders, Philadelphia, p 66–67
Berger A, Kolacny M, Passl R, Piza H 1980 Die Replantation ganzer Extremitäten — Pro und Contra. Hefte Unfallheilkunde 148: 557–564
Biemer E 1988 The organization of a central replantation center. In: Brunelli G (ed) Textbook of microsurgery. Masson, Milan, p 467–470
Biemer E 1982 Internationale Definitionen im Gebiet der Replantationschirurgie und Möglichkeiten eines Bewertungsschemas der funktionellen Ergebnisse. Handchirurgie Mikrochirurgie Plastische Chirurgie 14: 161–164
Biemer E 1979 Vein grafts in microvascular surgery. Annals Academy of Medicine 8: 382–386
Brown P W 1981 The rational selection of treatment for upper extremity amputations. Orthopedic Clinics of North America 12: 843–848
Brunelli G, Vigasio A, Brunelli F 1988 Muscular elementarization in replantation and revascularization cases of prolonged muscular ischemia or crush. In: Brunelli G (ed) Textbook of microsurgery. Masson, Milan, p 519–521
Brunelli C (ed) 1981 Ischaemia and replantation. Liviana, Padua
Burton R I 1981 Problems in the evaluation of results from replantation surgery. Orthopedic Clinics of North America 909–913
Burton R I, Beasley R W, Omer G, Meyer V E 1981 Organization for upper limb reattachment surgery. Orthopedic Clinics of North America 915–927
Chase R A 1970 The severely injured upper limb. To amputate or reconstruct: that is the question. Archive of Surgery 100: 382–387
Chen Zhong-Wei, Meyer V E, Kleinert H E, Beasley R W 1981 Present indications and contraindications for replantation as reflected by long-term functional results. Orthopedic Clinics of North America, 849–870
Doi K, Kawai S, Kotani H, Kuwata N 1983 Multiple organ failure after revascularization of lower limb. 7th Symposium of the International Society of Reconstructive Microsurgery, New York
Eger M, Schmidt B, Török G, Khodadadi J, Goldmann L 1974 Replantation of upper extremities. American Journal of Surgery 128: 447–450
Egloff D V, Narakas A 1983 Nerve anastomosis with human fibrin. Preliminary clinical report (56 cases). Annales de Chirurgie de la Main 2: 101–115
Eriksson E, Anerson W A, Reploge R L 1974 Effects of prolonged ischemia on muscle microcirculation in the cat. Surgical Forum 25: 254–255
Ferreira M C, Marquez E F, Azze R J 1978 Limb replantation. Clinics of Plastic Surgery 5: 211–221
Fujikawa S, O'Brien B McC 1975 An experimental evaluation of microvenous grafts. British Journal of Plastic Surgery 28: 244–246
Hales R, Pullen D 1982 Hypotension and bleeding diathesis

following attempted arm replantation. Anaesthesia and intensive care. Journal of the Australian Society of Anaesthetists 10: 359–361
Hayhurst J W, O'Brien B McC 1975 An experimental study of microvascular technique, patency rates and related factors. British Journal of Plastic Surgery 28: 128–132
Hunter J M, Schneider L A, Mackin E J, Callahan A D 1990 Rehabilitation of the hand: surgery and therapy. C V Mosby, St. Louis
Jabaley M E 1984 Technical aspects of peripheral nerve repair. Journal of Hand Surgery 9 B: 14–19
Jaeger S H, Tsai T M, Kleinert H E 1981 Upper extremity replantation in children. Orthopedic Clinics of North America 12: 897–907
Lanz O 1908 Die Transplantation betreffend. Zentralblatt für Chirurgie 35: 3–5
Mackinnon S E, Dellon A L 1988 Surgery of the peripheral nerve. Thieme, New York
Malcolm O P 1988 Compartment syndromes and reperfusion injury. Surgical Clinics of North America 68: 853–864
Matsuda M, Shibara H, Kato N 1978 Long-term results of replantation of 10 upper extremities. World Journal of Surgery 2: 603–612
May J W, Gallico G G 1980 Upper extremity replantation. (Current problems in Surgery) Year Book Medical, Chicago
McNeill J F, Wilson J S P 1970 The problems of limb replacement. British Journal of Surgery 57: 365–377
Messmer K 1973 Die Sauerstoffversorgung bei Blutersatz durch Kolloidlösungen. Infusionstherapie 1: 15–19
Meyer V E, Largiadèr J 1989 Injuries to the blood vessels In: Lamb D W, Hooper G, Kuczynski K (eds) The practice of hand surgery, 2nd edn. Blackwell Scientific Publications, Oxford 150–169
Meyer V E 1988 Restoration of peripheral nerves. In: Pho R W H (ed) Microsurgical technique in orthopedics. Butterworths, London
Meyer V E 1985a Upper extremity replantation. Churchill Livingstone, New York
Meyer V E 1985b Hand amputations proximal but close to the wrist joint: prime candidates for reattachment (long-term functional results). Journal of Hand Surgery 10A: 989–991
Meyer V E, Chen Zhong-Wei, Beasley R W 1981 Basic technical considerations in reattachment surgery. Orthopedic Clinics of North America 12: 871–895
Meyer V E 1981 Beitrag der Mikrochirurgie an die allgemeine Gefässtraumatologie. Angio Archiv 1: 163–164
Meyer V E 1979 Replantation surgery of the upper extremity: functional results. In: Lie T S (ed) Microsurgery International Congress Series 465: 24–27 Excerpta Medica, Amsterdam-Oxford
Meyer V E, Smahel J, Donski P 1980 Microvascular anastomosis using the telescope principle: experimental study. International Journal of Microsurgery 2: 81–86
Millesi H 1979 Microsurgery of peripheral nerves. World Journal of Surgery 3: 67–69
Nakayama K, Tamiya T, Yamamoto K, Akimoto S 1962 A simple new apparatus for small vessel anastomosis. Surgery 52: 918–922
Narakas A 1988 The use of fibrin glue in repair of peripheral nerves. Orthopedic Clinics of North America 19: 187–199
Nunley J A, Koman L A, Urbaniak J R 1981 Arterial shunting as an adjunct to major limb revascularization. Annals of Surgery 193: 271–273
Nylander G, Ragnarsson R, Berggren A, Oestrup L T 1989 The UNILINK system for mechanical microvascular anastomosis in hand surgery. Journal of Hand Surgery 14A: 44–48
Oestrup L T 1976 Anastomosis of small veins with suture or Nakayama's apparatus. Scandinavian Journal of Plastic and Reconstructive Surgery 10: 9–15
Piza-Katzer H, Partsch H, Urbanek A, Wenzel-Hora B I, Walzer R L 1987 Zur Frage der Lymphgefässregeneration nach Replantation und freier mikrovaskulärer Lappenplastik. Vasa 16: 60–66
Piza H, Millesi H, Piza F, Poigenfürst J 1977 Replantation einer samt Schulterblatt und Acromioclaviculargelenk ausgerissenen oberen Extremität. Vasa 6: 154
Russell R C, O'Brien B McC, Morrison W A, Pamamull G, McLeod A 1984 The late functional results of upper-limb revascularization and replantation. Journal of Hand Surgery 9A: 623–633
Smahel J, Meyer V E, Bachem U 1987 Glueing of peripheral nerves with fibrin: experimental study. Journal of Reconstructive Microsurgery 3: 211–218
Steinau H U 1988 Major limb replantation and postischemia syndrome. Springer, Berlin
Steinau H U, Elert O, Schneider M 1980 Prolongation of ischemia tolerance of amputated extremities by a stroma-free hemoglobin solution. Journal Thoracic and Cardiovascular Surgery 28: 35–38
Sunderland S 1978 Nerves and nerve injuries, 2nd edn. Churchill Livingstone, Edinburgh
Vogt B, Etter E, Ruetz A, Rüttimann A 1970 Lymphatic system in a case of reimplantation of upper limb after accidental total amputation. In: Viamonte M, Koehler P R, Witte M, Witte Ch (eds) Progress in lymphology II. Thieme, Stuttgart
Wynn Parry C B 1973 Rehabilitation of the hand. Butterworths, London

J. R. Urbaniak and J. S. Forster

5 Replantation in children

INTRODUCTION

The first successful replantation of an amputated extremity was performed on a 12-year-old boy in 1962 by Malt in Boston (Malt & McKhann 1964). Since that time, replantation and revascularisation have become effective treatment alternatives for complete and near complete amputations. Because of home and industrial injuries, most replantation surgery has been performed on patients in the third to fifth decades of life. Amputations in children are not rare, however. More than 10% of all replantations done at the Duke University Medical Center, Durham, N.C., since the first procedure in 1972 have been performed on patients less than 16 years of age.

As replantation surgery becomes more common, it becomes apparent from multi-centre studies that differences do exist when performing replantation on a child as compared with on an adult. Expectations of replant survival, patient selection, intraoperative and perioperative management, and, ultimately, long-term function can all differ in the paediatric patient.

SURVIVAL OF REPLANTED PARTS

With increasing experience, most major replantation centres are now able to achieve 80% survival of replanted parts (Beimer 1979, Ikuta 1975, Kleinert et al 1977, Lendvay 1973, O'Brien 1977, Tupper 1979, Urbaniak 1984). In children, successful replantations, as measured by survival, have consistently been lower, falling in many cases to below 70% (Urbaniak 1978).

In order to compare results between children and adults, it is necessary to define accurately what we mean by the term 'replantation'. A complete amputation occurs when a part has been totally severed from the body. The part is then replanted if it is reattached with microvascular repair. An incomplete amputation is only partially detached, but has no circulation. The connecting tissue may be skin, bone, tendon or nerve. Microvascular anastomosis is necessary to restore circulation. This procedure is called a revascularisation.

In children, as in adults, a revascularisation has a much greater chance of survival than a replantation, and involves a much shorter operating time, as there are fewer structures to repair. There may also be better venous drainage, which is important for survival. The degree of injury — complete versus incomplete — has been found, at Duke University, to be the major factor in predicting whether or not an amputated part will survive.

Amputations may also be classified by the mechanism of injury. Crush, avulsion, or sharp (guillotine) are all standard terms in use to classify amputations. Children tend to have a greater proportion of crush-avulsion injuries than do adults (Jaeger et al 1984, Urbaniak 1978). This is particularly true in the very young. Injuries by bicycle spokes, door hinges, horse bridles, and heavy objects falling on digits are all common mechanisms for amputations in children. In adults, various reports have determined that crush-avulsion injuries have a lower overall success rate due to the extent of injury. However, in one study which analysed the success rates of replantations of single digits in all age groups, there was no significant difference in the survival of digits when grouped by mechanism (Van Beek et al 1979). Nevertheless, in children, it would appear that the mechanism of injury — i.e. sharp versus crush-avulsion — is a prognostic factor, both in our experience and in that of others. Avulsion injuries in particular, no matter what the level at which they occur, tend to give poorer overall results (Stirrat & Seaber 1979). The level of amputation does not appear to make a significant difference to the survival expectation of an amputated part in either the child or the adult. One would think that the smaller overall size of a child would make vessel anastomosis more difficult, but vessel size in children does not correspond proportionately to the overall smaller size of the patient (Fig. 5.1). With skill, it should be possible for an accomplished microsurgeon to repair a 0.4 mm vessel (Urbaniak 1978).

Level may be a contributing factor to replant survival, in that amputations through the forearm, and above, contain more muscle, and therefore long ischaemia times cannot be tolerated before muscle necrosis begins. With digits, longer ischaemia times can be tolerated, because of the absence of skeletal muscle. As long as it remains reasonable, the degree of ischaemia does not appear to influence survival in a paediatric replantation. (See section on Storage of amputated parts below).

The number of arteries repaired during the replantation does not affect the final survival rate. As long as adequate flow is achieved, whether or not more than one artery is repaired in a digit does not appear to influence the final outcome. The number of veins repaired is, however, important, and is directly proportionate to success. This may help to explain why revascularisations have a higher success rate than replantations. Supporting evidence for the need for good venous patency is that the majority of failed replantations in paediatric patients at Duke University have been secondary to venous obstruction. Age does not affect the ability of a replanted part to survive. Decreased survival in patients less than 30 years of age or greater than 70 years has been noted (Van Beek et al 1979). The average age of the paediatric patients with failed replantations at Duke University is 7 years, whilst the average age for successful replantations is 8 years. This is not a significant difference.

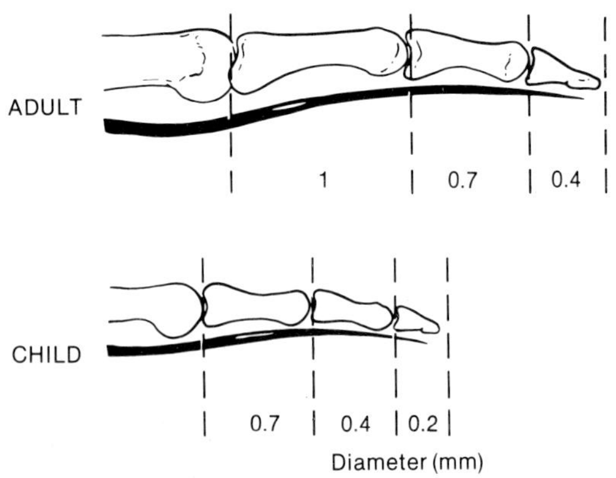

Fig. 5.1 Comparative size of digital artery in child and adult. Successful microsurgical repair is possible in a vessel 0.4 mm in diameter. (Reprinted with permission from Urbaniak 1984.)

While the degree and mechanism of injury, and the number of venous anastomoses are measurable parameters that affect the survival of replantations in children, other more difficult-to-measure factors certainly come into play. The higher level of anxiety in children, with the resulting persistent vasospasm in the perioperative period, appears to influence the ultimate outcome (Urbaniak 1984). Paradoxically, the prior knowledge that children tend to fare better in the long term than adults if a replantation is successful, may result in a decrease in survival statistics for children. A surgeon may be encouraged to attempt a more difficult replantation in a child, knowing that the final result may be better than would be expected in an adult, if the part survives.

PATIENT SELECTION

Despite experience with the replantation of more than 1000 amputated parts at the Duke University Medical Center, the decision to replant an amputated part is still not always easy (Urbaniak & Bright 1975). If the decision to replant is made, it must be done with the knowledge that considerable time, expense and emotional attachment to a replanted part will be invested by the patient, and his or her family. Particularly in the paediatric patient, the desire to salvage an amputated part may be heavily influenced by the obvious cosmetic deformity. However, a viable part is not always a functional part, as has been shown in both children and adults. As experience with replantations has increased, indications for what should, and should not, be replanted have been refined by assessing the long-term functional results (Jones 1982, Morrison et al 1978, Stirrat & Seaber 1979). This differs when considering children. General guidelines are listed in Table 5.1, comparing the indications for replantation in adults with the expanded list for children (Urbaniak 1983).

Table 5.1 Comparison of indications for replantation in adult and child

Adult	*Child*
Thumb	Thumb
Multiple digits	Multiple digits
Mid-palm	Mid-palm
Forearm to wrist	Forearm to wrist
Elbow and above	Elbow and above
Individual digit distal to sublimis	Individual digit
	Lower extremity

Thumb. No matter what the degree or mechanism of injury, an attempt at thumb replantation should be made in both the child and adult. Although good techniques for reconstruction of amputated thumbs have been developed, the patient's own thumb will give a better overall functional and cosmetic result with fewer procedures.

Multiple digits, mid-palm, wrist and forearm. Similarly, replantations of these parts have been shown to give good cosmetic and functional results in both adults and children (Urbaniak 1984, Urbaniak 1979). In the case of multiple digit amputations, if one or more of the digits is rendered non-replantable due to a severe injury, then the parts should be retained for potential use as tissue donor sites later during the procedure. The remaining parts, suitable for replantation, can then be attached to stumps other than their origin to give a more functional hand or a better cosmetic result.

Elbow and above. Amputations through the elbow and above give unpredictable results in both age groups (Stirrat & Seaber 1979, Weiland et al 1978). The mechanism of injury in both the paediatric and adult patient is usually a crush and/or avulsion with resultant damage to muscle, nerves and vessels, at multiple levels. The ischaemia time is also a consideration in these replantations, because of the danger of muscle necrosis. However, even in the adult patient, it is worthwhile to consider replanting an above-elbow amputation, if only to salvage an elbow (Urbaniak 1978). A below-elbow prosthesis will be easier for the patient to use than an above-elbow. In the child, the greater propensity for nerve regeneration can give a reasonable expectation of extrinsic, and perhaps intrinsic, muscle return of function if the part survives. Therefore, in a child, every attempt should be made to salvage an above-elbow amputation.

Lower extremity. Lower extremity amputations in adults are generally not replanted. There are several reasons for this: 1) excellent gait can be achieved with a well-fitted prosthesis; 2) amputations in adults are often crush injuries with resultant damage to nerves at multiple levels; 3) the propensity for reasonable neurologic return is poor; 4) the nerve injury will often lead to a painful dysaesthetic foot. In children, replantation in the lower extremity can give rewarding results. Although prosthetics in the lower extremity in children can result in reasonable gait, the low incidence of dysaesthesia and the greater propensity for useful neurological recovery in children makes lower extremity replantation in a child a worthwhile consideration. The additional problem of bony overgrowth in the paediatric amputation stump, requiring multiple revisions, is well known. The replantation of an amputated lower extremity can avoid the need for these revisions in the future, as well as maintain growth in the proximal and distal segments.

Single toes. The replantation of single toes is generally not advised, as the disability is minimal. Some consideration may be given to replanting an amputated great toe. Recent studies of patients who have had their great toe removed for transfer to the hand show minimal disability from this amputation (Lipton et al 1986). In general, the decision to replant a lower extremity part in a child is highly individual to the situation. The overall condition of the patient, as well as of the amputated part, will be a deciding factor.

Individual finger distal to sublimis. Replantation of an isolated finger distal to the flexor digitorum sublimis insertion can give good results in both the adult and the child (Kleinert et al 1977, Lendvay 1973, Van Beek et al 1979). Although level within the digit does not appear to make a difference to survival of the digit, adequate venous drainage needs to be maintained if a digit is to survive (Van Beek et al 1979). At least 4 mm of dorsal skin, with accompanying veins, proximal to the nail fold needs to be present if a microvascular venous repair is to be performed. Volar veins can be used, but in general the results of their repair is inconsistent and is not recommended unless no other veins can be located. If no distal veins are present for repair (proximal veins are always present), one distal artery may be anastomosed to a proximal vein (A–V fistula). Another method of attempting to salvage a distal replantation without available distal veins is to remove the nail plate, and encourage bleeding with frequent dressing changes with heparin-soaked sponges (every 2 hours). Repeated massaging of the digit to relieve venous congestion is rarely successful. The use of medical-grade leeches to extract the venous blood is not common in the United States.

For very distal amputations in the child, which cannot be replanted due to a lack of artery or veins to repair, the part may be applied as a composite graft. The chance of survival of such a part is greatly diminished but, as compared with the adult, may have a greater chance of survival by inosculation.

Individual finger proximal to sublimis. Replantation of an isolated digit amputated proximal to the sublimis insertion in adults is generally not advised because of the limited excursion of the tendons that frequently results (Van Beek et al 1979). In children, however, a good functional range of motion is likely, and cold intolerance and dysaesthesias are uncommon. Two-point discrimination in a replanted digit in a child will usually approach 4 mm (Gelberman et al 1978). Therefore, even considering the decreased chance of survival in a child, the overall results in the parts salvaged will be better than in the adult (Jaeger et al 1984, Urbaniak et al 1984, VanGiesen et al 1983).

Injuries to the epiphyseal plate are a concern, because of the propensity for growth retardation at that site. If the injury does not involve the epiphyseal plate directly, there is potential for retardation of growth as a result of hypoxia or anoxia. Recent studies have demonstrated that reasonable growth, achieving 80–100% of normal, may be anticipated (Donski et al 1979, Jaeger et al 1984, O'Brien 1977). If an injury involves a joint, every attempt should be made to preserve the joint. If this is not possible, a fusion is still acceptable for a child. Reconstructive procedures can later transfer a joint from a toe, if this is desired. Primary silicone implants, although employed in adult replantations, are not recommended in children.

Our 15-year experience with more than 1200 replantations has influenced us to become more selective of our candidates for replantation in adults. However, despite the lower survival rate of replanted parts in children, the functional outcome is generally better than in adults. Therefore, only in the most mutilating injuries should replantation of an amputated part of a child not be attempted. However, the treatment must be highly individual to each patient. (Figs 5.2 to 5.4)

PREOPERATIVE MANAGEMENT

Storage of amputated parts

An amputated extremity can survive 6 hours if not cooled, but if cooled will survive up to 12 hours. Beyond that point, irreversible necrosis begins, and attempts to restore circulation are usually fruitless. The muscle of the amputated limb is the limiting factor. There are reports of digits surviving 33 hours of warm ischaemia (Chiu & Chen 1984). In general, digits will survive longer, as no muscle is present in the detached part. Nonetheless, all efforts should be directed towards minimising the warm and cool ischaemia times.

Two methods of preserving parts are in common use. The first is the immersion technique, in which the part is placed in a bag of lactated

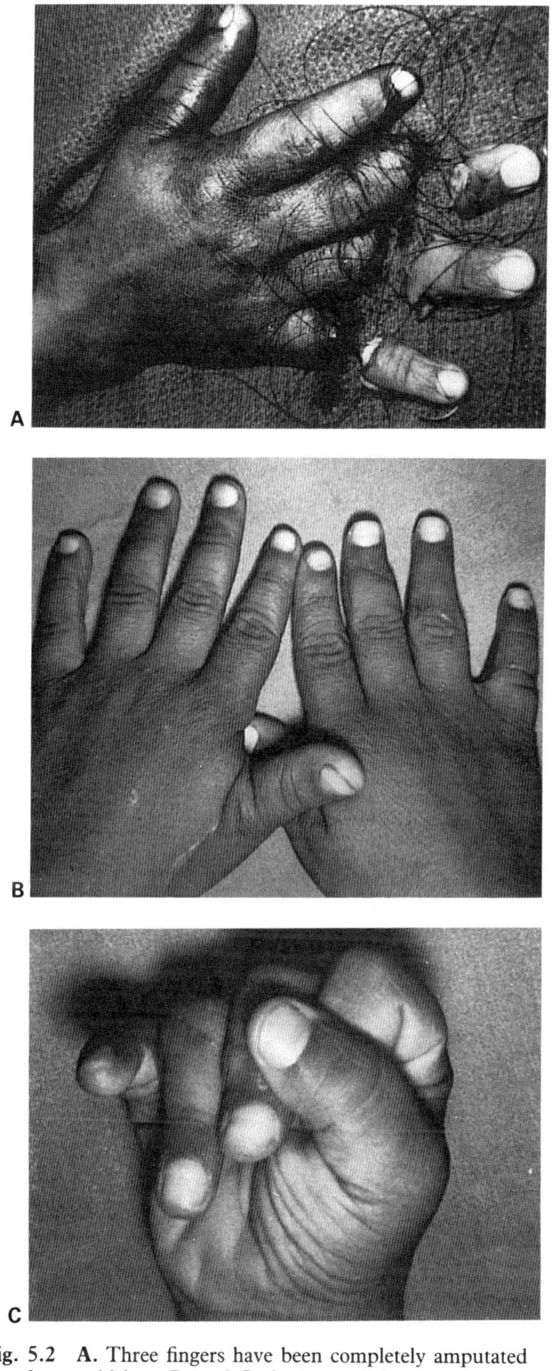

Fig. 5.2 **A.** Three fingers have been completely amputated in a 3-year-old boy. **B.** and **C.** At 2 years after successful replantation, the child has satisfactory flexion and extension, continued digital growth, and 4 mm of two-point discrimination in the replanted digits. (Reprinted with permission from Urbaniak 1984.)

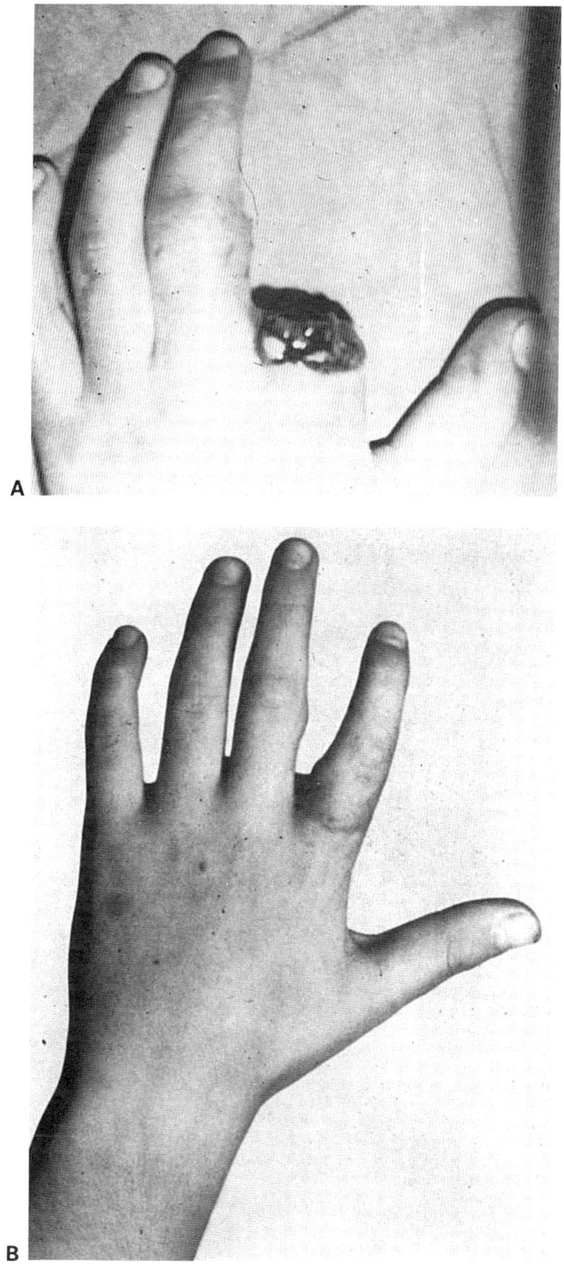

Fig. 5.3 **A.** The index finger of a 6-year-old child was amputated in an electric fan. **B.** Successful replantation resulted in 6 mm of two-point discrimination and a good range of motion in the index finger. A similar amputated part would usually not be replanted in an adult. (Reprinted with permission from Urbaniak 1984.)

A

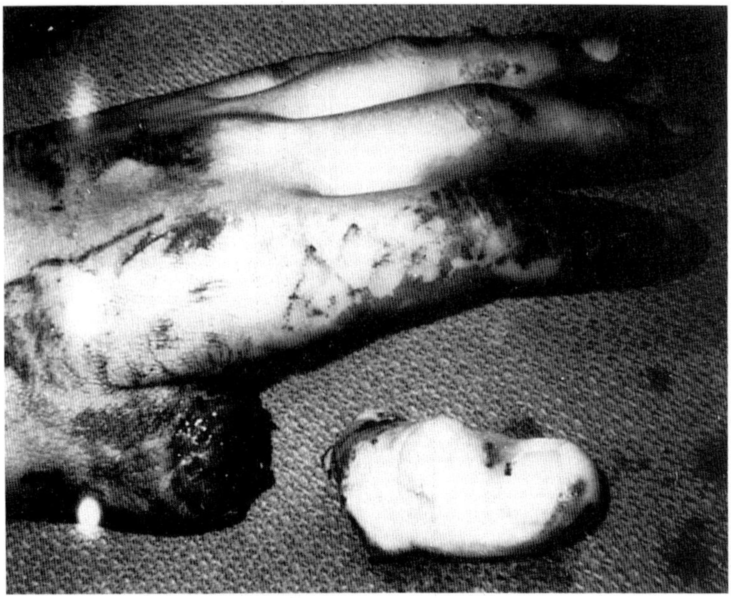

Fig. 5.4 **A.** A 12-year-old boy sustained complete amputation of the thumb in a motorcycle accident. **B.** and **C.** The thumb was replanted, and useful motion was achieved at the metacarpo-phalangeal and interphalangeal joints. Growth has continued in the replanted portion, and two-point discrimination was 4 mm. (Reprinted with permission from Urbaniak 1984.)

B C

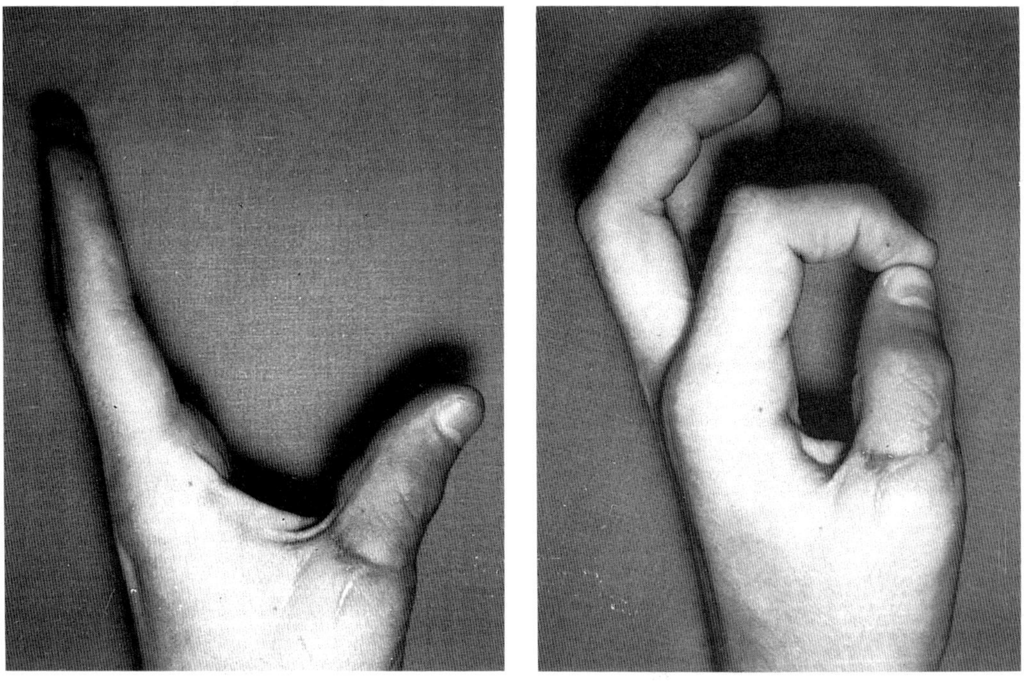

Ringer's solution or saline and the bag then surrounded by ice (Urbaniak 1979). The second method involves wrapping the part in a moist sponge and placing it in a plastic bag which is put on ice (Kleinert et al 1977, Morrison et al 1977, Tamai 1978).

Our laboratory studies have shown that both methods are adequate for the preservation of parts (Wang & Yong 1981). In general, the first method is preferable; with this method the part is less likely to come in direct contact with ice, which may precipitate frostbite. At least one of the failed replantations in the paediatric patients at Duke University was for this reason. Particularly with children, the small parts are prone to become entangled or strangulated in gauze. Maceration using the immersion technique has not occurred, and the instructions to the referring physicians are simplified.

If the amputation is incomplete, it is not advisable to instruct the primary care physician to complete the amputation in order to lessen the ischaemic time. We do not recommend placing ice around the partially amputated part, as this may induce further vasospasm and ischaemia.

Instruments for surgery

Instruments for replantation in the child differ little from those used in adult replantation (Bright 1979, Daniel & Terzis 1977, Meyer 1985, Stirrat et al 1978). A basic hand and tendon repair set is essential, as are power tools for the insertion of pins and wires, as well as a wide variety of pins, K-wires, plates and screws. The range of instruments used during the microvascular repair need not be extensive, and the choice depends in large part upon the individual surgeon's preference. Certain basic requirements should be met. The instruments should be at least 10 cm long to allow the handles to rest on the thumb-index web. The handles should be rounded, to allow fine digital manipulation rather than excessive movement of the wrist and forearm. The needle holders should be of the non-ratchet type to allow easy release. For paediatric replantation, it helps to have fine tips for use on very small distal veins. Jeweller's forceps, micro-irrigators and microtip dilators should be available in a variety of sizes. Clamps should have a closing pressure of no greater than 30 g. A microtip bipolar coagulator is essential to avoid the propagation of thermal damage to intima that would be caused by unipolar diathermy or cautery. Likewise, small haemoclips for both haemostasis and tagging of structures in the initial exploration are helpful.

Above all, magnification is needed. While the initial exploration of vessels is generally done with 3.5 × to 4.5 × loupes at our institution, for the very small amputated parts of a child, a microscope is desirable. The microscope should have a maximum magnification of at least 20 times and preferably of 30 times. A diploscope to provide for an assistant, powered focusing and zoom magnification change, and horizontal X–Y movement are strongly recommended.

Suture size differs little in the child from that in the adult. Monofilament nylon is preferable to polypropylene, as it is easier to handle and knot. Standard suture and needle sizes which may be used in a paediatric patient are given in Table 5.2.

Table 5.2 Appropriate needle and suture size for microvascular repairs in upper extremity of a child

Location	*Needle size (μm)*	*Suture size*
Wrist	135–150	9–0 to 10–0
Palm	75–135	10–0
Proximal digit	50–75	10–0 to 11–0
Distal digit	40–50	11–0 to 13–0

Patient preparation

Two teams are highly preferable for replantation surgery (Urbaniak 1978). When the patient arrives in the emergency department, one team takes the amputated part to the operating room. After adequate cleansing of the part with an antiseptic solution, the vessels and nerves are identified via lateral incisions which are placed slightly dorsal to permit easier location of the veins. The exploration is performed as previously described, using loupe magnification or a microscope in the case of very small amputated parts. Arteries and nerves are identified in the volar compartment, while the dorsal veins are identified in the sub-dermal space. An alternate approach to be used for vein identification in the small parts of a child is to delay this until the arterial repair has been performed. Distension and back flow will then help to identify very small veins that would otherwise be difficult to see.

Debridement of dirty tissue should be thorough, but care should be taken to avoid excessive removal of bone, and to avoid damaging the already identified neurovascular structures. In general, for both adults and children, shortening should be done on the amputated part. In the event that the replantation fails, more length is retained with the patient. This may differ in the child (see Method of bone repair). Distal bone fixation on the amputated part may be performed at this time.

While the part is being prepared, the child is made ready for surgery. A thorough physical examination is made, and a history, both present and past, is taken. Appropriate X-ray examinations are made. A blood count, urinalysis, blood type and cross-match, and an activated partial thromboplastin time are necessary tests, in addition to others that might be dictated by the patient's condition. Intravenous fluids are started, and antibiotics (usually a cephalosporin) are given. One luxury in the care of a child is that sedation may be given to the patient before informed consent is given by the parents or guardians.

The patient is then taken to the operating room. In adults, most replantations are done with an axillary block, with the triple benefit of no general anaesthesia, less need for other medication for postoperative pain relief, and peripheral vasodilatation. In-dwelling catheters in the axillary sheath are generally contraindicated, because of the increased risk of bleeding at the catheter site if heparin or other anticoagulants are used (Nunley et al 1987). While an axillary block is not contraindicated in children, its use as a primary anaesthetic for replantation in the very young child is limited. In a patient less than 10 years of age, the lack of ability to cooperate and the resultant anxiety and motion will make replantation surgery difficult. Therefore, a general anaesthetic is recommended for children less than 10 years of age. The axillary block may be given after the child is asleep for peripheral vasodilatation or for pain management in the immediate postoperative period.

A long procedure is the general rule and, therefore, a urinary catheter should be inserted at this stage. A tourniquet is applied to the arm and is inflated if necessary to diminish the bleeding.

SURGICAL PROCEDURE

Method and order of surgery

The method of surgery varies according to level. There are also some basic differences between adults and children in the methods for digital or hand replantation. The order of surgery progresses as follows:

1. Location and tagging of vessels
2. Debridement
3. Shortening and fixation of bone
4. Extensor tendon repair
5. Flexor tendon repair
6. Arterial anastomosis
7. Nerve repair
8. Venous repair
9. Skin coverage.

Identification and tagging of vessels has been described in a previous section. Debridement should be thorough, with necrotic muscle removed as necessary. Pulsating jet lavage may be helpful.

Bone fixation

Arterial, venous and nerve repairs should never be performed under tension (Urbaniak 1983). To achieve a patent anastomosis, either bone shortening, to effectively lengthen vessels, or vein grafting should be performed. The preferences of individual microsurgeons vary. Some state that it is rarely necessary to shorten bone to achieve a tension-free anastomosis (Urbaniak 1979). It has been our policy to shorten bone to allow a more thorough debridement, particularly in severe crush or avulsion injuries. In individual digits, up to 8 mm of bone may be taken. Whereas fusion of injured joints is often performed in the adult, an effort is made to reconstruct the joint in a child. In the forearm, 2–3 cm of bone may be resected to achieve adequate bone alignment and to allow tension-free anastomoses without vein grafting. The epiphyseal plates should be preserved and protected, and a vein graft is selected rather than shortening the epiphyseal area.

As stated previously, most of the resected bone should be taken from the amputated part when feasible (i.e. epiphysis not involved). A knowledge of the location of the epiphyseal plates of all digits and the thumb is essential.

Arthrodesis of a joint may be necessary occasionally in the child. When this is performed, the epiphysis should be preserved to maintain growth.

The method of skeletal fixation in the child varies with the site of amputation. Ease of insertion of a fixation device diminishes intraoperative time, and ease of removal eliminates the need for subsequent surgery for removal of devices. The fixation should not require a large mass of bone, because of the small bones of a child. The fixation device should not require excessive stripping of tissues, which may injure already compromised structures. Rigidity of fixation is important if early motion is desired. Finally, the fixation device should not damage the epiphyseal plate.

Multiple methods of fixation for replantation have been used, and the application of any one technique may depend greatly on the location of the replantation site. These methods are (Fig. 5.5):

1. Kirschner wires, longitudinal or oblique
2. Intra-osseous wiring
3. Intramedullary screw fixation
4. Plates and screws.

Kirschner wires have been the method favoured at Duke University for replantation. Particularly in the digits, we have found this method to be the most successful for the following reasons: 1) they are quick to insert and easy to remove; and 2) less bone exposure and skeletal mass is needed than with the other methods. A single smooth K-wire placed longitudinally is very unlikely to damage an epiphyseal plate. If rotational control is needed, then a single oblique wire can be placed.

Intra-osseous wiring is favoured by some surgeons (Lister 1978). This method requires more time, but removal is not necessary. It requires more stripping but little bone stock for insertion, and is useful near the articular surfaces. Plating is the method of choice for replantation proximal to the wrist because of the rigidity obtained. The use of mini-plates and screws in the small bones of the hand in children is very limited, because of the small size of the bones. Small plates may be used for metacarpals; however, since they require a second procedure for removal, their use in children is limited.

Intramedullary screws require almost no dissection for insertion, but do require good bone stock (Urbaniak 1984). Their usefulness is limited to areas where no angulation at the fixation site is needed, as in the thumb. Of course, they are impossible to remove and therefore should be used with caution in the severely contaminated wound.

Silicone implants may be used for joint replacement in the adult, but we have not inserted them in children.

Extensor tendon repair

Primary repair of extensor tendons is always advisable for both children and adults. In digital replantation, all components of the extensor hood should be carefully reconstructed over the metacarpo-phalangeal joint. The lateral bands are

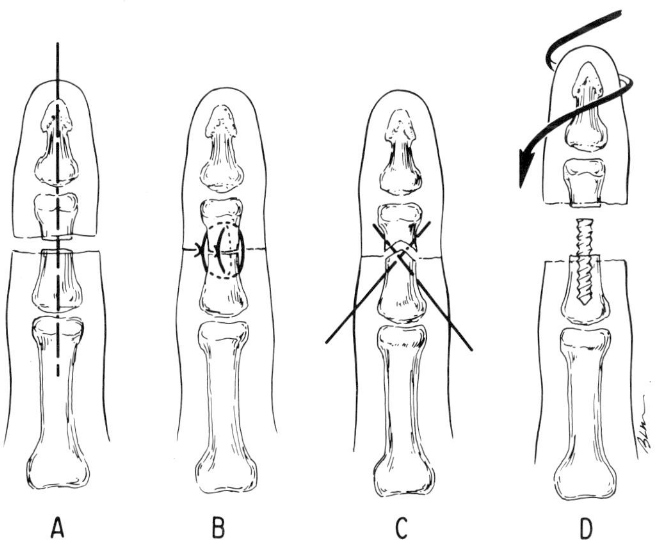

Fig. 5.5 Common methods of bone fixation in replantation. **A.** Single longitudinal intramedullary pin (most common). **B.** Intramedullary wires. **C.** Cross-Kirschner wire fixation. **D.** Screw with head removed. (Reprinted with permission from Urbaniak 1984.)

repaired to obtain maximum extension of interphalangeal joints of the digit. If no tendon is available for repair, as in a severe avulsion injury, then secondary tendon grafting or transfer may be necessary. Repair is accomplished quickly with the use of one or two sutures of non-absorbable material in a mattress fashion. 4–0 suture is the usual size; however, 5–0 suture may be necessary in the very small child.

Flexor tendon repair

Primary flexor tendon repair should be attempted for most replantations. Secondary repair is usually difficult, with scar about the nerves and vessels, and re-injury of the neurovascular structure may occur. When performed as a secondary procedure, the use of a silicone rod is often necessary. While good results with the use of silicone rods have been reported in children, two procedures and a level of cooperation for therapy not possible for small children are required.

As in all flexor tendon surgery, care should be taken while retrieving proximal tendon stumps. Injudicious use of tendon grabbers can cause injury to the remaining sheath. Particularly in the revascularisation of an incompletely amputated part, care should be taken not to retrieve tendons blindly from the palm, as the vascular arch may be injured. 'Milking' the forearm, making proximal incisions, the gentle insertion of a suction catheter into the sheath and the application of suction, are all techniques that can be used to retrieve flexor tendons.

Primary repair may be done with a 4–0 polyester suture, but in the very young child, a 5–0 suture may be used. The Tajima repair is an excellent method for use in replantation surgery (Fig. 5.6) (Tamai et al 1978). It is not only strong, but also achieves tagging of both proximal and distal tendon stumps prior to the arterial repair (Urbaniak et al 1985). Once arterial repair has been performed, then the final tendon suture can be tied into place. This allows greater exposure in the small digits of a child for a difficult arterial repair, particularly at the proximal phalangeal region.

Postoperative care of flexor tendon injuries in the replantation patient requires longer periods of immobilisation than would be used in an adult patient with no vascular compromise. For children who cannot co-operate with early passive motion techniques, routine flexor tendon repairs are also held for four weeks with the wrist and metacarpophalangeal joints in flexion. Thus, postoperative

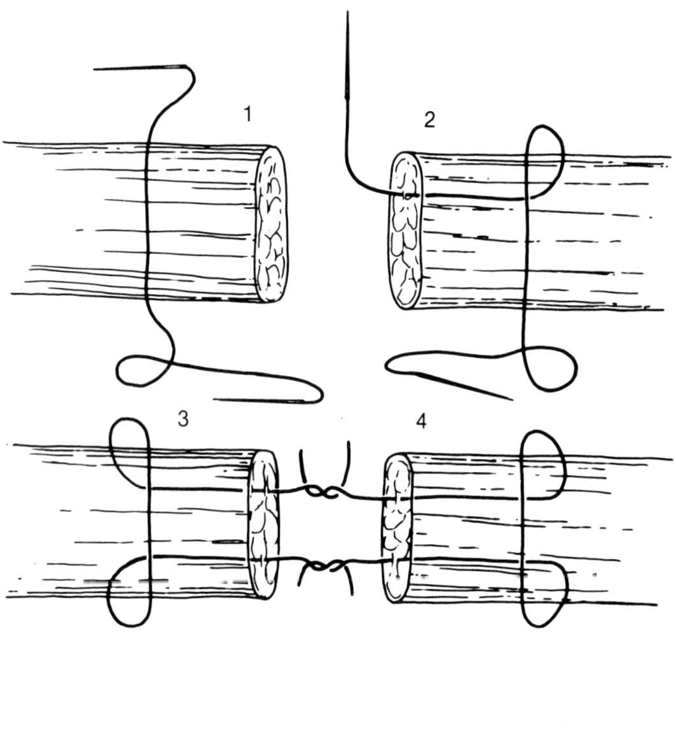

Fig. 5.6 The Tajima method of tendon repair is particularly useful in replantation of amputated digits.

management of the tendon repair for the paediatric patient is essentially the same with or without the vascular repair. If tenolysis is to be performed in a child after replantation, it is generally advised to wait at least three, and perhaps six, months to achieve maximum passive motion.

Arterial repair

Standard principles for vascular repair are used for both children and adults. No major differences exist in the actual technique of repair, with the exception that the very small distal vessels in children require fewer stitches. In individual digital amputations, one vessel or two may be repaired, depending on the surgeon's preference, the time involved, the number of remaining parts to be revascularised, and the availability of suitable vessels. Multiple techniques, such as transposing vessels or the use of Y vein grafts, are helpful (Jones & Jupiter 1985).

Arteries should be freed from surrounding subcutaneous tissue for 1.5–2 cm. Branches should be coagulated with a bipolar coagulator to avoid damaging intima. Normal intima should be visualised in both proximal and distal stumps under magnification. No tension should be present at the anastomotic site. If there is tension, then at this stage a vein graft should be used. Normal intima repaired to normal intima in a vessel without tension, and the skill of the microsurgeon, are the main determining factors for the success of an anastomosis.

After preparation of the vessel, the proximal end should be dilated. This should allow a flow of blood reaching 10 cm which lasts for 20–30 seconds. If this is not sustained, then there is either a problem with the vessel intima requiring more resection, or a vasospastic problem. This can be due to hypovolaemia, acidosis, hypothermia or a response to pain. These problems should be corrected, and the vessel then irrigated with warm, heparinised, lactated Ringer's solution to aid in relief of vasospasm. If spasm still persists, the vessel may be irrigated with a papaverine solution, but this should be done with caution. Vasospasm may be only temporarily relieved by this measure, and a false sense of security may be gained.

Two vascular clamps of appropriate size applying no greater than 30 g of pressure are then applied, but should be retained for no longer than 30 minutes. After dilatation of the vessel ends, heparin (3000 units dosage, adjusted for the size of the child) is given intravenously prior to beginning the anastomosis. Throughout the procedure, the pneumatic tourniquet may be inflated and deflated for short periods of time, to avoid excessive damage to vessels by prolonged use of microclips and to diminish blood loss.

Nerve repair

Primary direct nerve repair in replantation surgery is generally easy to perform. Grafts are seldom needed to bridge gaps, except perhaps in the severe avulsion injury. However, in the child, and particularly in digital replantation, the small size of the bone with the accompanying epiphyseal plates may limit bone resection. Therefore, grafts may be needed to repair nerves with tension-free suture lines. Secondary repair is acceptable and may give similar results to primary repair, but is more difficult, requires a second general anaesthetic and risks injury to repaired vessels (Urbaniak 1983).

The nerve is trimmed to pouting fascicles, geographic alignment of groups of fascicles is obtained with the aid of magnification, and the nerve ends are approximated without undue tension. Standard epineurial sutures are used to reconnect most nerves. In the digits of a small child, only two sutures are usually necessary to achieve adequate alignment. In general, 8–0 to 10–0 suture material is used for the repair.

Venous repair

The ability to achieve adequate venous drainage is essential to the survival of an amputated part. In the Duke University experience with paediatric replants, inadequate venous drainage has been the leading mechanism of failure. Therefore, at least two veins should be reconnected for each artery that is repaired. Vein grafting or vein transposition should be performed to achieve a patent, tension-free anastomosis.

Techniques of vein identification have been discussed above. Some microsurgeons prefer to anastomose veins first so that back bleeding is prevented and a drier field is achieved (Daniel & Terzis 1977, Morrison et al 1978, Russell et al 1984). It has been our policy to repair arteries first. This is done for two reasons. Firstly, after an artery has been repaired, the back flow can be used for the identification of small veins. This is particularly helpful in the small dorsal veins of a child. Secondly, the surgeon does not waste valuable time repairing veins only to discover subsequently that arterial repair is impossible. In order to achieve a bloodless field, intermittent use of the pneumatic tourniquet is beneficial.

In replantations at, or distal to, the distal interphalangeal joint, occasionally no dorsal veins are available for repair. 'Artery only' replantations may be successful by using one of the following methods:

1. Repair of volar veins, which is more difficult, as the veins are smaller with thinner walls.
2. Removal of the nail plate and periodic scrapping of the raw nail bed, with application of heparin-soaked pledgets to encourage bleeding.
3. Anastomosis of the second distal artery to a vein in the proximal stump, to allow back flow from the artery to the vein (A–V fistula).
4. Periodic massaging by medical personnel or family member.
5. Medical-grade leeches (not popular in some societies).

Despite the reported variable success of these methods, successful repair of dorsal veins provides the best chance of survival.

Skin coverage and dressing

After all structures have been repaired, meticulous haemostasis is achieved. The skin is closed with interrupted, loosely placed nylon sutures. If the closure of any wound is too tight over any vessel anastomosis, then the skin should be left open and the wound allowed to drain. Skin coverage is desirable over a repaired vessel, and may be obtained by using a local flap or a small skin graft. Fasciotomies are performed where indicated, to allow for swelling and venous drainage. Frequently, the longitudinal incisions in the digit are not closed.

The dressing should be bulky and compressive but not restrictive. The limb should be elevated to allow venous drainage. Fingertips should be left exposed to allow inspection and the application of the monitor of choice. Plaster splints may be incorporated in the dressing to avoid motion, which is particularly important in the child. It has been our policy not to change the dressing for two weeks, as vasospasm secondary to anxiety or pain may lead to failure of the replant. One situation in which a dressing change is indicated, is the formation of a 'blood cast' from bleeding into the dressing. This will inhibit venous drainage and is one of the first areas that should be checked when inadequate venous drainage is apparent.

POSTOPERATIVE MANAGEMENT

Postoperative management of the replantation can be as challenging as the surgery itself, particularly in the paediatric age group. Postoperative care begins in the operating room. In most children, especially if they appear to be anxious, a 20 gauge silicone catheter (No. 5 ureteral) is placed adjacent to the median and/or ulnar nerves, depending on the digit which has been replanted. This is for the later injection of a dilute solution of local anaesthetic (0.25% bupivacaine) every 6–8 hours. This will aid in the relief of vasospasm by means of a regional sympathetic block. It has the advantage of always being available, and does not require the administration of a second axillary block, which is emotionally traumatic to a child.

The replanted part, and the patient should be kept warm. The room temperature should be at least 22°C and the patient should be kept well hydrated. No caffeine-containing foods or beverages are allowed, and smoking is strictly prohibited in the patient's room.

Anticoagulation is a matter of surgeon's preference (Daniel & Terzis 1977, Kleinert et al 1977, Morrison et al 1978, Tamai 1978, Tupper 1979, Urbaniak 1979).

In general, heparin is used for more severe crush or avulsion injuries. The dosage is in the range of 15 units/kg per hour, and is monitored by maintaining the activated partial thromboplastin time at approximately two times normal. The heparin is administered for a week. Dextran or aspirin may be given to the patients with sharp amputations. The use of dipyridamole for platelet inhibition and vasodilatation in the adult may be helpful, but is not recommended in the very young child. Chlorpromazine as both a vasodilator and a sedative is helpful in the adult population, but its use in the child should be with extreme caution because of the danger of hypotension, dystonic reactions, and a lowered seizure threshold.

We have found the use of temperature monitors to be reliable. They are easily applied, cause little discomfort to the patient and, for a child who does not like hospital personnel touching his or her fingers, they provide a means of continuous monitoring without disturbing the patient. The normal ambient skin temperature is 31–35°C. We feel that a drop below 30°C or a drop of greater than 2° below that of a normal digit is significant. Others have reported similar success but using different parameters (Lu Shiuh-Yen et al 1984).

Antibiotics are administered for one week. Children are kept sedated and in bed for at least four days. As stated, it is our policy not to change the dressing for 2–3 weeks unless the part shows signs of vascular compromise. Earlier dressing changes have, in our experience, resulted in significant vasospasm, and in some cases loss of the replanted part.

MANAGEMENT OF THE FAILING REPLANT

A failing replant, as measured by any of a number of parameters, is an emergency. All parameters should be checked in a systematic fashion in an attempt to salvage a replanted part. Monitor failure, as in a probe falling off, is common. If the monitor is not at fault, then the patient should be checked for the presence of circumstances predisposing to vasospasm, such as hypovolaemia, ingestion of caffeine-containing foods, pain, and smoking in the room. The dressing should be checked for the presence of excessive blood soaking, which can create an obstruction to first venous and then arterial flow. A dressing change, as mentioned, should be done with great care in the early stages of replantation, because of the risk of vasospasm just from the dressing change itself. The patient should be sedated, and in the case of a young child, return to the operating room may be necessary.

An injection of bupivacaine may be given via the nerve catheter to relieve vasospasm. Although its fibrinolytic effect is questionable, a bolus of heparin may be given intravenously in an attempt to salvage a part.

If all the above measures are unsuccessful, then exploration and re-anastomosis is indicated. A vein graft to artery or vein may be needed. Thrombectomy of an artery may be successful, but in general, local resection to normal intima and placement of a vein graft is preferred.

SUMMARY AND CONCLUSIONS

Most major replantation centres are now achieving nearly 90% survival for amputations in adults, while lower rates are common in children. Major contributing factors have been the degree of injury, the mechanism of injury and the adequacy of venous drainage. The desire of the microsurgeon to replant any amputation in a child, and the tendency of the child to become more anxious and vasospastic, may also be contributing factors.

A skilful microsurgeon, using the techniques set forth, should be able to maintain patency in vessels down to 0.4 mm in diameter in children. At least a 60% success rate can be achieved in children. The long-term outcome for the child is expected to be better because (Fig. 5.7):

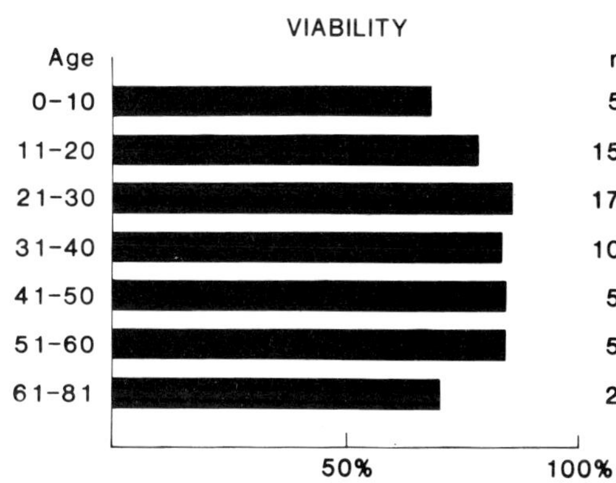

Fig. 5.7 Viability rates from the Duke experience.

1. Nerve recovery will approach normal two-point discrimination.
2. Motor recovery will be similar to that achieved by a comparable peripheral nerve repair. This is usually much better in the child than in the adult.
3. Joint motion can be at least 50% of normal.
4. Cold intolerance is usually not present in the child.
5. Near normal growth can be achieved. The growth potential of an undamaged epiphyseal plate averaged 80% of normal in our series of replantations. If damage to a plate occurs, then growth inhibition and deformity may occur at that site.
6. Cosmetic acceptability of the hand will be better than any amputation.

REFERENCES

Biemer E 1977 Replantation von Fingern und Extremitatenteilen, Technik und Erge bnisse. Chirurg 48: 353

Bright D S 1979 Techniques of microsurgery. In: AAOS symposium on microsurgery: practical use in orthopaedics. C V Mosby, St. Louis, p 40

Chiu Haw-Yen, Chen Ming-Ting 1984 Revascularisation of digits after thirty-three hours of warm ischaemia time. A case report. Journal of Hand Surgery 9A: 63

Daniel R, Terzis J 1977 Reconstructive microsurgery. Little, Brown and Company, Boston

Donski P K, Carwell G R, Sharzer L A 1979 Growth in the revascularised bone graft in young puppies. Plastic and Reconstructive Surgery 64: 239

Garrett W E, Seaber A V, Boswick J, Urbaniak J R, Goldner J L 1984 Recovery of skeletal muscle after laceration and repair. Journal of Hand Surgery 9A: 683

Gelberman R H, Urbaniak J R, Bright D S, Levin L S 1978 Digital sensibility following replantation. Journal of Hand Surgery 3: 313

Gordon L, Leitner D, Buncke H, Alpert P 1985 Partial nail plate removal after digital replantation as an alternate method of venous drainage. Journal of Hand Surgery 10A: 360

Ikuta Y 1975 Microvascular surgery. Lens Press, Hiroshima

Jaeger S H, Tsai T M, Kleinert H R 1984 Upper extremity replantation in children. Orthopedic Clinics of North America 12: 897

Jones J M, Schenck R R, Chesney B 1982 Digital replantation: comparison of function. Journal of Hand Surgery 7A: 183

Jones N F, Jupiter J B 1985 The use of Y-shaped interposition vein grafts in multiple digit replantations. Journal of Hand Surgery 10A: 675

Kleinert H E, Juhala C A, Tsai T M, Van Beek A 1977 Digital replantation: selection, technique and results. Orthopedic Clinics of North America 8: 309

Lendvay P G 1973 Replacement of the amputated digit. British Journal of Plastic Surgery 26: 398

Lipton H, May J, Simpson S 1986 Preoperative and postoperative gait analysis of patients undergoing great toe to thumb transfer. Presented American Society for Surgery of the Hand, New Orleans

Lister G 1978 Interosseous wiring of digital skeleton. Journal of Hand Surgery 3: 427

Lu Shiuh-Yen, Chiu Haw-Yen, Lin Tzo-Wu, Chen Ming-Ting 1984 Evaluation of survival of digital replantation with thermometric monitoring. Journal of Hand Surgery 9A: 805

Malt R A, McKhann C 1964 Replantation of severed arms. JAMA 198: 716

Meyer V 1985 Upper extremity replantation. Churchill Livingstone, Edinburgh

Morrison W A, O'Brien B M, MacLeod A M 1977 Evaluation of digital replantation. A review of 100 cases. Orthopedic Clinics of North America 8: 295

Morrison W A, O'Brien B, MacLeod A N 1978 Digital replantation and revascularisation. A long term review of one hundred cases. Hand 10: 125

Nunley J A, Spiegl P V, Goldner R D, Urbaniak J R 1987 Longitudinal epiphyseal growth after replantation and transplantation in children. Journal of Hand Surgery 12: 274

O'Brien B M 1977 Microvascular reconstructive surgery. Churchill Livingstone, Edinburgh

O'Brien B M, Franklin J D, Morrison W A, MacLeod A 1980 Replantation and revascularisation in children. Hand 12: 12

Russell R, O'Brien B M, Morrison W et al 1984 Late functional results of upper limb revascularisation and replantation. Journal of Hand Surgery 9A: 623

Stirrat C R, Seaber A V, Urbaniak J R, Bright D S 1978 Temperature monitoring in digital replantation. Journal of Hand Surgery 3: 342

Stirrat C R, Seaber A V 1979 The microsurgery laboratory. In: American Academy of Orthopaedic Surgeons, Symposium on microsurgery: practical use in orthopaedics. C V Mosby Company, St. Louis

Tajami T 1976 Personal communication

Tamai S, Hon Y, Tasumi Y et al 1978 Microvascular anastomosis and its application in the replantation of amputated digits and hand. Clinical Orthopaedics and Related Research 133: 106

Tamai S 1978 Digital replantation: analysis of 163 replantations is an eleven year period. Clinics in Plastic Surgery 5: 195

Tupper J W 1979 Vascular defects and salvage of failed vascular repairs. In: American Academy of Orthopaedic Surgeons. Symposium on microsurgery: practical uses in orthopaedics. C V Mosby Company, St. Louis

Urbaniak J R, Bright D S 1975 Replantation of amputated digits and hands in children. Inter-Clinic Information Bulletin 14: 1

Urbaniak J R 1978 Replantation of amputated hands and

digits. In: American Academy of Orthopaedic Surgeons; instructional course lectures, Vol 27. C V Mosby Company, St. Louis
Urbaniak J R 1979 Digital and hand replantation. Current status. Neurosurgery 4: 551
Urbaniak J R 1979 Replantation of amputated parts: technique, results and indications. In: American Academy of Orthopaedic Surgeons. Symposium on microsurgery: practical use in orthopaedics. C V Mosby Company, St. Louis
Urbaniak J R 1983 To replant or not to replant? That is not the question. Editorial. Journal of Hand Surgery 8: 507
Urbaniak J R 1984 Replantation in children. In: Serafin D, Georgiade N (eds) Paediatric plastic surgery. C V Mosby Company, St. Louis
Urbaniak J R, Roth R H, Nunley J A, Goldner R D 1985 The results of replantation after amputation of a single finger. Journal of Bone and Joint Surgery 67A: 611
Urbaniak J R, Cahill J D, Mortensen R Tendon suturing methods. Analysis of tensile strength. In: American Academy of Orthopaedic Surgeons. Symposium on tendon surgery in the hand.
Van Beek A L, Wavak P W, Zook Z G 1979 Microvascular surgery in young children. Plastic Reconstructive Surgery 63: 457
VanGiesen P J, Seaber A V, Urbaniak J R 1983 Storage of amputated parts prior to replantation. Journal of Hand Surgery 8A: 60
Wang S A, Yong K F 1981 Replantation of severed limbs. Clinical analysis of 91 cases. Journal of Hand Surgery 6: 311
Weiland A J, Villareal-Rios A, Kleinert H E et al 1978 Replantation of digits and hand. Analysis of surgical techniques and functional results in 71 patients with 86 replantations. Journal of Hand Surgery 2: 1

H. J. Buncke, F. A. Valauri and G. M. Buncke

6 Toe-to-thumb transfer

'We ought to define a hand as belonging exclusively to man . . . corresponding in sensibility and motion with that of ingenuity which converts the being who is the weakest in natural defenses to the ruler of all mankind.'

(BELL, 1934).

The importance of the hand is self-evident. The dexterity of the hand, unlike other species, allows the human the ability to perform several unique functions (Boyes 1970b).

Man has learned to manipulate and control his environment through the combined use of his hand and brain. The hand functions not only as a prehensile organ but also as a tactile one providing a prime mechanism for sensory perception (Beasley 1981).

The prehensile function and its relationship to the activities of the thumb have been discussed by Napier (1956). These are indeed important; however, the hand is also a critical part of body image, because like the face it is an 'exposed' part of our body which interfaces with our social as well as physical environment (Buncke 1981). Therefore, the significance of the aesthetics of the hand should be recognized, particularly in our competitive society where prejudice and intolerance associated with damaged hands may be socially devastating to the affected individual (Beasley 1971). Thus, physical impairment alone is only a part of the deficit, and aesthetic qualities must also be considered. Appearance is related not only to anatomical deficit, but also to the fluidity of motion. For example, awkward manoeuvring may draw more attention and be more cosmetically unacceptable than partial absence of a digit alone. A suitable reconstruction is one which permits more natural-appearing movement of the hands, as well as improved static appearance. Bearing these broader concepts in mind, let us now review the functions of the hand with a better understanding of the ramifications of the deficits sustained when a thumb has been lost.

The function of the hand is largely dependent on the thumb, as it accounts for 40 to 50% of total hand function (Bunnell 1931); in the mutilated hand, the thumb takes on an even greater role, providing prehension to an otherwise fairly useless extremity (Fig. 6.1 A–D).

Mobility of the thumb is essential for strategic positioning which permits opposition; and maximal opposition to the little finger requires flexion rotation and abduction of the metacarpophalangeal joint of the thumb (Flatt 1961). In turn, opposition permits large and small object grasp. The strength of the thumb is conferred by both the intrinsic and extrinsic muscles (Boyes 1970a). By virtue of the strength and mobility of the thumb, power grip and twist grip are possible. Nail pinch, key pinch, pulp pinch and chuck pinch all require coordinated mobility of the thumb with one or more of the other digits.

Additionally, nail pinch requires a maximum interphalangeal joint flexion of the thumb. Fine manipulation represents the culmination of mobility, joint flexion and sensibility, where sensibility is dependent upon the unique pulp padding, the stable glabrous skin and the nail plate. The nail plate functions as exoskeleton, the terminal phalanx with its septal attachments to the pulp skin magnifies the sensation through the nail bed nerve plexus, and the stabilised pulp skin allows the nail pinch needed for fine manipulation of objects (Zook 1980). Thus, the relationship of mobility and function to the variety of combinations of digital opposition with varying motion of individual joints in these digits must be recognised in planning hand reconstruction (Fig. 6.2).

Before embarking on a reconstruction, several factors must be considered (Hentz 1985). These include:

1. *The level of amputation.* This helps to define the deficit, whether it is only of pulp tissue, as in a very distal amputation, or whether it is a more proximal, and thus more complex, injury requiring restoration of length, nail bed, bone, pulp, joint and nerve elements.
2. *Patient age.* For example, the need for growth potential in a child, or the likelihood of stiffness in a replanted or reconstructed digit in an older patient must be considered, and thus, in part, dictates the choice of operation.

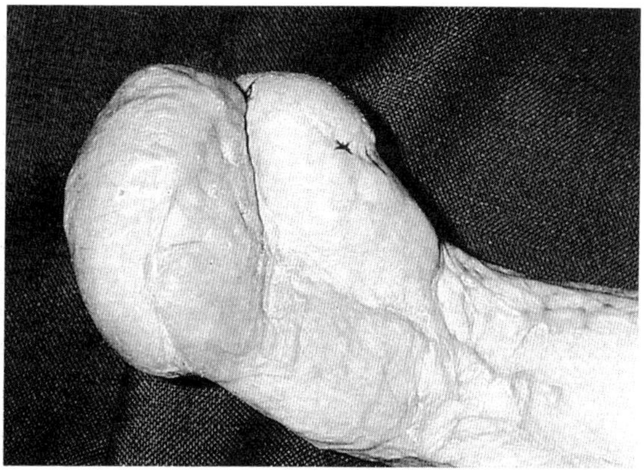

A

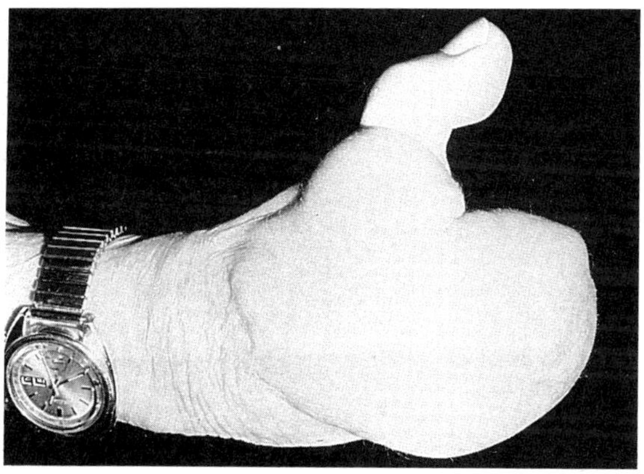

B

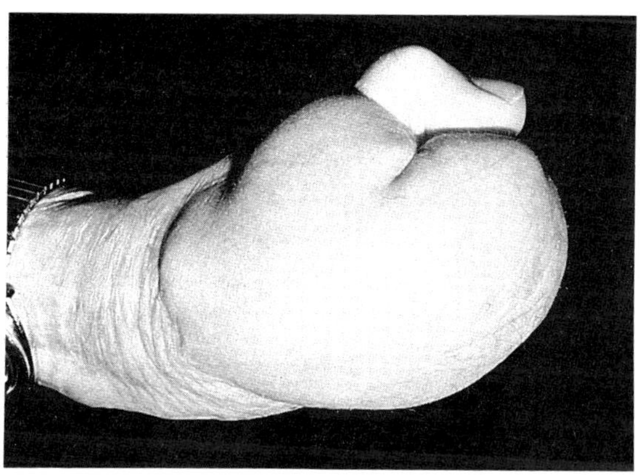

C

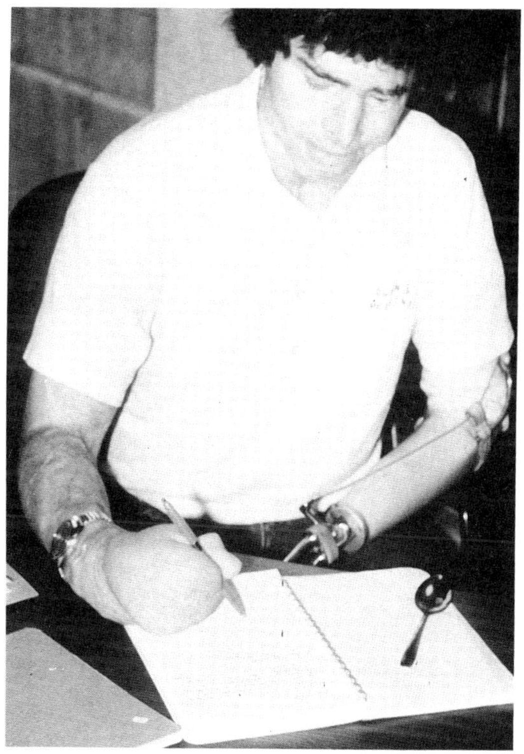

D

Fig. 6.1 **A.** Severe burn crush injury to the right hand and complete loss of the left hand at the elbow level. **B.** After great toe transfer – extension. **C.** Flexion. **D.** Prior to great toe transfer, the patient was dependent on others for hygiene. Post-transplantation, the patient is now independent.

A

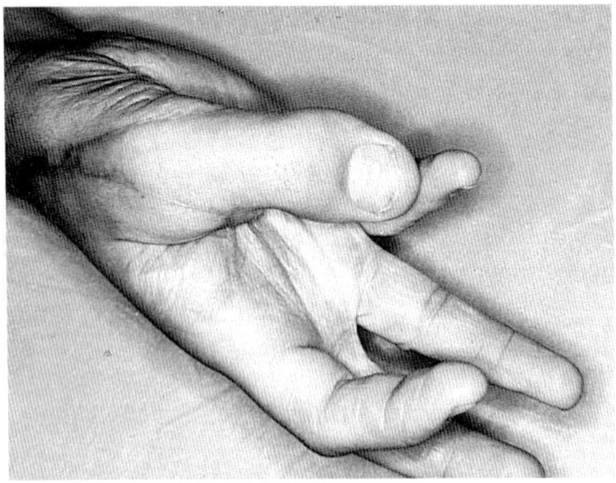

B C D E F

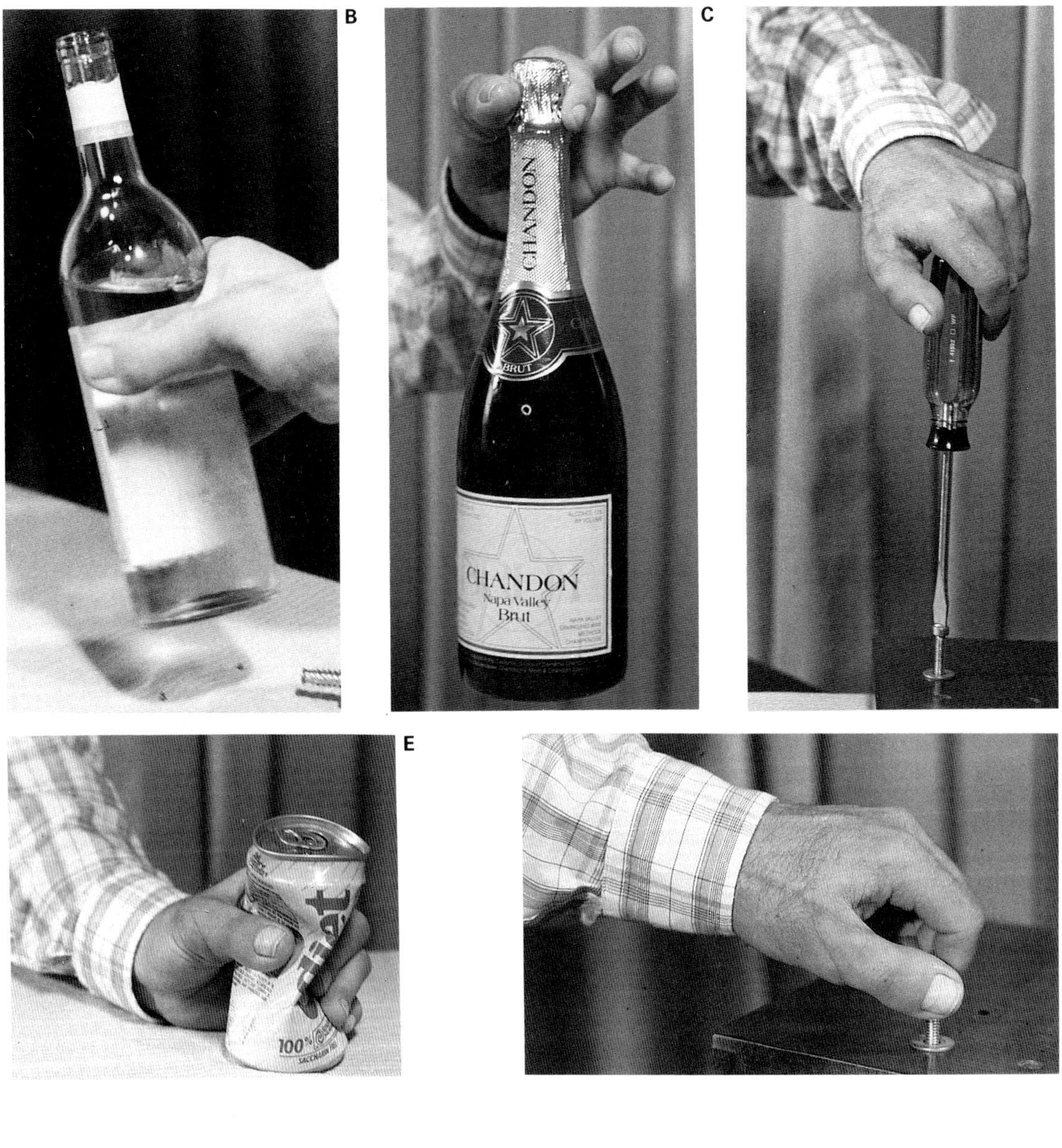

Fig. 6.2 Hallux transfer patient demonstrating: **A.** Opposition; **B.** Large object grasp; **C.** Small object grasp; **D.** Twist grip; **E.** Power grasp; **F.** Fine manipulation.

3. *The patient's vocational and avocational needs.* A labourer would require a powerful yet stable hand, whereas in a technician, dexterity and increased sensibility may be of greater importance. Additionally, cosmetic considerations must always be taken into account, particularly in patients, such as receptionists, for whom appearance and contact with the public is extremely important.

4. *The status of the contralateral limb.* An example would be the patient with bilateral injury, where prehension is essential for useful function. This brings to mind Bunnell's admonition, 'when you have nothing, a little is a lot'.

5. *The dominance of the injured hand.* An injury may be better tolerated by the non-dominant hand, or injury to the dominant hand may require a change of dominance in order to achieve maximum function.

6. *The status of the other digits.* The loss of the thumb is clearly the most significant, but the loss of other digits, and in particular the combination of other digits, such as those needed for opposition to the thumb, may also constitute a severe disability.

7. *Patient motivation* (Brown 1978). This is critical for the success of any reconstructive effort, as these procedures generally require intensive physical therapy, and additional revision surgeries are often helpful in optimising the final results.

All these factors need to be taken into account and weighed very carefully in making the final assessment and decision on the choices for reconstruction.

After defining the exact nature of the deficit, both anatomically and functionally, a distinction between anatomical and functional deficit must be considered. It is important to understand that the functional result does not necessarily follow anatomical restoration of the deficit. However, in those situations where anatomical reconstruction is desirable, it is important to clearly define the nature of the deficit. Noting which structures are absent, for example bone, joint, tendon, pulp or nail, and the selection of the proper operation for reconstruction, must be judged against these requirements and the procedure's ability to restore the lost tissues and functions. The deficit created by the donor site must also be carefully considered.

The theoretical reconstructive ideal would be to restore all of the missing structures in such a way that they would function as well as an undamaged thumb, and there would be no donor deficit. Recalling the functional importance of structures such as the nail plate, IP joint and the septated, stable, sensate glabrous skin with unique gripping properties essential for fine manipulation and pinch grip, or the enhancement of power grip imparted by IP flexion with intrinsic and extrinsic muscle motors, the critical importance of these anatomical attributes is clear.

Clarification of the arguments over reconstructive alternatives are brought into focus by reviewing the present techniques and their ability to meet the criteria of restoration with minimal donor disability.

Littler (1976) has chronicled the history of conventional thumb reconstruction in detail. A brief review will provide some valuable insight into the development of various techniques, their attributes and deficiencies.

Phalangisation was introduced by Huguier in 1874, and might be helpful where distal amputations have occurred and deepening of the web space will improve the ability to grasp larger objects. However, these circumstances are usually quite limited. A number of recent papers have again advocated the use of this technique (Tubiana & Roux 1974).

Bone lengthening (Buck-Gramcko 1971, Matev 1979 and 1980) has gained renewed interest in the past several years, but distraction is limited by the soft tissues, and often results in a stiff and unaesthetic thumb.

Nicolandoni (1897) introduced the use of bone graft and thoracic skin flap. This was the forerunner of the present day osteoplastic techniques (Biemer & Stock 1983, Chase 1969) which are now often innervated by neurovascular skin island flaps, usually from the ulnar side of the ring or middle fingers or from the first web space of the foot (Tubiana & Duprac 1961, Verdan 1968, Doi 1981). These reconstructions, however, offer no replacement of the absent joints, and are often bulky and unaesthetic. Additionally, bone graft resorption has been observed, and in the case of attached neurovascular skin flaps, cerebral transfer may not be achieved (Murray 1967).

Guermonprez in 1887 suggested the transfer of the adjacent digit to the thumb stump, and several surgeons have since made contributions to this and related procedures. Joyce in England in 1918 attempted transfer of the ring finger, and Noesske in 1919 performed the first pollicisation of the index finger. Dunlop (1933), Guelette (1930), Iselin (1937), Zsulyevich (1938), Hilgenfeldt (1950), Kleinschmidt (1920), Gosset (1949), Le Tac (1952) and Sels (Gosset & Sels 1964) all advanced transposition techniques.

During and after World War II, Bunnell (1952), Littler (1953 and 1966) and Peacock (1966) refined digital transposition and neurovascular island techniques. Pollicisation is the procedure of choice in a child with a congenital four-fingered hand. However, this technique results in a 50% reduction in grasp leverage, and 20% reduction in grip strength (Murray 1967); thus it may be functionally deficient. It is often thin, and therefore may be an unaesthetic substitute for a thumb. Gillies (1955) introduced the 'cocked-hat' procedure for amputations distal to the metacarpo-phalangeal joint.

In 1900, Nicolandoni successfully performed two-staged toe-to-thumb transfers. These were essentially cross toe-to-thumb flaps, where the donor hand and recipient foot were held in position by casting or bandages until the division of the toe's vascular pedicle on the foot, and the completion of the transfer. This technique, although successful, was not readily accepted, as it demanded rather uncomfortable immobilisation of the patient, and interest in transposition techniques was mounting.

The Nicolandoni toe transfer was later resurrected by Freeman (1956), Clarkson (1955), Byars (1952) and Blair (Blair & Byars 1940).

In 1966, Buncke, using 'micro-miniature' (vessel diameter less than 1 mm) techniques, performed the first single-staged transference of the great and second toes to the thumbs of a Rhesus monkey. Cobbett (1969) and then Buncke (Buncke et al 1973) each followed with their first clinical great toe-to-thumb transfers. Interest in the new technique soared, and multiple authors have described a variety of refinements (May & Bartlett 1985).

Concern over the size of the transferred great toe and the donor site morbidity prompted development of the wrap-around flap as favoured by Morrison (Morrison 1980, Morrison et al 1983) and Urbaniak (1985). However, this operation may be inferior in its reconstructive goals, in that it fails to provide the distal toe joint, and the distal phalanx, which supports the nail plate and pulp critical to important sensory and gripping features of the digit, is absent. Although some modifications include the dorsal portion of the distal phalanx of the great toe, the key attachments of the phalanx to the pulp skin are still disrupted.

In cases where a bone graft is utilised, resorption has been noted (Urbaniak 1985); and in more proximal amputations, the interphalangeal joint is not replaced, thus eliminating the possibility of nail pinch manipulation. Furthermore, to facilitate donor site closures, most surgeons removed the distal half of the great toe distal phalanx, thus wasting valuable bone stock (Leung & Ma 1982, Tomita et al 1983). Some authorities (Morrison 1980) routinely perform cross toe flaps from the second toe to resurface the plantar aspect of the great toe. This necessitates a later procedure for division of the flap and entails surgery on the second toe.

The Chinese Yang (Yang & Gu 1979) and Leung (1983) prefer the second toe transfers for thumb reconstruction, because of both concern about the size discrepancy of the great toe, and cultural considerations. It is important to recognise that in Oriental cultures, the absence of the great toe is unacceptable aesthetically as well as functionally, as footwear is usually of the open toe style and requires a first web space for proper fit of the sandal. The use of the second toe for restoration of the thumb may be appropriate in children or women with a small thumb where the size of the great toe is excessive. Second toes do, however, have a rather bulbous-appearing pulp, especially when in the thumb position, and may require later tailoring procedures. The toe transfer also has a tendency towards hyperextension deformity of the metacarpo-phalangeal joint, and flexion deformity of the distal interphalangeal joint (Fig. 6.3 A, B). There is decreased strength on power grip when compared to the hallux transfer for thumb reconstruction. The second toe is probably best suited for digital reconstruction other than the thumb.

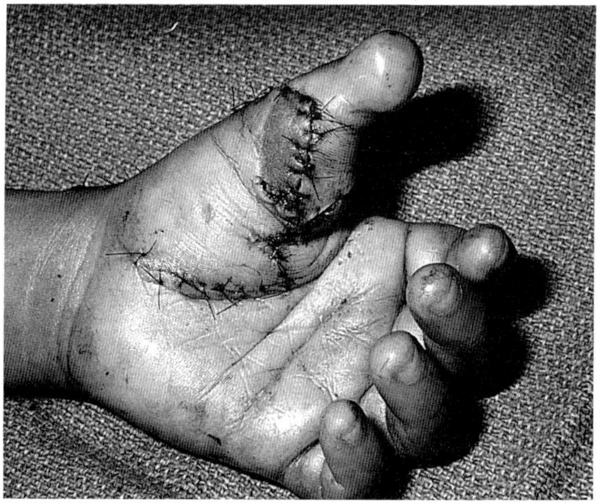

A

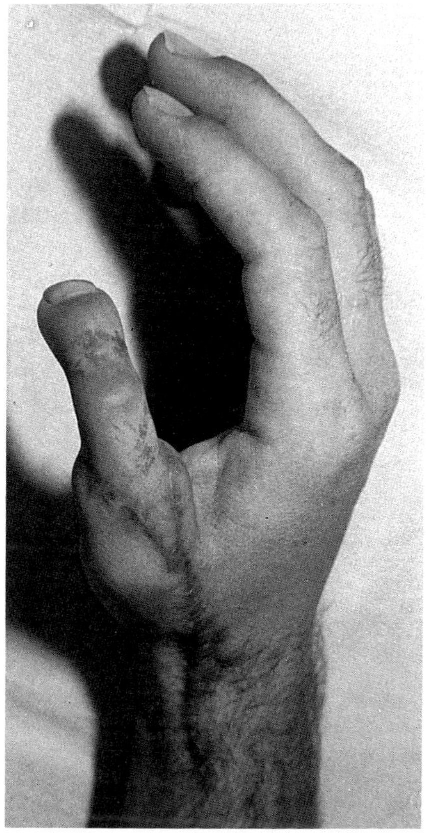

B

Fig. 6.3 Example of second toe transfer for thumb reconstruction. **A.** Note hyperextension deformity of the MP joint and flexion deformities of the PIP joint. **B.** Note bulbous tip and narrow digital appearance.

Recently, the French (Foucher et al 1980), apparently discontented with the appearance of their toe transfers to the thumb position, have utilised great toe wrap-around flaps in combination with a second toe neurovascular flap.

Controversy over the most appropriate techniques for reconstruction still continues, and technical refinements are being made to address these concerns. Ideally, reconstruction of the damaged hand would be best accomplished by regeneration or allotransplantation, as these techniques would replace all of the absent structures with little or no donor disability. Although these techniques are not feasible today, they may be possible in the future. Of the available techniques, the hallux transfer offers the best reconstructive alternative for thumb restoration.

Anatomically, the great toe is very similar to the thumb (Fig. 6.4). Harvesting may be accomplished in a variety of ways to accommodate amputations at several levels and, unlike other techniques, toe transfers allow for replacement of the absent metacarpals as well as the metacarpo-phalangeal joints. They provide stable glabrous skin, and a nail plate complex which closely mimics that of the thumb. The long flexors and extensors of the toe are anatomically analogous and provide the same important power and mobility to the hand which has suffered a thumb amputation; also, except for very proximal amputations, intrinsic function is maintained. Anatomical studies show that while the metacarpo-phalangeal joints of the great toes tend to be hyperextension joints and the thumb metacarpo-phalangeals tend to be flexion joints, these problems can be adequately addressed by angled osteotomy, capsuloplasty and also by the natural tendency of post-transferred toes to assume a more flexed attitude (May & Bartlett 1985). Additionally, the skeletal anatomy of the great toe, while somewhat heavier than that of the thumb, does bear a marked similarity in length and joint configuration.

In considering the hand, as described by Brand (1985), as the 'hand machine', there are three major aspects which he describes: 1) the motor or muscles; 2) the transmission of tendons, bones or joints; and 3) the application or skin and pulp tissue with gripping and sensory capabilities.

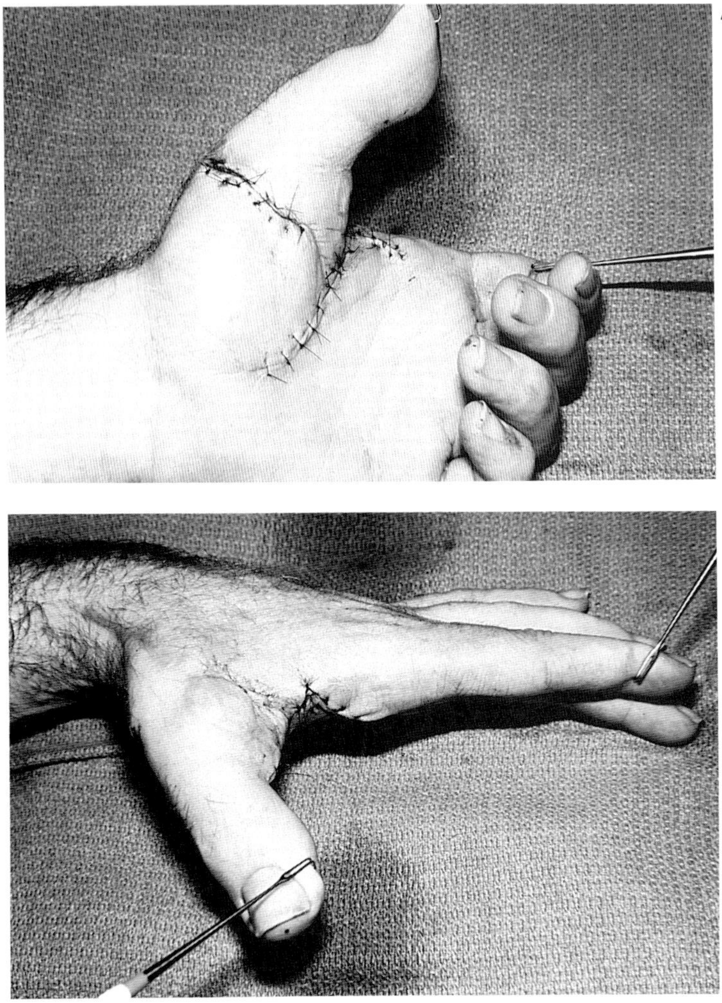

A

B

Fig. 6.4 **A.** and **B.** Appearance of great toe-to-thumb transfer.

Analysis of the toe transfers (Buncke 1976) on this basis reveals, with regard to motors, that except for very proximal amputation with loss of intrinsics, the motors are identical to those that normally would motor the digits of the hand. 'Transmission', of the tendons, bones and joints, provided by toe transfers are nearly identical to those of the lost pollex; and with regard to 'application,' certainly the toe skin, pulp and nail tissue are anatomically similar to those of the lost thumb, and thus may provide the same gripping and sensory capabilities. Additionally, the toe transfer offers the benefit of bringing the defect from the hand to the foot, where it is generally better accepted and well tolerated.

GREAT TOE TRANSFERS

Physical examination to determine the presence or absence of pulses in both the donor foot and the involved hand are performed. Doppler and angiogram studies are obtained as indicated.

In a recent study (Buncke et al 1986) of 102 toe-to-hand transfers an evaluation of plantar versus dorsal dominance was made using preoperative Doppler and angiogram comparing these results with the intraoperative surgical findings. Contrary to earlier studies (Wang 1983, Leung 1983, Gilbert 1976), dorsal dominance was found in only 58% of cases. A high correlation was found between Doppler, angiogram and intraoperative surgical

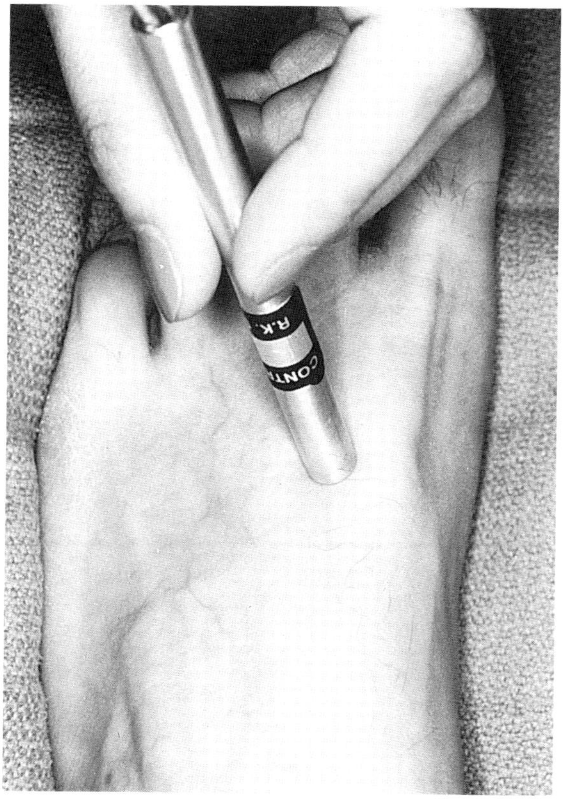

A

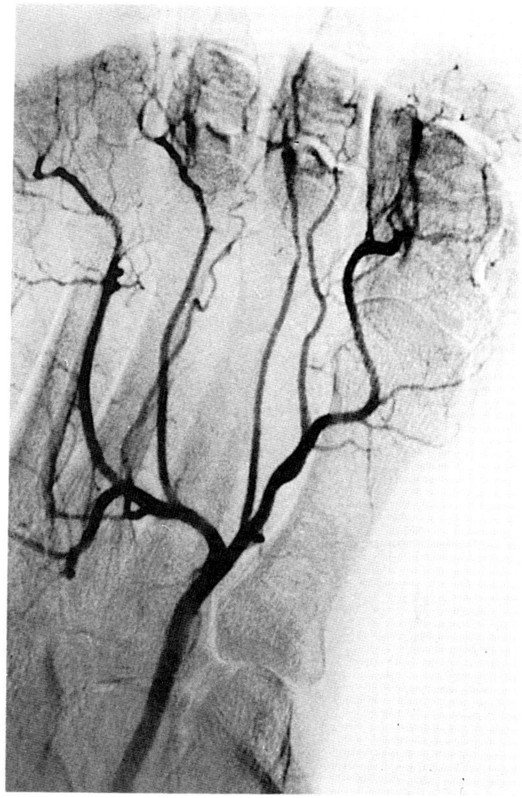

B

anatomy. Due to this high correlation, angiogram is felt to be necessary in patients with inconclusive preoperative Doppler examinations or prior foot trauma (Fig. 6.5 A–F). If an angiogram is necessary, the use of Hexabrix (Mallinckrodt) angiogram dye and intra-arterial tolazoline (Ciba) at the time of the dye injection greatly reduces the incidence of arterial spasm during the angiogram procedure. The majority of angiograms to the donor and recipient areas were performed the day prior to surgery without any evidence of intimal damage when examined intraoperatively (Peimer & Echkert 1982).

Indications

The primary indication for great toe transfer is for restoration of the missing thumb, as it preserves the breadth of the palm and, particularly with interphalangeal flexion, restores strong opposable pinch and grasp (Fig. 6.6 A and B).

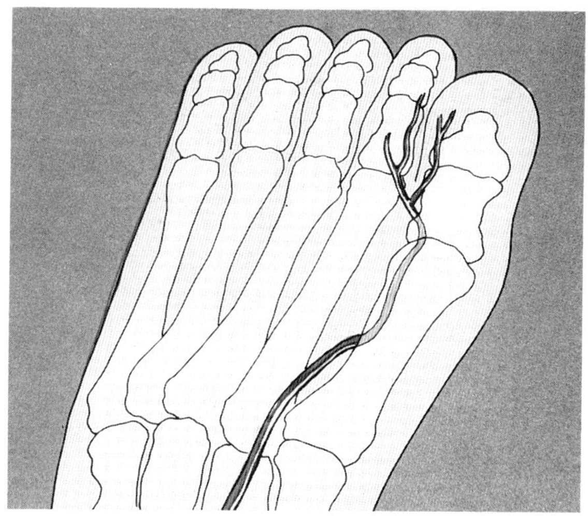

C

Fig. 6.5 Correlation of Doppler and angiographic studies. **A.** The doppler signal is followed distally along the dorsalis pedis artery. If the signal is not present distal to the level of the base of the first and second metatarsal, then the donor vessel is considered plantar. **B.** and **C.** Angiogram of plantar dominant foot; note that the vascular supply to the toe runs under the metatarsal shaft.

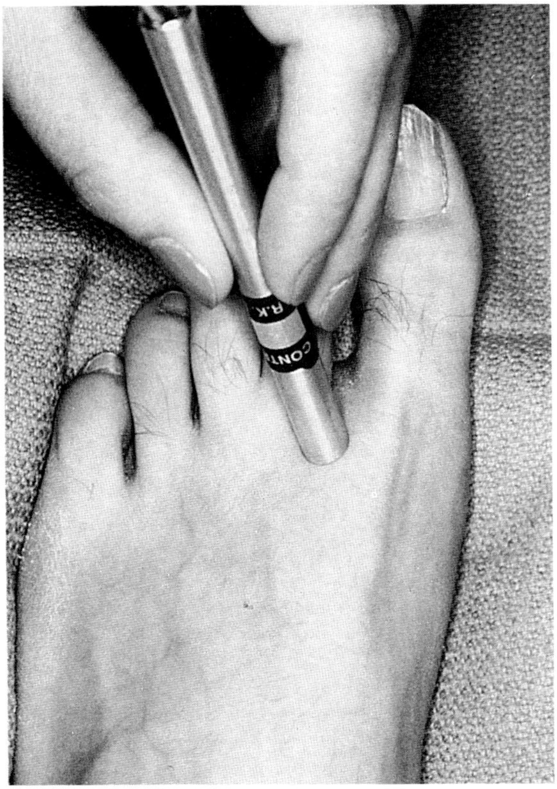

D

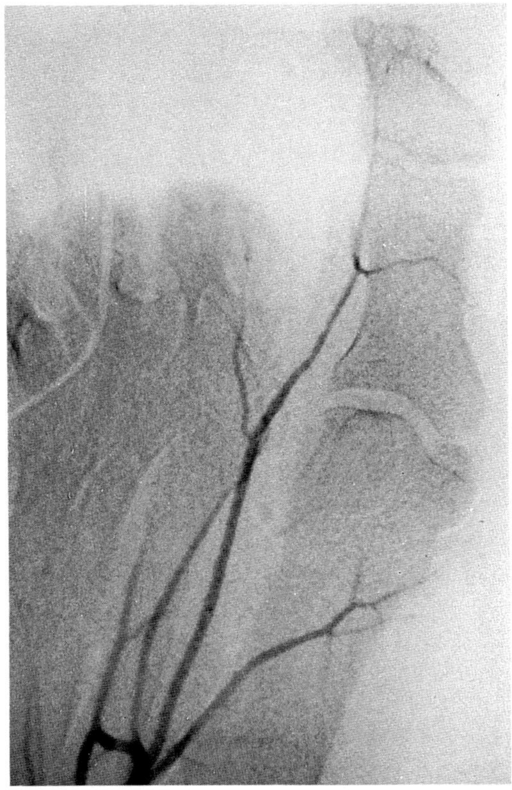

E

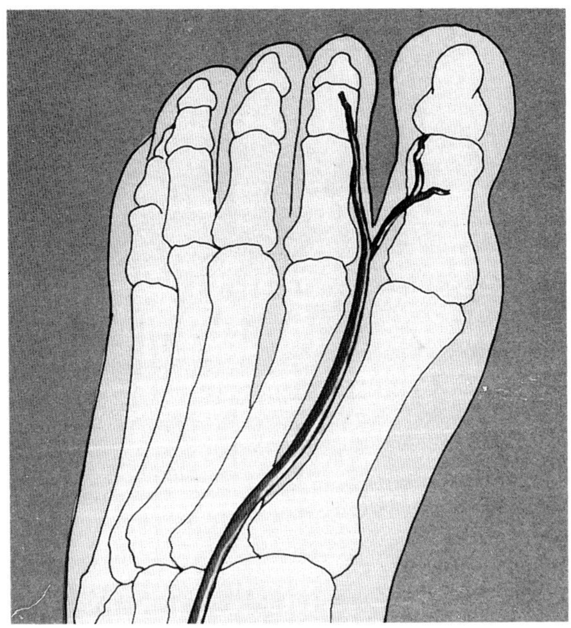

F

Fig. 6.5 (cont) **D**. If Doppler signal can be followed to the distal metatarsal, the donor toe is dorsal dominant. **E.** and **F.** Angiogram of dorsal dominant foot; note the dominant vessel runs in the middle of the first metatarsal space on the A.P. view.

Operative sequence

The vascular anatomy of the hand must be well understood when planning the great toe-to-thumb operation (Parks et al 1978). If Doppler is not adequate in identifying the vessels in the usual recipient areas (i.e. dorsal radial artery, digital arteries, or radial or ulnar arteries at the wrist), then a preoperative angiogram of the hand is necessary, as might be the case in a massively traumatised hand.

Clay models of the great toe will help in planning skin incisions and in determining the length of toe needed for adequate pinch. The model also gives the patient a clearer understanding of final function and aesthetic results (Buncke & Shah, 1979) (Fig. 6.7 A and B).

The operation is performed with two operating

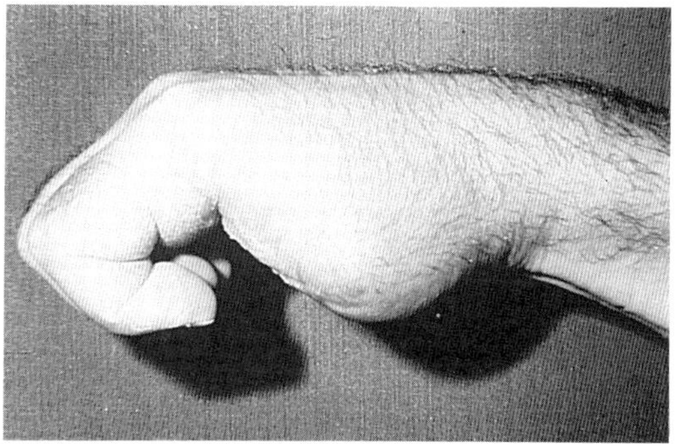
A

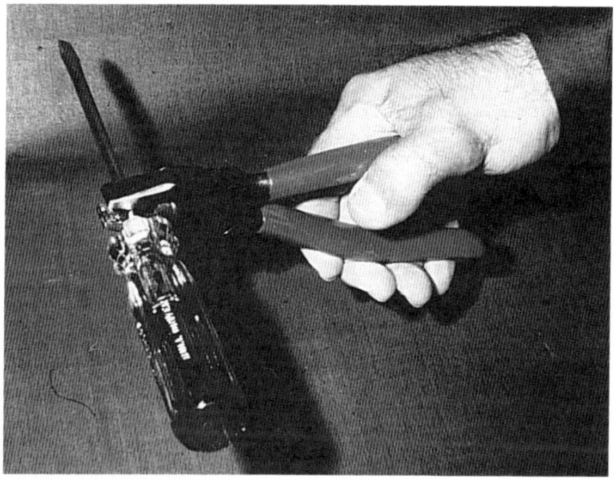
B

Fig. 6.6 **A.** Inability of thumb amputation patient to grasp. **B.** Ability to grasp after hallux transfer.

teams, one dissecting the hand and the second removing the toe. The team working at the recipient site will measure the length of the artery, nerve, vein and tendon needed, and will relay that information to the operative team working at the donor site. The ipsilateral toe is most often used, so that the donor dorsal metatarsal artery will lie near the dorsal radial artery at the time of transfer.

Recipient tendons in the hand are usually available, unless initial trauma involved avulsive injury with loss of the long flexors or extensors. In such cases, the index proprius on the extensor side, the palmaris longus or flexor carpi radialis on the flexor side should be used as motors. Preferably, tendon repairs should be performed at the wrist well away from the area of osteosynthesis, in order to avoid adhesions. Exposure of the donor long flexor is most easily accomplished through an incision along the medial side of the instep, where the flexor is found deep to the abductor hallucis muscle.

Recipient nerve neuromas are usually found at the level of the amputation scar. If nerves were originally avulsed, exposure of the median nerve in the forearm is necessary to locate the proximal neuromas. Nerve transfer from the ulnar side of the ring and long fingers may be necessary. Occasionally, adequate functional sensation can be achieved by anastomosing the donor digital nerve to the dorsal radial sensory nerve, if the thumb volar digital nerves are not present.

When dissecting the donor arterial pedicle, all vascular structures must be kept on the great toe side in order to avoid inadvertently damaging the pedicle. A long arterial pedicle can be obtained in the dorsal dominant foot. However, in the plantar dominant foot, the pedicle is frequently short, since dissection along the plantar surface of the foot is precarious and frequently causes donor foot problems (i.e. haematoma, neurapraxia). Interpositional vein grafts for plantar dominant toes can be used to extend the pedicle (Buncke et al 1978, Fujikawa & O'Brien 1975).

Once the donor soft tissue structures have been mobilised and the length of the various structures have been matched to the recipient defect, the toe is amputated through the metatarso-phalangeal joint leaving the vascular pedicle intact. At this juncture, the tourniquet is released and haemostasis is obtained. If the toe does not pink-up immediately, one must examine the pedicle under magnification. The most common cause of vascular spasm is an untied or unsatisfied arterial branch on the pedicle. Segmental spasm can also be treated with topical warm bupivacaine or papaverine solution placed directly on the vessel.

Once adequate circulation to the great toe is assured and the recipient site is ready, the pedicle is transected. Osteosynthesis is performed expeditiously to avoid prolonged ischaemia. Wide bony contact is made with step osteotomies or bone pegs in the hand fitted to a hollowed-out proximal phalanx. Bony stabilisation is assured with longitudinal K-wires or interosseous wires (Fig. 6.8). When possible, the metacarpo-phalangeal joint of the thumb should be reconstructed using the proximal phalanx of the toe to the

A

B

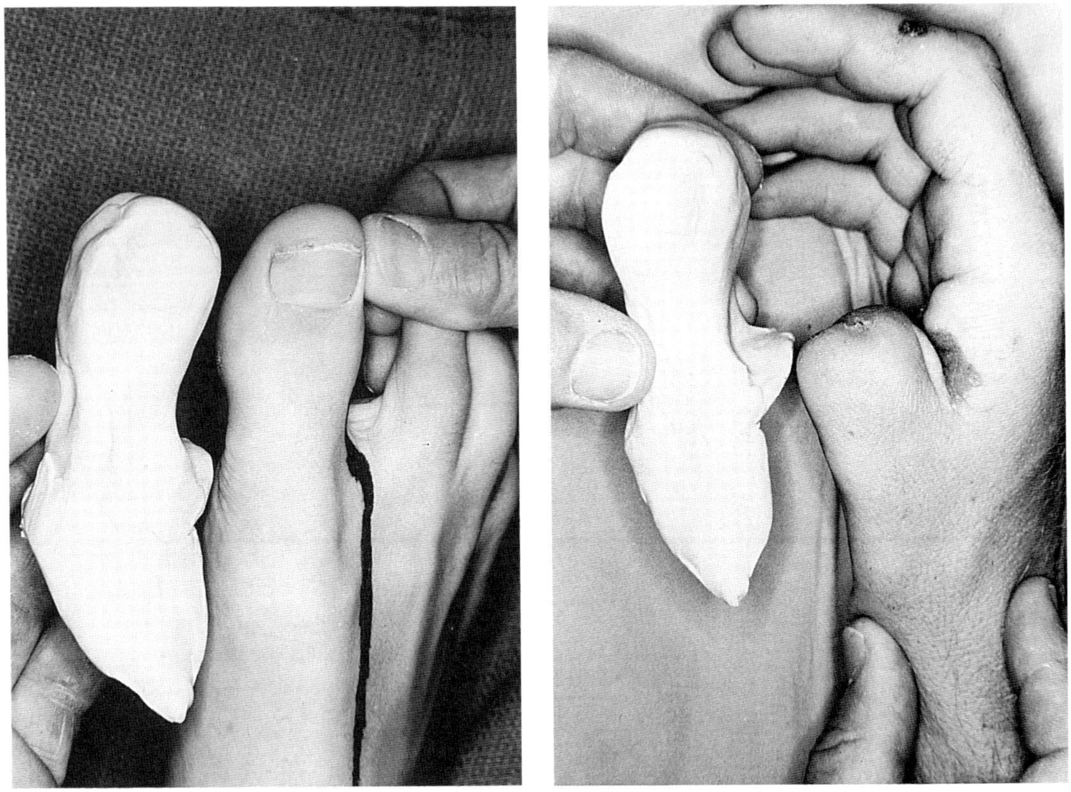

Fig. 6.7 A. and B. Clay models of proposed toe transfer.

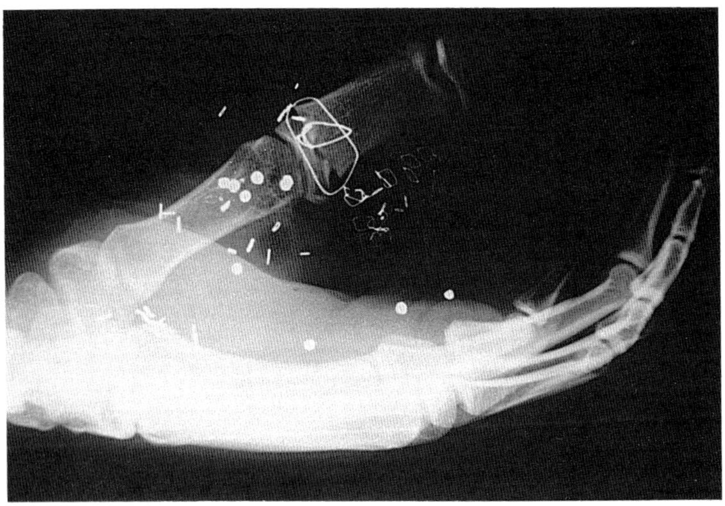

Fig. 6.8 X-ray demonstrating interosseous wiring technique of osteosynthesis.

metacarpal head of the thumb. Tendon repairs should be performed next. Arterial repairs are performed under the operating room microscope. If the toe is dorsal dominant, then the long arterial pedicle can be anastomosed to the dorsal radial artery in an end-to-end or end-to-side fashion. If the toe is plantar dominant, the pedicle is usually shorter and will probably require a vein graft to lengthen the pedicle such that the anastomosis can be performed to a recipient artery outside the zone of injury (Alpert et al 1978). Nerves are repaired in a standard microsurgical fashion. Veins are repaired on the dorsum (Fig. 6.9 A–G). Skin closures should be loose. Skin grafts to the hand are preferable to tight wound closure, even if it is necessary to place the grafts directly on the anastomosis (Gingrass et al 1973, McDonald & Buncke 1981). The hand should be placed in a loose, bulky absorbent dressing and elevated on pillows, thus avoiding trauma and compression.

Operating times for hallux transfers were seven hours on average (Buncke 1986). Hospitalisation was 13 days. Adjunctive surgery for soft tissue coverage was performed in only 18% of the cases in contrast to other studies (Lister 1985). This may reflect the more prevalent use of skin grafts in our series.

Postoperative monitoring is accomplished by physical examination, fluoroscanning and pulse oximetry. The physical examination of the digital pulp for turgor and nail bed colour, as well as the presence and nature of capillary filling, are assessed. Capillary refill with one or two-second delay is normal, whereas rapid refill or blue colour indicates venous congestion or venous obstruction. The loss of turgor or lack of capillary filling indicates arterial occlusion.

Fluoroscanning (Graham et al 1985) is a washout technique which involves the intravenous injection of fluorescein. A 'baseline' skin fluorimetry is made of the transferred toe, and then the fluorescein injected. At a ten-minute interval, a second fluorimetry reading is made and an increase in the fluorescence should be noted if arterial flow is present. If no rise is noted, then arterial obstruction should be considered. A third reading is taken one hour after the fluorescein injection, and should reveal a decreased reading approaching the pre-injection level. If not, venous congestion or possible occlusion must be considered.

Pulse oximetry (Buncke et al 1986) requires no administration of medications, and rapidly detects the loss of pulse as well as changes in oxygen saturation. If the signal is lost, then arterial occlusion may have occurred, and if oxygen saturation decreases then possible venous occlusion should be investigated.

In the event of venous congestion, loosening or even removal of the dressing should be performed as well as elevation of the reconstructed hand. If congestion is not relieved within several minutes, reoperation and redo of the venous anastomosis or additional venous grafting should be considered. In some cases, partial or total removal of the nail plate and abrasion of the nail bed allows for relief of venous congestion, and nail bed bleeding may be maintained by heparin soaks for about four days, at which time the nail bed heals (Gordon et al 1985). Leeches have also been useful for this purpose (Foucher et al 1980).

Arterial spasm may present similarly to occlusion, and manoeuvres such as median and ulnar nerve blocks at the wrist should be considered, as well as the use of pharmacological agents such as nifedipine (Nilsson et al 1984). If prompt resolution of the arterial insufficiency is not evident, one must reoperate.

Additionally, the hand is kept elevated and in a warm environment, either by the use of a heating pad or a warm room temperature. Dressings are bulky and absorbent but loose, thus protecting the thumb from trauma. All dressings should be split in the immediate postoperative period to prevent compression.

Pharmacological agents

Interest in the use of pharmacological agents (Ketchum 1978) to enhance flap survival has developed, and several medications have been advocated for a variety of these effects. Our series reflects the use of some of these agents, and some general statements can be made. Cephalosporin antibiotics (Monson & Nelson 1984, Neu 1984) are used routinely in the perioperative period, and have significant experimental and clinical data to support their use. Aspirin is an effective antiplatelet drug; with appropriate dosage, it can selectively block only vasoconstricting prostaglandins (Pederson & Fitzgerald 1984). Aspirin is used for two months as part of our postoperative routine. Isoxsuprine (Finseth & Adelberg 1973) and chlorpromazine (Buncke & Blackfield 1963, Bibi et al 1986) have been investigated many times, and several beneficial attributes have been proclaimed. Clinically, we have not found definitive effects and

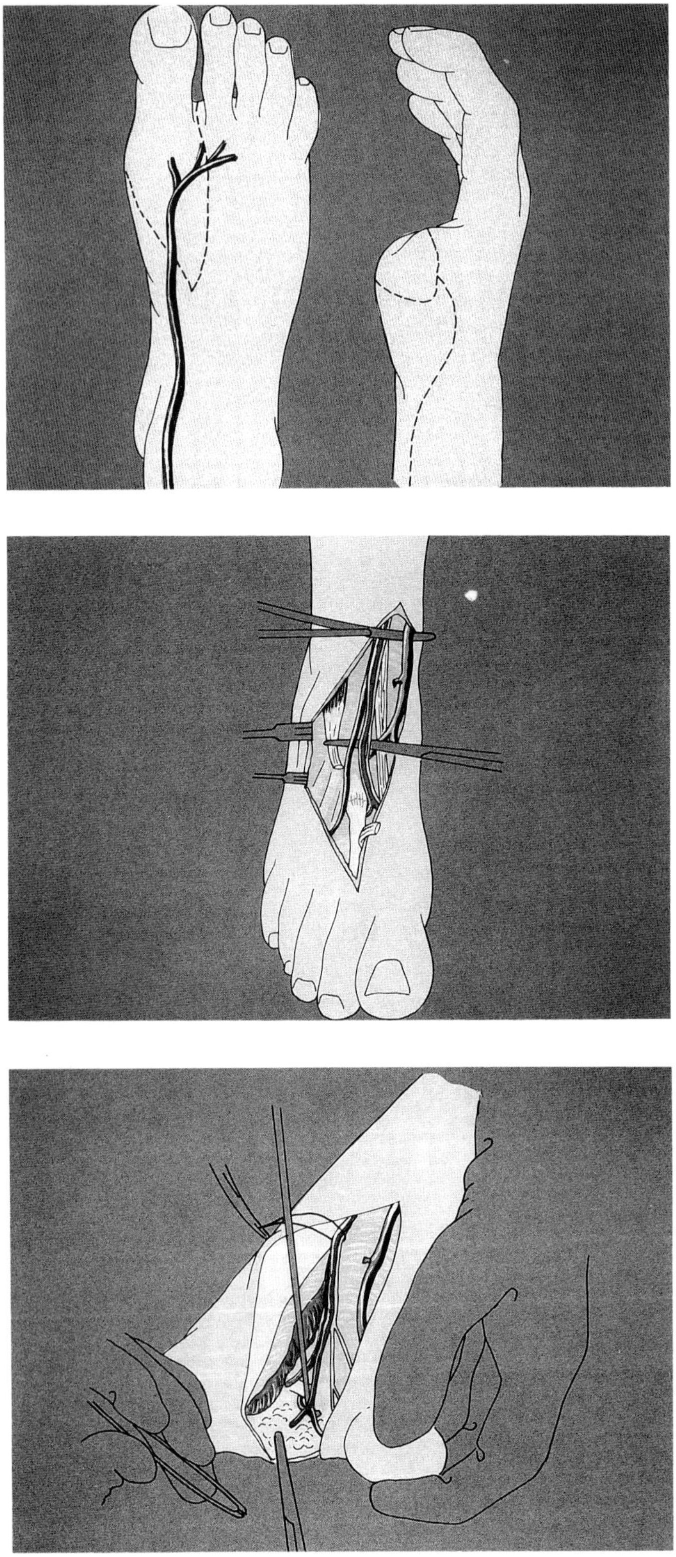

A

B

C

Fig. 6.9 **A.** Skin markings for great toe-to-thumb transfer; note course of greater saphenous vein. **B.** Through a dorsal skin incision, the extensor hallucis brevis is transected and retracted exposing a dorsalis pedis neurovascular pedicle. **C.** The vascular pedicle is followed distally to the great toe. The lateral branch of the second toe is ligated.

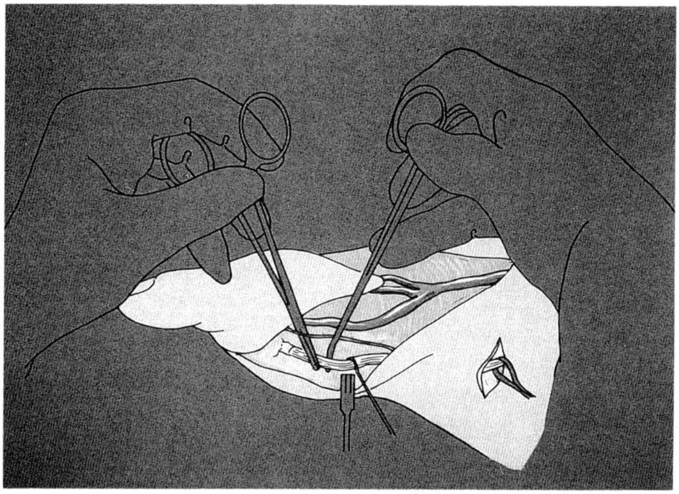

D

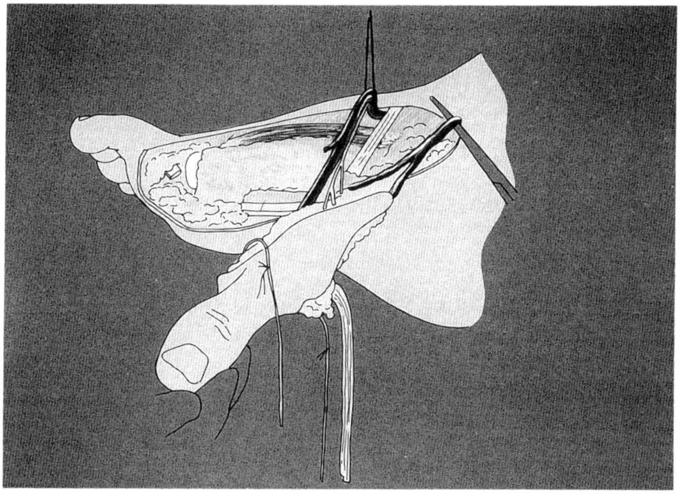

E

Fig. 6.9 (cont) **D.** Through a medio-plantar incision, the flexor tendon to the great toe is identified and followed proximally. **E.** The great toe is amputated through the metatarso-phalangeal joint. The plantar nerves and flexor tendon are followed as far proximally as possible and then transected. The vascular pedicle is left intact until the time of transfer. The extensor tendon is left intact to protect from accidentally avulsing the vascular pedicle. **F.** Dorsal dominant great toe ready for transfer with critical structures labelled. **G.** Osteosynthesis is performed such that the metacarpal is pegged into the proximal phalanx of the toe.

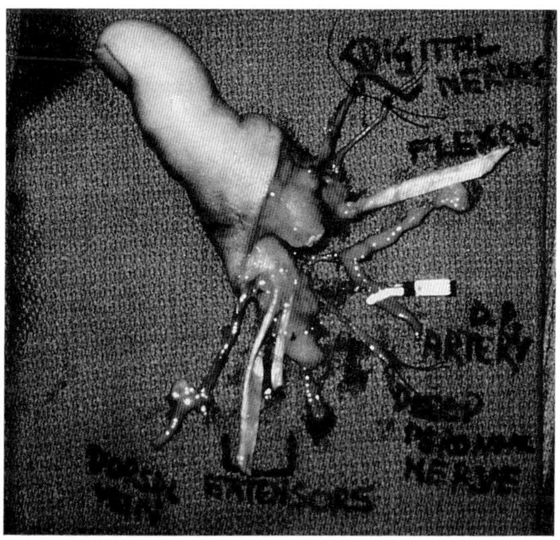

F

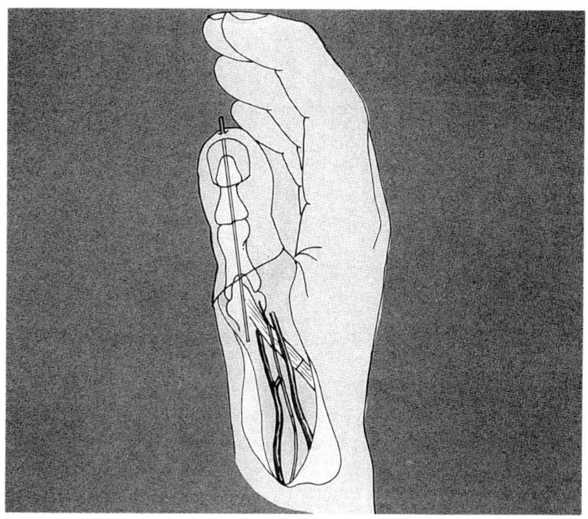

G

have decreased their use. Dextran (Bryant et al 1964, Moncrief et al 1963, Winfrey & Foster, 1964) is used in all of our cases, usually for five postoperative days. Heparin is used in cases where very small vessels are present, and sometimes after revision of an anastomosis is performed for thrombosis (Elcock 1972). Regional wrist blocks with bupivacaine may be used occasionally to provide pain relief and reduce the possibility of vasospasm.

Nifedipine (procardia), a calcium blocker, may be useful in preventing vasospasm, but further investigation is needed.

These medications are adjuncts and not substitutes for well done microsurgical anastomoses. Thus, because high patency rates are expected, it is difficult to judge their effectiveness and appreciate their value in the clinical setting.

Hand therapy

The patients are carefully followed by a staff of specially trained hand therapists, and a post-toe-transfer protocol has been established (Robbins & Reece 1985). The goals of physical therapy after toe transfer are: 1) to protect the repaired structures; 2) to restore the range of motion to the joints; 3) to restore tendon gliding; and 4) to restore strength. This is accomplished by a programme consisting firstly of protective splinting, and secondly of individualised gentle progressive joint mobilisation, which is determined by the type of bony fixation, the vascular status of the hand and concomitant injuries of the hand. Usually this programme is instituted at the tenth postoperative day. Progressive resistive exercises are begun after two months in order to increase strength. Additionally, monitoring of the sensory return and recording of the range of motion is carried out at intervals throughout the period of therapy and follow-up.

Postoperative function

Analysis of our series (Valauri et al 1986), as well as review of the literature, reiterates the very favourable results obtained by great toe-to-thumb transfer in properly selected cases. Our experience consists of 55 hallux-to-thumb transfers in 55 patients; 79% were male and 21% were female. The follow-up period averaged 37 months. Average ages for the great toe-to-thumb patients was 31 years for both men and women. It is of interest that the non-dominant hand is most often injured. Perhaps this is because of the use of the non-dominant hand as a 'helping hand' holding an object while the dominant hand operates the saw, cutting blade or press machine, thereby placing the non-dominant hand in a position of greater jeopardy.

Bilateral injuries were commonly severe in nature, often multi-digital and unreplantable. The lost digits cause varying disabilities, depending on the dominance of the hand injured as well as the specific digits damaged. For example, proximal injuries to the digits were almost always more disabling than distal injuries, and the loss of the thumb at any level created the greatest single digit disability. It is interesting to note, however, that our series revealed that, with hallux transfer patients for thumb restoration, the level of amputation has less influence on grip and pinch strength than might be predicted (Chase 1960, Srinivasan & Landsmeer 1982). Patients with thumb amputations through the proximal phalanx had similar pinch and grip strength to those with amputations distal to the interphalangeal joint when stratified according to the dominance of the injured hand and the number of injured digits. Recall that flexor pollicis longus provides much of the power, grip and pinch, and, in more proximal amputations, may compensate for the loss of intrinsic function (Brand 1985).

The function of the transplanted toes is generally excellent (Frykman et al 1986). Power grip and pinch are summarised in Table 6.1. Two-point discrimination for great toes was 14, with ranges from 5 to 25 mm, and improvement which plateaued by 18–24 months. Additionally, two-

Table 6.1 Strength of great toe-to-thumb transfer

Function	*Side of injury*	*Strength (% of uninjured side)*
Pinch	Dominant	85.1 (50–110)
	Non-dominant	45.3 (20–60)
Grip	Dominant	78.4 (50–130)
	Non-dominant	51.2 (25–70)

point discrimination in children appears to be better than that of older patients.

Range of motion is a complex problem because reconstruction may or may not restore the interphalangeal or metacarpo-phalangeal joint, depending upon the level of injury. Thumb mobility is the product of all three thumb joints working together in concert.

The evaluation of thumb mobility was simplified by measuring the distance from the pulp of the thumb to the palmar surface of the fifth metacarpal head. All patients in our series were within 3 cm of this point, with 40% within 1 cm and 10% making contact. Average interphalangeal motion was 55° ranging from 10/90 to 35/60 (Fig. 6.10 A and B).

Patients often later decline tenolysis and capsuloplasties, as they feel their function is adequate and desire no further surgery. However, the importance of interphalangeal flexion for nail pinch and small object manipulation should be recognised, and revision surgery to improve interphalangeal function is encouraged.

Complications

The complications of great toe-to-thumb transfer (Valauri et al 1986) are summarised in Table 6.2.

Recipient site

There was no instance of total necrosis of a transfer. Partial loss was noted in two patients. Both of these cases underwent re-exploration and vein grafting to restore blood flow.

Cigarette smoke is hazardous to the survival of

A B

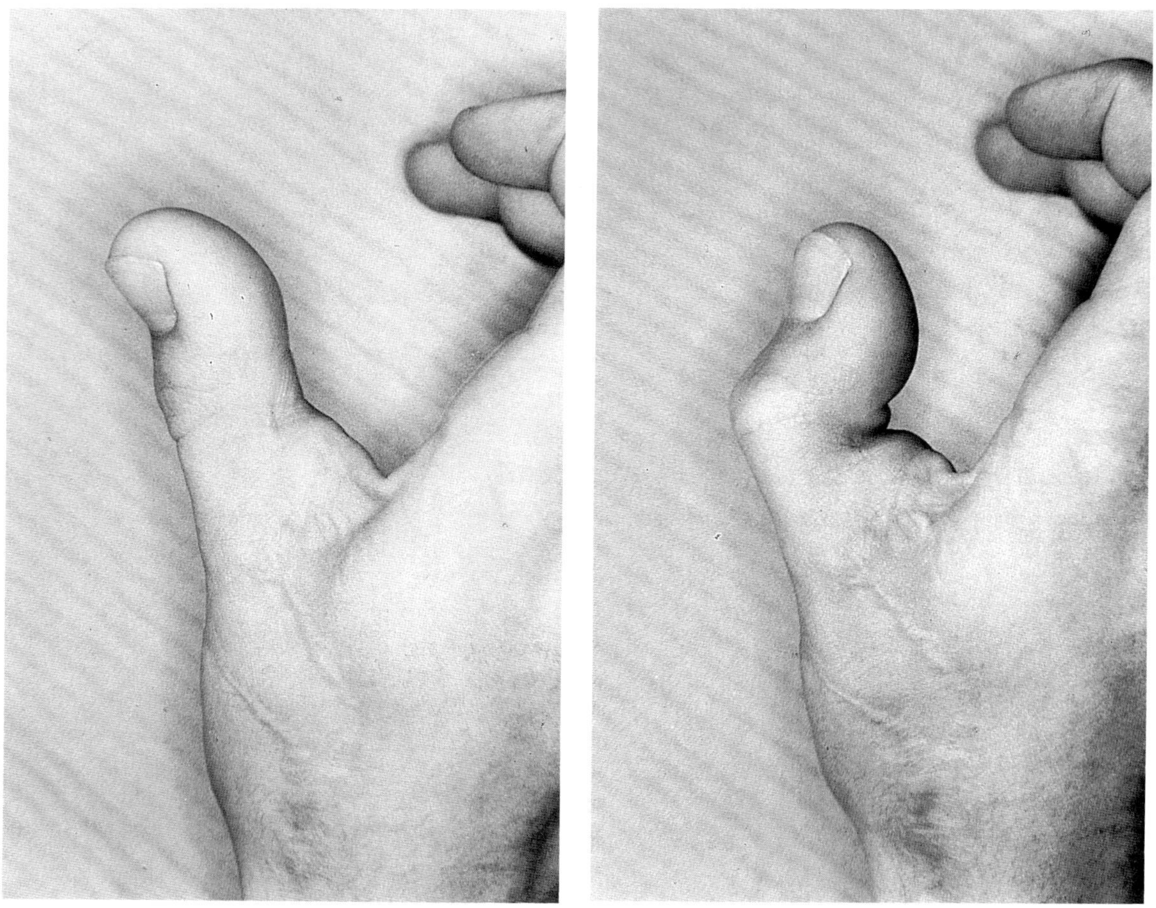

Fig. 6.10 **A.** and **B.** Interphalangeal flexion after hallux transfer.

Table 6.2 Great toe complications (Valauri et al 1986)

Site	Complication	Frequency
Recipient	Total loss	0/55 = 0%
	Partial loss	2/55 = 3.6%
Donor	Wound infection	4/55 = 7.3%
	Delayed healing (>4 weeks)	12/55 = 21.8%
	Cold weather aching	28/55 = 50.9%
	Lack power push-off	2/48 = 4.2%
	Returned to previous activity level	45/48 = 93.9%

a toe transfer, as nicotine is a potent vasoconstrictor and the smoke itself may also significantly reduce oxygenation (Harris et al 1980, Sarin et al 1974). Smoking was felt to be a significant factor in the partial loss of a transfer in one of these patients.

No cases of recipient site infection were noted. Cold intolerance was present in 10% of these patients, but this did not represent a significant problem to these patients. In fact, one of our patients uses a diving glove when he goes skiing and finds that this eliminates the problem.

Donor site

Great toe donor site morbidity in our series consisted of delayed healing (greater than four weeks) for 22% of the patients, and development of minor wound infections in four patients. All wounds were healed within three months. The hallux donor site required skin grafting to achieve final coverage in four patients. One-half of the great toe transfers had an aching sensation in their donor foot in cold weather.

Patient satisfaction is high, with a return to work by most patients within an eight month period. Most have returned to their near normal activities within as short a time as six weeks after operation.

Contrary to some reports (Lister 1985), athletes tolerated the great toe transfers very well. Two of our patients play college football, and one half of our patients participate in vigorous activities, including hiking, skiing, mountain climbing, tennis, basketball and football (Poppen 1981, 1983).

CONCLUSION

Toe transfer is a safe, reliable and effective means of reconstruction which restores hand function to a high degree, utilising anatomically similar tissue to those which have been lost. This is accomplished with minimal donor site disability (Fig. 6.11).

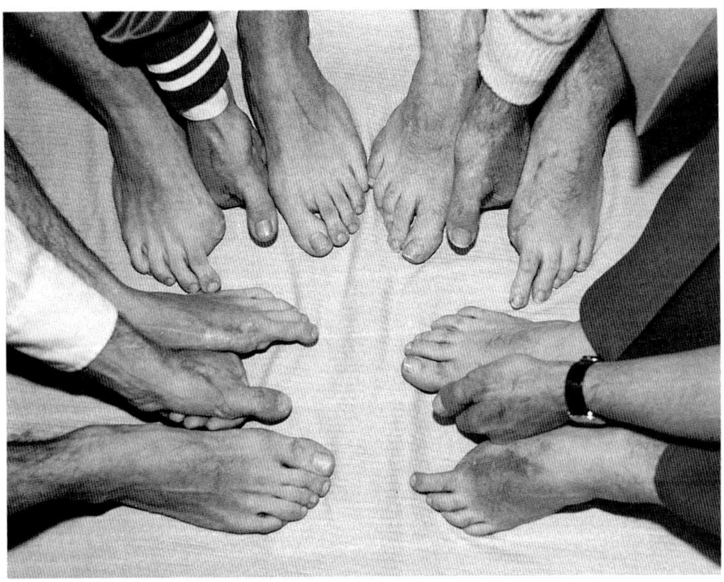

Fig. 6.11 Four great toe-to-thumb transfers; donor and recipient sites.

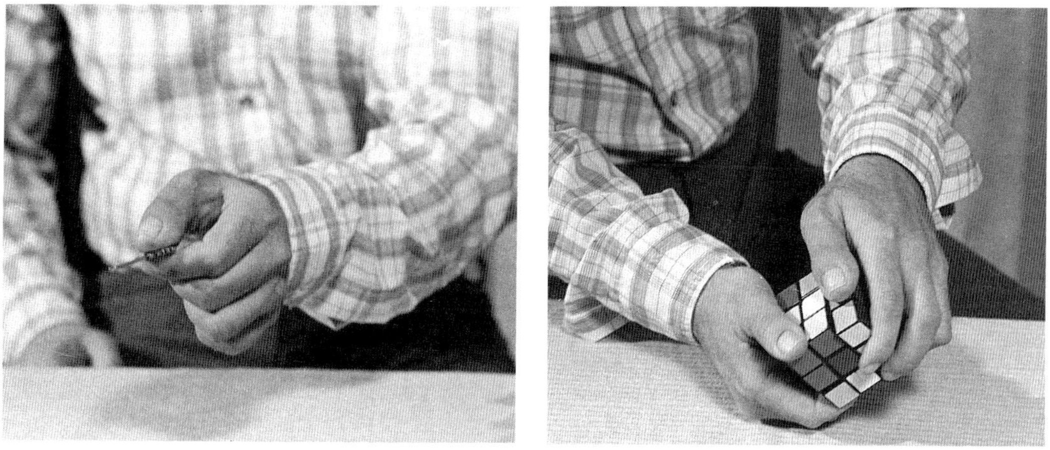

A B

Fig. 6.12 **A.** and **B.** Great toe-to-thumb transfer.

Because of this 'anatomical reconstruction of the hand, toe transfers restore the attributes of the specialised tactile qualities of its glabrous skin, the excellent sensibility, dexterity, mobility, power, appearance and growth potential. While not the perfect solution, the toe transfer does provide this unique combination which other methods cannot achieve (Fig. 6.12 A and B).

REFERENCES

Alpert B S, Buncke H J, Brownstein M 1978 Replacement of vessels with vein grafts when replanting crushed amputated fingers. Plastic and Reconstructive Surgery 61: 171

Beasley R W 1981 Introduction to hand injuries. W B Saunders, Philadelphia PA p 1–6

Beasley R W 1971 Cosmetic considerations in surgery of the hand. Surgical Clinics of North America 51: 2

Bell Sir Charles 1934 Bridgewater thesis IV, London

Bibi R, Ferder M, Strauch B 1986 Prevention of flap necrosis by chlorpromazine. Plastic and Reconstructive Surgery 77(6) June: 954–959

Biemer E, Stock W 1983 Total thumb reconstruction: one-stage reconstruction using an osteo-cutaneous forearm flap. British Journal of Plastic Surgery 36: 52–55

Blair V P, Byars L T 1940 Toe to finger transplant. Annals of Surgery 112: 287

Boyes J H 1970a Chapter 1 The normal hand, mechanics of muscle and tendon action. In: Bunnell's surgery of the hand, 5th edn. Lippincott, Philadelphia p 9–20

Boyes J H 1970b Chapter 2 Phylogeny and comparative anatomy primate hand and thumb. In: Bunnell's surgery of the hand, 5th edn. Lippincott, Philadelphia p 50–52

Brand P W 1985 Mechanics of individual muscles at individual joints. In: Brand P W (ed) Clinical mechanics of the hand. Mosby, St Louis, p 222–255

Brown P W 1978 The role of motivation in patient recovery. Connecticut Medicine 42

Bryant F M et al 1964 Study of antithrombotic properties of dextran of large molecular weight. Journal of Cardiovascular Surgery 5: 48–52

Buck-Gramcko D 1971 Lengthening of first metacarpal in cases of loss of thumb and several fingers. In: Transactions of fifth international congress. Butterworths, Australia, p 553

Buncke G M, Buncke H J, Valauri F A, Brooksher R, Alpert B S, Hing D N 1986 Review of 102 toe-to-hand transfers: correlation of preoperative angiograms and surgical anatomy. Presented at the Fourth Annual Residents' and Fellows' Hand Surgery Conference, February 1986, New Orleans

Buncke H J 1981 Aesthetic aspects of hand surgery. Clinics in Plastic Surgery April 8: 2

Buncke H J, Shah K G 1979 Toe digital transfers. In: Serrafin D, Buncke H J (eds) Microsurgical composite tissue transfers. C V Mosby, St Louis 573–586

Buncke H J, Alpert B S, Shah K G 1978 Microvascular grafting. Clinics of Plastic Surgery 5: 185

Buncke H J 1976 Toe digit transfer. Clinics of Plastic Surgery 3: 49

Buncke H J et al 1973 Thumb replacement: great toe transplantation by microvascular anastomosis. British Journal of Plastic Surgery 26: 194

Buncke H J, Buncke C M, Schulz W P 1966 Hallux-to-hand transplantation utilizing microvascular anastomoses. British Journal of Plastic Surgery 19: 332

Buncke H J, Blackfield H M 1963 The vasoplegic effects of chlorpromazine. Plastic and Reconstructive Surgery 31(4): 353

Bunnell S 1952 Digit transfer by neurovascular pedicle. Journal of Bone and Joint Surgery 34A: 772.

Bunnell S 1931 Physiological reconstruction of a thumb after total loss. Surgery Gynecology and Obstetrics 52: 245

Byars L T 1952 Toe to finger transplant — final result. Plastic and Reconstructive Surgery 9: 274

Campbell-Reid D A 1980 The Gillies thumb lengthening operation. Hand 12: 123

Chase R A 1969 An alternative to pollicization in subtotal thumb reconstruction. Plastic and Reconstructive Surgery 44(5): 421–429

Chase R A 1960 Functional levels of amputations in the hand. Surgical Clinics of North America 40: 415

Cherry G W 1979 The differing effects of isoxsuprine on muscle flap and skin flap survival in the pig. Plastic and Reconstructive Surgery 64(5) November 670–672

Clarkson P 1955 Reconstruction of hand digits by toe transfer. Journal of Bone and Joint Surgery 37A: 270

Cobbett J R 1969 Free digital transfer. Report of a case of transfer of a great toe to replace an amputated thumb. Journal of Bone and Joint Surgery 51B: 677

Cooney W P, Chao E V S 1977 Biomechanical analysis of static forces in the thumb during hand function. Journal of Bone and Joint Surgery 59A (1): 27–36

Doi K 1981 New procedure on making a thumb — one stage reconstruction with free neurovascular flap and iliac bone grafts. Journal of Hand Surgery 6 (4) July 346–350

Dunlop J 1933 Use of index finger for a thumb. Journal of Bone and Joint Surgery 5: 99

Elcock H W 1972 The effect of heparin on thrombosis at microvenous anastomosis sites. Archives of Otolaryngology 95: 68

Finseth F, Adelberg M G 1973 Prevention of skin flap necrosis by a course of treatment with vasodilator drugs. Plastic and Reconstructive Surgery 61: 738

Flatt A E 1961 Kinesiology of the hand. In: The American Academy of Orthopedic Surgeons: instructional course lectures, vol 18. Mosby, St Louis p 266–281

Foucher G, Merle M, Maneaud M, Michan J 1980 Microsurgical free partial toe transfer in hand reconstruction: a report of 12 cases. Plastic and Reconstructive Surgery 65(5) May: 616–625

Freeman B S 1956 Reconstruction of the thumb by toe transfer. Plastic and Reconstructive Surgery 17: 393

Frykman G K, O'Brien B, Morrison W A, MacLeod A M 1986 Functional evaluation of the hand and foot after one-stage toe-to-hand transfer. Journal of Hand Surgery 11A(1): 9–17

Fujikawa S, O'Brien B M 1975 One experimental evaluation of microvenous grafts. British Journal of Plastic Surgery 28: 244–246

Gilbert A 1976 Composite tissue transfers from the foot: Anatomic basis and surgical techniques. In: Danillier A I, Strauch B (eds) Symposium on microsurgery. C V Mosby, St Louis

Gillies H, Reid D A C 1955 Autograft of the amputated digit. British Journal of Plastic Surgery 7: 338

Gingrass R P, Cunningham D S, Palletta F X 1973 Skin grafting of exposed arterial vein grafts: a clinical and experimental study. Journal of Trauma 13: 951

Gordon L, Leitner D W, Buncke H J, Alpert B S 1985 Partial nail plate removal after digital replantation as an alternative method of venous drainage. Journal of Hand Surgery 10A: 360–364

Gosset J, Sels M 1964 Technique, indications et résultats de la pollicisation du 4e doigt. Annales de Chirurgie de la Main 18: 1005

Gosset J 1949 La pollicisation de l'index. Journal de Chirurgie 65: 403

Graham B H, Gordon L, Alpert B S, Walton R, Buncke H J, Leitner D W 1985 Serial quantitative skin surface fluorescence: a new method for postoperative monitoring of vascular perfusion in revascularized digits. Journal of Hand Surgery 10A: 226–230

Guelette R 1930 Pollicisation de l'index, étude critique des procédés de restauration du pouce. Journal de Chirurgie 36: 1

Guermonprez F 1887 Notes sur quelques resections et restaurations du pouce. P Asselin, Paris

Harris G D, Finseth F, Buncke H J 1980 The hazard of cigarette smoking following digital replantation. Journal of Microsurgery 1: 403

Hentz V 1985 Reconstruction of individual digits. Hand Clinics 1: 2 (May)

Hilgenfeldt C 1950 Operativer daumenersatz, Ferdinand Enke Verlag, Stuttgart

Huguier P C 1874 Replacement du pouce par son metacarpien, par l'agrandissement du premier espace interosseux. Archives of General Medicine (Paris) 1: 78

Iselin M 1937 Reconstruction of the thumb. Surgery 2: 619

Joyce J L 1929 Results of a new operation for substitution of a thumb. British Journal of Surgery 16: 362

Joyce J L 1918 A new operation for the substitution of a thumb. British Journal of Surgery 5: 499

Ketchum L D 1978 Pharmacological alterations in the clotting mechanism: use in microvascular surgery. Journal of Hand Surgery 3(5): 407

Kleinschmidt O 1920 Ueber daumenplastik unter verwendung des ubrauchbaren mittelfingers. Brun Beitrage Klinische Chirurgie 120: 589

Le Tac R 1952 Reconstitution du pouce détruit par pollicisation de l'annulaire ou du 5e doigt, Annales de Chirurgie de la Main 78: 262

Leung P C, Wong W L 1983 The vessels of the first metatarsal web space. Journal of Bone and Joint Surgery 65A (2): 235

Leung P C 1983 Thumb reconstruction using second toe transfer. Hand 15: 21

Leung P C, Ma F Y 1982 Digital reconstruction using the toe flap: report of 10 cases. Journal of Hand Surgery 7: 366–370

Lister G D 1985 The choice of procedure following thumb amputation. Clinical Orthopaedics and Related Research 195:49–50

Littler J W 1976 On making a thumb: one hundred years of surgical effort. Journal of Hand Surgery 1(1) July: 35–51

Littler J W 1966 Digital transposition. In: Adams J P (ed) Current practice in orthopaedic surgery, vol 3. Mosby, St Louis

Littler J W 1953 Neurovascular pedicle method of digital transposition for reconstruction of the thumb. Plastic and Reconstructive Surgery 12: 503

Matev I B 1979 Thumb reconstruction after amputation at the interphalangeal joint by gradual lengthening of the proximal phalanx — a case report. Hand 11: 302

Matev I B 1980 Thumb reconstruction through metacarpal bone lengthening. Journal of Hand Surgery 5: 482

Matev I B 1979 Thumb reconstruction after amputation at the MP joint by bone lengthening. Journal of Bone and Joint Surgery 52A:957

May J W, Bartlett S P 1985 Great toe-to-hand free tissue transfer for thumb reconstruction. Hand Clinics 1(2) May: 271–284

McDonald H D, Buncke H J 1981 Split thickness skin grafts in microvascular surgery. Plastic and Reconstructive Surgery 68(5): 731

Michon J, Merle M, Bouchon Y, Foucher G 1985 Thumb reconstruction pollicization or toe-to-hand transfers. A comparative study of functional results. Annales de Chirurgie de la Main 4(2): 98–110

Moncrief J A, Darin J C, Canizardo P C, Sawyer R B 1963 Use of dextran to prevent arterial and venous thrombosis. Annals of Surgery 158: 552

Monson T P, Nelson C L 1984 Microbiology for orthopaedic surgeons: selected aspects. Clinical Orthopaedics and Related Research 190: 14–22

Morrison W A 1980 Thumb reconstruction with a free neurovascular wrap-around flap from the big toe. Journal of Hand Surgery 5: 575

Morrison W A et al 1983 Experience with thumb reconstruction. Journal of Hand Surgery 9B(3) October: 223

Murray J F et al 1977 Transmetacarpal amputation of the index finger: a clinical assessment of hand strength and complications. Journal of Hand Surgery 2: 471

Murray J F 1967 The neurovascular island pedicle flap. Journal of Hand Surgery 49A: 1288

Napier J R 1956 The prehensile movements of the human hand. Journal of Bone and Joint Surgery November 38B(4)

Neu H C 1984 Cephalosporin antibiotics as applied in surgery of bones and joints. Conical Orthopaedics and Related Research. 90: 50–63

Nicolandoni C 1900 Daumenplastik und organischer ersatz der fingerspitze (Anticheiroplastik und daktylo-plastik), Archiv für Klinische Chirurgie 6: 606

Nicolandoni C 1897 Daumenplastik, Klinische Wochenschrift Wien

Nilsson H, Jonasson T, Ringqvist I 1984 Treatment of digital vasoplastic disease with the calcium-entry blocker nifedipine. Acta Medica Scandinavia 215(2): 135–9

Noesske K 1920 Ueber ersatz des bamt metakarpus verlorenen daumens durch operative. Umstellung des zeigefingers, Medizinische Wochenschrift Munchen 16: 465

O'Brien J R 1968 Salicylates and platelets. Lancet 1: 779

Parks B J, Arbelaez J, Horner R L 1978 Medical and surgical importance of the arterial blood supply of the thumb. Journal of Hand Surgery 3(4): 383

Peacock E E Jr 1966 Reconstruction of the thumb. In: Flynn J E (ed) Hand surgery. Williams & Wilkins, Baltimore, M D

Pederson A K, Fitzgerald G A 1984 Dose-related kinetics of aspirin. New England Journal of Medicine 311: 1205

Peimer C A, Echkert B S 1982 Microvascular response to angiography. Journal of Hand Surgery 7(1): 4

Poppen H K, Norris T R, Buncke H J 1983 Evaluation of sensibility and function with microsurgical free tissue transfer of the great toe to the hand for thumb reconstruction. Journal of Hand Surgery 8(5): 516

Poppen H K, Mann R A, O'Konski M O, Buncke H J 1981 Amputation of the great toe. Foot and Ankle 1: 333–337

Robbins F, Reece T 1985 Hand rehabilitation after great toe transfer for thumb reconstruction. Archives of Physical Medicine Rehabilitation 66(2): February 109–112

Sarin C L, Austin J C, Mickel W 1974 Effects of smoking on digital blood-flow velocity. Journal of American Medical Association. 229: 1327

Srininvasan H, Landsmeer J M F 1982 Internal stabilization in the thumb. Journal of Hand Surgery 17(4): 371–375

Tomita Y, Kurota K, Okubo K 1983 Wrap-around flap with tip of distal phalanx. Presented at the Seventh Symposium of the International Society of Reconstructive Microsurgeons, June, New York

Tubiana R, Roux J 1974 Phalangization of the first and fifth metacarpals. Journal of Bone and Joint Surgery 56A(3): 447–457

Tubiana R, Duprac J 1961 Restoration of sensibility in the hand by neurovascular skin island transfer. Journal of Bone and Joint Surgery 43A: 474

Urbaniak J R 1985 Wrap-around procedure for thumb reconstruction. Hand Clinics 1 (2) May

Valauri F A, Buncke G M, Buncke H J 1986 Hand reconstruction with toe-to-hand transfers: a comprehensive review. Presented to the American Society for Reconstructive Microsurgery, February, New Orleans

Verdan C 1968 The reconstruction of the thumb. Surgical Clinics of North America 48: 1033

Wang W 1983 Keys to successful second toe-to-hand transfers: a review of 30 cases. Journal of Hand Surgery 8(6): 902

Winfrey E W, Foster J H 1964 Low molecular weight dextran in small artery surgery. Archives of Surgery 88: 110

Yang D, Gu Y 1979 Thumb reconstruction utilizing second toe transplantation by microvascular anastomoses: a report of 78 cases. Chinese Medical Journal 92: 295

Zook E G, Van Beek A L, Russell R C, Beatty M E 1980 Anatomy and physiology of the perionychium: a review of the literature and anatomic study. Journal of Hand Surgery 5(6):528–536

Zsulyevich I 1938 Ein fall von plastischem daumenersatz. Chirugie 10: 433

P. C. Leung

7 Toe transplantations in hand reconstruction

INTRODUCTION

Function of the hand is maintained by the integrity of its components, namely, the thumb and fingers, and adequate lengths of these components are essential for their proper performance. When losses of these components occur, either completely or partially, serious impairment of hand function results. It is, therefore, not uncommon to find many difficult problems in the attempt to restore hand function when partial or complete loss of the components is the cause of the functional impairment. Such losses are usually the result of trauma, or occasionally, may be manifestations of congenital malformations.

Trying to restore the missing length of the thumb and fingers has been a challenge to surgeons for decades, and many conventional methods have been used. The more popular ones include: pollicisation for thumb loss; distraction lengthening of individual digits, especially the thumb; reconstruction with a central core of bone and a pedicled skin flap, etc. (Buck-Gramco 1971, Marter 1972, Reid 1960).

All these conventional methods have defects and fail to fulfil the ideal of restoring a digit, not only with good motor and sensory function, but also with reasonable external appearance. Since the advent of microsurgical techniques, new areas have opened for reconstruction. Missing components may now be restored by transplanting composite tissues from the foot. The reconstructed digits possess not only the desired length, but also a sensitive pulp and a nail.

In this chapter, different varieties of hand reconstruction using composite transfers from the toes are presented. These procedures include reconstruction of the thumb, single fingers, pincer components and double fingers. The presentation and discussions are based upon the author's personal experience of over 120 toe transplants and similar procedures.

THUMB RECONSTRUCTION USING THE SECOND TOE

Since the choice of the transplant and the technical considerations depend on the level of the thumb loss, a good classification of the type of amputation is necessary to simplify and standardise the indications. When thumb loss is distal to, or at the interphalangeal joint of, the thumb, reconstruction is not necessary because the residual stump should be long enough for essential thumb function. Any amputation proximal to the interphalangeal joint will benefit from second toe transplantation. Four types of amputation are identified (Fig. 7.1):

1. Type 1 Amputation at proximal phalanx or metacarpo-phalangeal joint
2. Type 2 Amputation at the first metacarpal
3. Type 3 Loss of the whole first metacarpal and thenar eminence
4. Type 4 Loss of the thumb together with one or two radial fingers.

Different planning is necessary for different types of amputation (Leung 1983). For Types 1 and 2, the donor toe need not include the metatarsal bone, because either the metacarpo-phalangeal joint is still intact (Type 1) or the residual metacarpal is sufficiently long to give an effective

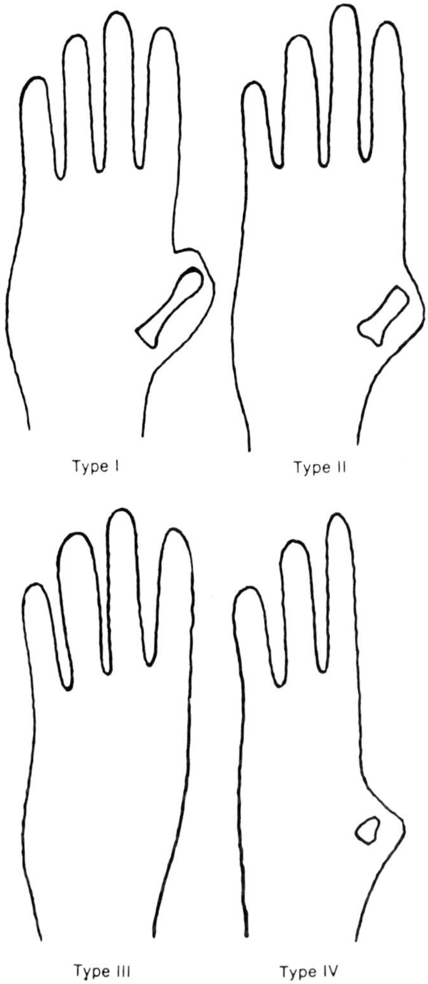

Fig. 7.1 Four different types of thumb amputations indicated for toe transplants.

new thumb using the second toe without the metatarsal. For Type 3 and 4 amputations, it is better to take the metatarso-phalangeal joint together with the second toe, so that not only is the new thumb longer, but its function will be better. When there has been extensive soft tissue damage and losses in either Type 3 or 4 amputations, a large skin flap may be raised together with the donor toe, so that the metatarsal bone may be adequately covered (Leung 1985) (Fig. 7.2).

Technical considerations

In principle, the second toe, together with its

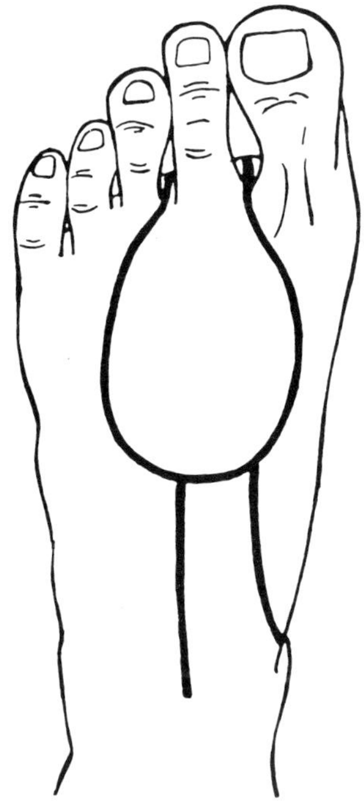

Fig. 7.2 Large skin flap transferred together with second toe.

feeding artery and draining veins, sensory nerves, and extensor and flexor tendons, is removed from the donor foot with as little trauma as possible, and this graft of composite tissues is transplanted to the recipient site. Its blood supply is re-established, and respective donor and recipient structures joined. The following technical points need to be considered.

(1) Preparation of the veins

Preparation of the veins is the first step and should be completed before any other procedure is undertaken. The long saphenous vein is always available. An extra vein may be included from the short saphenous side, or from the middle of the dorsal arch (Leung 1980, Leung & Wong 1983). The main patterns of the superficial dorsal veins are shown in Figure 7.3. All the tributaries of the veins should be tied or clipped. A thin layer of adventitia may be left around the veins, but near the expected site of anastomosis, the vessel wall should be cleared of areolar tissue as much as possible. The veins are traced proximally to give the required lengths.

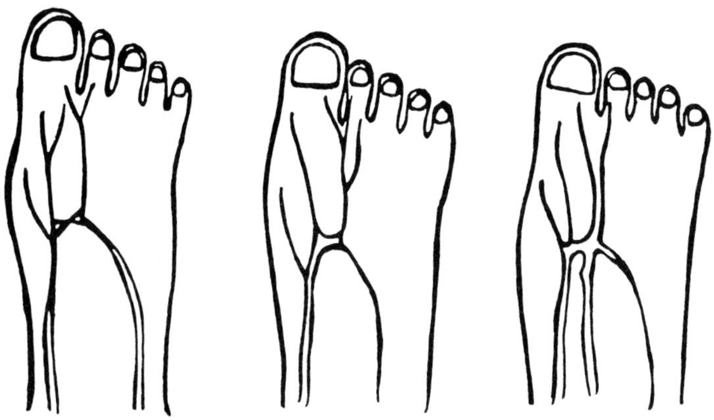

Fig. 7.3 Three main patterns of superficial veins from the second toe.

(2) Preparation of the artery

Although the digital artery has been used as the feeding vessel, it is much safer to use the dorsalis pedis artery, because it is of much larger dimension and it is constant. The isolation is usually started on the dorsum of the foot, and it may be thoroughly exposed by cutting the tendon of extensor hallucis brevis and retracting the small muscle upwards and proximally by pulling on the cut tendon. The tendon may later be left or attached to the extensor of the great toe.

The different patterns of distribution of the terminal branches of the dorsalis pedis artery must be realised during the isolation of the second toe. These different patterns have been analysed by the author and others (Leung & Wong 1983, Yang 1979, Gilbert 1976) and are shown diagrammatically in Figure 7.4.

There have been arguments about whether angiographic examination is necessary to identify the actual pattern of the artery so that its isolation may be facilitated. A series of 20 angiograms indicated that the study was useful in confirming the presence and origin of the first dorsal metatarsal artery, which is the terminal branch of the dorsalis pedis artery, but was not useful in demonstrating the depth of the artery. Therefore, what may be accomplished by angiographic study is apparently achievable by careful clinical examination alone. In fact, with the help of an ultrasound Doppler stethoscope, the first dorsal metatarsal artery is easily detected in the first three types of arterial pattern. Failure to detect the arterial bruit indi-

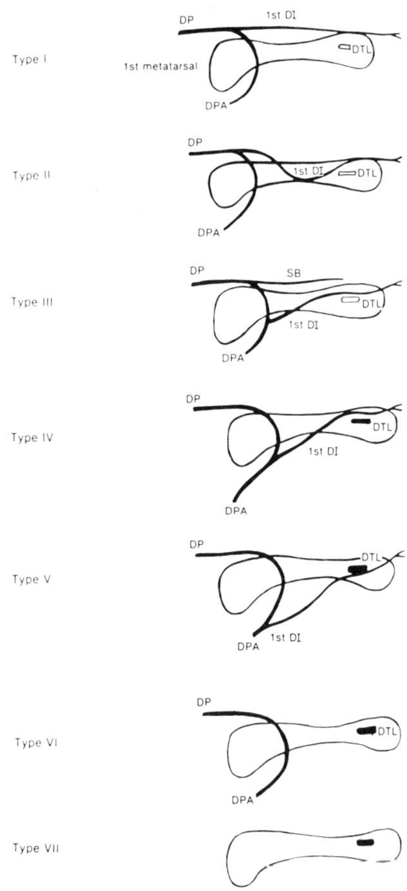

Fig. 7.4 Different patterns of the first dorsal metatarsal artery.

cates that the first dorsal metatarsal artery is either absent, very deep or is arising from the deep plantar arch.

Isolation of the artery is done in the same way as the veins, except that as much sharp dissection as possible is done, and as much adventitia as possible is removed. Blunt manoeuvres easily introduce constricting bands around the artery. If adventitial tissues are cleared from the artery, vasoconstriction after anastomosis may be minimised.

For the superficial types of arterial pattern, retraction of the soft tissues is sufficient to expose the first dorsal metatarsal artery. For the deeper types, however, osteotomy of the second metatarsal bone near its base may be necessary to enable lateral retraction of the metatarsal so that there is a good view deep down the first metatarsal space. Ligation of the connection between the dorsalis pedis artery and the deep plantar arch is usually left until a late stage, when isolation is completed.

When a small superficial artery is available at the same time as a main one deep to the interosseous muscles, it may be better to sacrifice it, as its reliability cannot be guaranteed.

(3) The extensor tendon

The long extensor tendon to the second toe marks the plane between the superficial veins and the muscular layer. During the isolation of the artery, the tendon may have to be cut proximally at its required length, and lifted upwards to facilitate exposure. Isolation of this tendon is simple and straightforward. The short extensor tendon is usually sacrificed.

(4) The plantar dissection

A long triangular flap of skin based on the proximal phalanx is raised before the neurovascular structures are isolated. The plantar skin is very thick and is associated with a deep layer of fatty areolar tissue which needs to be removed.

The digital nerves need to be carefully dissected. They occupy a deep plane 2 mm to each side of the flexor tendons amongst dense areolar tissue. At a variable distance from the toe webs, each digital nerve arises from a common metatarsal nerve supplying the web. With careful dissection, the digital nerves to the second toe may be separated from the adjacent component, so that sensation in the remaining toe is not affected. This is particularly true for the great toe. However, if the common metatarsal nerve to the second web is too small to be separated into two, the whole nerve may be taken to ensure better sensory recovery of the transplanted second toe.

The flexor tendons occupy a position plantar to the second metatarsal bone, and are the last structures to be tackled in the isolation process. Usually, only the long flexor is taken to give flexion of the distal interphalangeal joint, but occasionally, to give more strength, both tendons are used. Long lengths of these tendons are difficult to obtain, as they give origin to the short muscles of the foot at mid-plantar level. In situations where long donor tendons are required for wrist level anastomosis, this problem will be inevitable. As far as possible, bridging tendon grafts are to be avoided.

(5) The recipient site

For Type 1, 2 and 4 amputations, the terminal branch of the radial artery at the anatomical snuff box is used as the recipient artery, and the cephalic vein on the radial side of the wrist, together with one other dorsal vein, are used as the draining veins. These vascular structures are approached through a curving incision on the dorsum of the wrist. Using artery and veins on the dorsum has the definite advantage not only of convenience, but that gentle dorsiflexion of the wrist will relax the rejoined structures during the postoperative period. For Type 3 amputations, or when the terminal branch of the radial artery has been damaged, the radial artery on the volar surface of the wrist may have to be used. Under such circumstances, the end-to-side method of anastomosis is preferred unless a carefully performed Allen's test has confirmed that the blood supply from the ulnar artery is satisfactory. When the arterial and venous anastomoses occupy different surfaces of the wrist, postural splinting to relax the various anastomosed vessels becomes difficult, and extra care needs to be taken. When there is extensive scarring from the previous trauma, the structures being isolated need to be carefully freed so as to ensure that the scarring will not hinder their future function. In cases of thick, hard scarring, one might have to consider the use of an extended skin flap taken together with the second toe. Subcutaneous tunnels should be made as wide as possible, so as to allow compression-free passage of the vessels during the postoperative period of bleeding and oedema (Leung 1979).

(6) The transplantation

The vascular pedicle of the completely isolated toe is left intact in the foot. The tourniquet is released and the circulation to the toe is checked. Usually, there is a slow return of blood flow. If this does not occur, the feeding artery is checked carefully for adventitial bands, all of which should be freed by sharp dissection. If better flow is not achieved in spite of these manoeuvres, and after the application of local vasodilating agents, such as papaverine, magnesium sulphate or lignocaine, the artery may be cut proximally at the desired length, or one of the major ligated branches may be re-opened. Irrigation with heparinised saline or diluted blood through the opened artery may then be done to ensure good distal filling.

The right length of bone is prepared before the isolated toe is transferred to the hand for transplantation. In the majority of cases (Types 1 and 2), the base of the proximal phalanx of the second toe is denuded of cartilage and prepared for fixation. Occasionally, when a new metacarpophalangeal joint is to be reconstituted, long capsular flaps need to be included with the transfer. The intramedullary bone peg fixation method is preferred by the author (Leung 1981) (Fig. 7.5). This method has the following advantages: it is technically simple; it allows quick stable fixation; it controls rotation well; it requires no additional fixation; and it does not cause fractures.

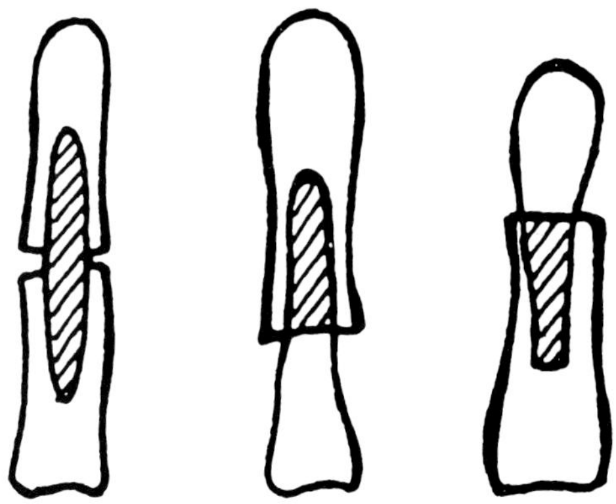

Fig. 7.5 Intramedullary bone peg for osteosynthesis.

The arterial anastomosis is preferably done in an end-to-end fashion, because the high pressure thus generated in the blood flow to the transplanted toe is a good safeguard to its survival.

The digital nerves of the toe are joined to the digital nerves of the thumb at different levels, so that cross-scarring is not readily formed. Careful epineural suturing should be as satisfactory as microscopic fascicular suturing for these purely sensory nerves.

The simplest and safest means of tendon anastomosis should be performed, otherwise the already long operation will be even further prolonged. Since the toe flexor and extensor tendons are always smaller than the recipient tendons, the 'fish-mouth' technique done by embracing the smaller tendon within the split larger tendon is suitable and quick. There is a tendency to overflexion at the proximal interphalangeal joint of the transplanted toe because of a stronger flexor pull, and because of the basic fact that the proximal interphalangeal joint is the most mobile joint in the toe. In order to minimise this unwanted deformity in the transplanted toe, the extensor tendon needs to be put under some extra tension, so as to counteract the strong flexor pull (Leung 1985).

After completion of the anastomoses, the circulation should be checked again and again. Usually, the volar structures are joined before the hand is turned, and then the dorsal structures are tackled. The artery is the first structure to be anastomosed on the dorsal side, so that after its completion, there are still 40–60 minutes before the entire operation is completed. This period allows sufficient time for observing the transplant's circulation, so that if kinking or compression occur, circulatory arrest will be revealed before the completion of the operation.

After the completion of all the anastomotic procedures, and when the circulation is satisfactory, closure of the incisions is begun. No tension should be allowed. Raw areas should be covered with split-thickness skin grafts. Similarly, any suture line causing tension or pressure on the vascular structures should be released, and skin grafts applied.

(7) Postoperative monitoring

Dressings should be very loose, and circumferential woollen coverings are not desirable. The wrist is kept slightly dorsiflexed when arterial anastomosis is performed in the anatomical snuff box, and neutral when volar anastomosis has been done. A strong plaster-of-Paris slab, outside a bulky woollen dressing, serves the splinting purpose well.

The tip of the transplanted toe is left exposed outside the dressing and under constant clinical observation, half-hourly for four hours, then hourly for 3–4 days. Clinical observation is the most useful and reliable means of detecting circulatory problems.

The first indication of a possible circulatory problem is venous congestion, which usually results from oedema, tight stitching, bandaging or faulty positioning. Early venous congestion may be detected by eliciting the 'throbbing sign': squeezing the tip of the toe causes blanching; gradual release of pressure enables the squeezing fingers to feel throbbing before there is return of colour. The throbbing indicates good arterial input without adequate drainage. This is a warning, but not a sign of immediate danger (Leung 1979). Inspection and adjustment of the dressings and positioning should be made so as to avoid further deterioration. The throbbing usually persists for a few days and then spontaneously subsides.

Healing is usually achieved by primary intention, although partial loss of skin grafts may call for secondary grafting (normally by using stored split-thickness skin grafts).

The wrist splint is retained for at least three weeks, whilst the transplanted toe is allowed to move actively under close supervision after the first week. More intensive motor training is started after three weeks (Leung et al 1981).

Results

Survival

Of 45 cases of thumb reconstruction using second toe transplantation done by the author in 8 years (1977–1984), there were only cases of partial failure. A total of nine cases underwent rescue operations, all performed within the first 48 hours after operation. Seven toes were totally revascularised, and two underwent distal segment gangrene, as a result, probably, of embolic phenomena.

Motor function

The grasping and pinching functions of the reconstructed hand were observed, and compared with those of the opposite hand. Each function was graded according to the efficiency of performing standard tests. Grasping was evaluated by having the patient grip the examiner's two fingers tightly, and pinching was assessed by having the patient pinch together the thumb and its adjacent finger and resisting the examiner's finger pull. Performances as efficient as those of the normal hand were classified as 'excellent', those that were obviously clumsy and weak were graded as 'fair'. Performances that were between 'excellent' and 'fair' were considered to be 'good'.

All those of our patients with Type 1 amputation had excellent grasping function. Eight of the 14 patients with Type 2 thumb loss also had excellent results, and the remaining six individuals had good results. However, none of the patients with Type 3 or 4 amputations had excellent function. Grasping was considered fair in all cases. Pinching was good in five Type 3 thumbs and two Type 4 thumbs. Two other Type 3 patients and six other Type 4 patients had fair pinch only (Fig. 7.6)

As for the two patients with partial survival, the surviving proximal stumps were rigid and stiff, but they served as a short opposing digit with sensation for both grasping and pinching actions.

The joint movements of the transplanted toes were examined. For Type 1 and Type 2 transfers, the metacarpo-phalangeal joints of the toes were not transplanted. Since the distal phalanx of the

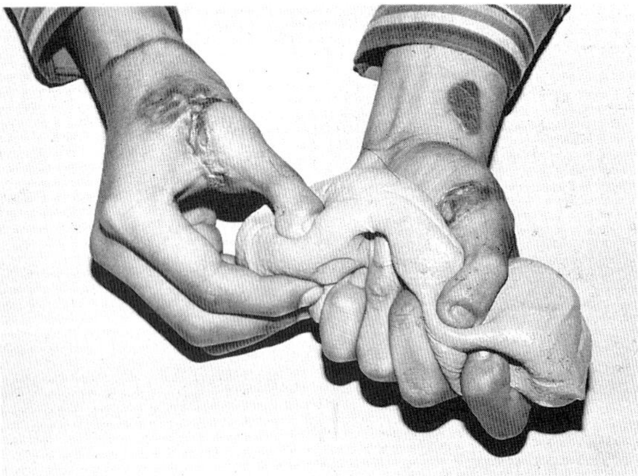

A

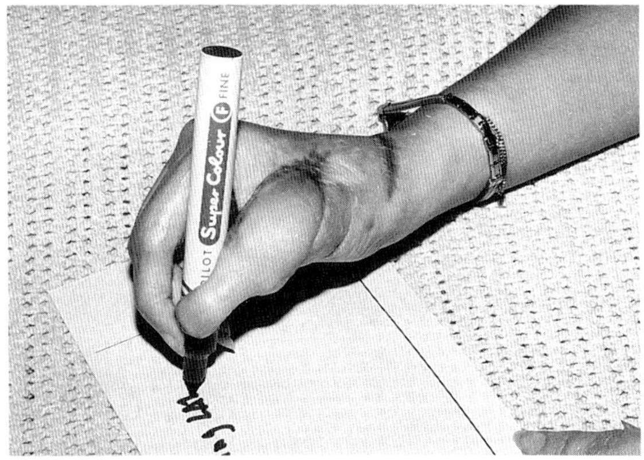

C

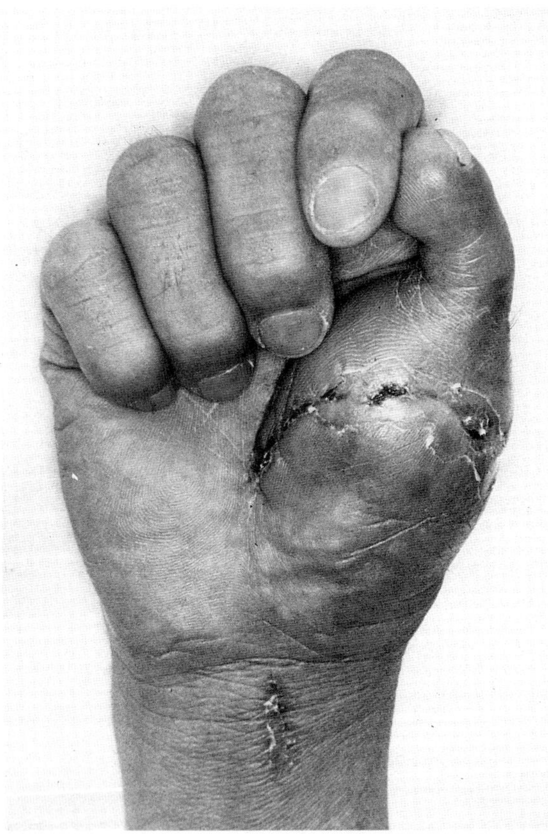

B

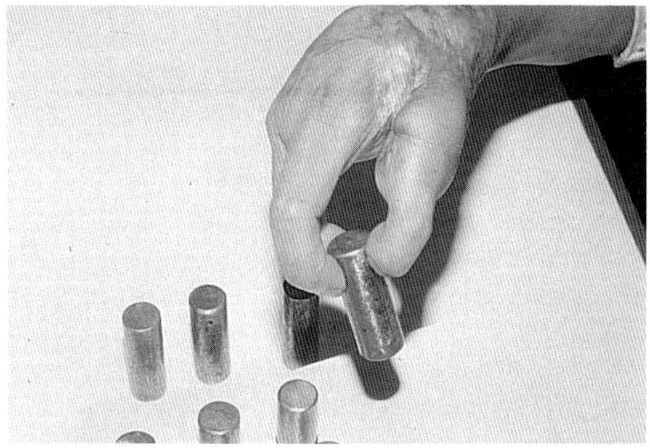

D

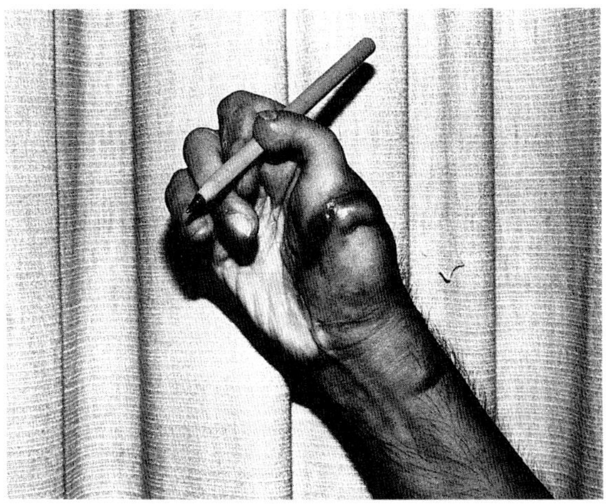

E

Fig. 7.6 Function of reconstructed thumbs is demonstrated. **A.** and **B.** Type I; **C.** Type II; **D.** Type III; and **E.** Type IV.

second toe was very short, movement at the distal interphalangeal joint was always minimal and insignificant (less than 10° was demonstrated on measurement). The mobility of the transplanted toe depended on its proximal interphalangeal joint, and on the movement of the intact elements of the recipient thumb. Measurements of the former joint showed 70–110° of flexion (average 90°).

As for Type 3 and 4 transfers, the metatarso-phalangeal joints of the toes were also transplanted, and the movements of these joints were limited to 30–40° only. The proximal interphalangeal joint movements of these transplanted toes were not as good as those of Type 1 and 2 transfers. They were limited to 30–90°, with an average of 50°. These joint measurements actually explain why Type 1 and 2 reconstructions had excellent-to-good grasp and pinch, whereas Types 3 and 4 were rated considerably lower. Excellent-to-good function depended very much upon the integrity of the joints of the recipient digit, namely the carpo-metacarpal joint in all of the patients, and the metacarpo-phalangeal joint in four individuals. The latter four patients demonstrated the best motor function amongst the whole group of patients.

Sensory assessment

Two tests were used for the tips of all the transplanted toes. The pin-prick test was used for painful sensation, and the Moberg two-point discrimination test for touch sensation.

Pain detection was present in all the transferred toes, although three Type 3 and four Type 4 digits obviously had some impaired pain sensation. The two-point discrimination test might serve as a quantitative indicator of the relative attainment of sensory nerve regeneration. The test was positive at 2–5 mm for 10 patients, 6–8 mm for 28, 9–15 mm for 4, and over 15 mm for 3 patients. Type 1 and 2 transfers all had good results, whereas all of the poor results were in Type 3 and 4 transfers.

THUMB RECONSTRUCTION USING WRAP-AROUND FLAPS

Morrison and O'Brien (Morrison et al 1980) described the vascular pedicle 'wrap-around' free flap from the great toe for reconstruction of thumb amputations distal to the thumb metacarpo-phalangeal joint. A varying amount of skin, soft tissue and nail is taken as a composite graft based on the dorsalis pedis artery and long saphenous vein. Thumb bone elements are replaced by inserting a bone graft into the proximal phalanx, and the soft tissue composite graft is used to form a cover for the bone graft peg. Vascular anastomoses are secured between the radial and dorsalis pedis arteries and the cephalic and the long saphenous veins.

Indication

Thumb reconstruction using wrap-around flaps is indicated for amputation through the distal 1 cm of the proximal phalanx of the thumb with an uninjured metacarpo-phalangeal joint. The carpo-metacarpal joint of the thumb should also be normal.

Recipient site

The amputated end of the proximal phalanx is prepared for a bone peg by clearing out the medullary cavity.

The bone graft measures 5 cm, 2 cm being inset into the medullary cavity of the thumb proximal phalanx, and 3 cm projecting distally. Holes are drilled in the graft to encourage revascularisation, and one or two wire loops fix the graft to the phalanx. The lateral digital nerve, the radial artery and the cephalic vein are isolated and prepared to receive their respective tissue mates from the great toe.

Donor site

The dorsalis pedis artery and long saphenous vein are traced to the first metatarsal space where a large branch is given off to the great toe. Three-quarters of the soft tissue circumference of the great toe (starting at the level of the metatarsophalangeal joint) are removed with the pedicle. This soft tissue composite transfer contains skin, subcutaneous tissue and the nail of the great toe. 0.5 cm of nail and 1–2 cm of skin and pulp over the medial side of the great toe are left untouched over the phalanges. Proximal dissection isolates the lateral digital nerve, which is taken with soft tissue as a composite graft (Fig. 7.7).

The dissection is done in a bloodless field, then the tourniquet is deflated to check the circulatory state of the composite graft. Haemostasis is secured and, after skin closure, the remaining toe defect is covered with a free skin graft.

Transfer

The composite graft from the foot is transferred to the thumb by wrapping the graft around the bone peg. The radial artery is anastomosed to the dorsalis pedis artery, and the cephalic vein to the long saphenous vein. The respective digital nerves are joined. Any skin defect is covered with a split-thickness skin graft, and the composite graft is stitched very loosely around the bone graft, so that postoperative bleeding will drain rather than collect under the graft.

Results

The transferred grafts survived without complications in all but one of 15 cases. In four other cases, impending ischaemia required re-exploration and revision of the arterial anastomoses.

A

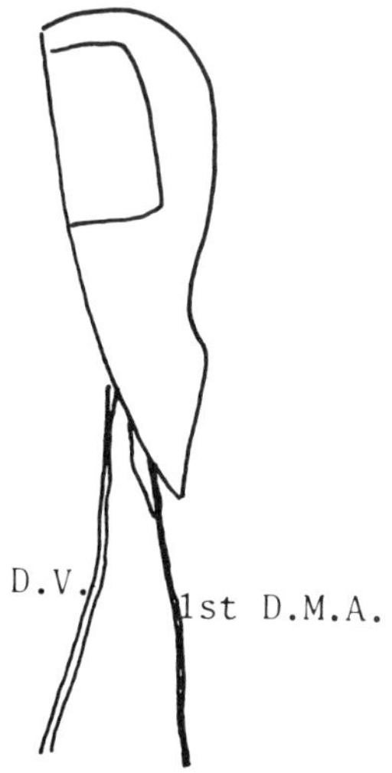

B

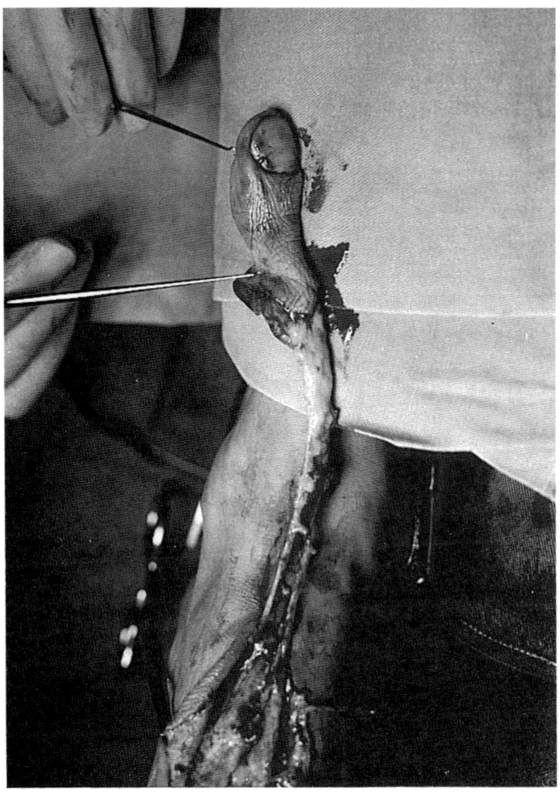

C

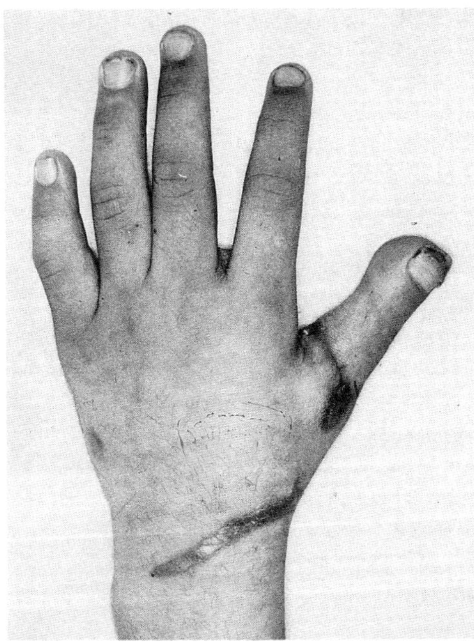

Fig. 7.7 **A.** and **B.** Composite tissue graft consisting of three-fourths of pulp and nail of great toe and vascular pedicle — the wrap-around flap. DV = dorsal vein; 1st DMA = first dorsal metatosal artery. **C.** Reconstructed thumb, using wrap-around flap.

At six months, thumbs reconstructed by the wrap-around procedure had good opposition from the carpo-metacarpal joint, and averaged 45° motion at the metacarpo-phalangeal joint. The appearance of the thumbs' wrap-around graft was good, and two-point sensibility averaged 9 mm.

Great toe soft tissue healing required one month, and a special shoe with foam-rubber padding helped walking. Scarring on the dorsum of the foot was marked when the second toe and the wrap-around flap were removed together.

Bone graft resorption, and even fracture, occurred in the first few cases (Leung & Ma 1982) and regrafting was required. However, when a small segment of the distal end of the distal phalanx of the great toe is removed, together with the wrap-around flap, and used as a cap on the bone graft, revascularisation occurs at both the proximal and distal ends of the bone graft, and resorption and fracture may thus be prevented. Subsequent operations using this technique avoided such complications.

FINGER RECONSTRUCTION

During the period 1977–1983, 40 cases of second toe transplantations were performed for the reconstruction of a finger. Thirty five of these patients were male, and five female (Leung, in press).

Finger reconstruction was done for those hands where, after mutilating injury, all fingers had been amputated, or when one finger remained but was stiff and functioning poorly. There was one case where operation was performed for cosmetic reasons.

In most of the patients, (30, i.e. 75%), the finger to be constructed still retained its metacarpo-phalangeal joint. Under such circumstances, no metatarsal was taken. In the remaining patients (10, i.e. 25%), the fingers were amputated proximal to the metacarpo-phalangeal joint and, for such patients, the metacarpo-phalangeal joint of the second toe with a short segment of second metatarsal were transplanted together.

Table 7.1 Indications for toe transplantation (based on 40 cases of second toe transplantation performed between 1977 and 1983; see p. 113)

Indication	*No. of cases*
Four fingers amputated	31
Three fingers amputated	8
Cosmetic replacement	1

Since the purpose of the transplantation was for the re-establishment of pinch function, the second toe was placed on either the second or third ray to give an index or middle finger. The choice between an index or middle finger depended on whether or not the thumb was capable of maintaining an effective side pinch with either the stump of the amputated index or the second metacarpal head. When this side pinch, though defective, was maintained, the second toe was placed onto the third ray. After this transplantation, an effective tip pinch was achieved, in addition to the existing side pinch. When no side pinch was present, the transplantation was put on the second ray, to give side pinch and tip pinch (Fig. 7.8). Table 7.2 indicates the number of index and middle fingers reconstructed.

The bone fixation at the transplantation site was achieved by using an intramedullary bone peg passing into the medullary cavities of the adjacent bones, in the fashion described previously by the author. Slight radial rotation of the transplanted toe was necessary to give an effective pinch with the thumb. Other surgical procedures closely followed thumb reconstruction.

Results

Although vascular problems were not uncommon, survival of the transplanted toe has not been a major problem. Twelve of the 40 transplantations showed early signs of arterial occlusion within 48 hours of the surgery, and re-exploration, irrigation and re-anastomosis had to be carried out. The causes of the arterial occlusion included vasospasm, venous congestion and kinking of the artery. Re-exploration usually rescued the transplanted toe, although some underwent gangrenous changes, probably as a result of emboli washed distally into the transplanted toe during the process of irrigation. These gangrenous portions had to be amputated later, and the transplantations

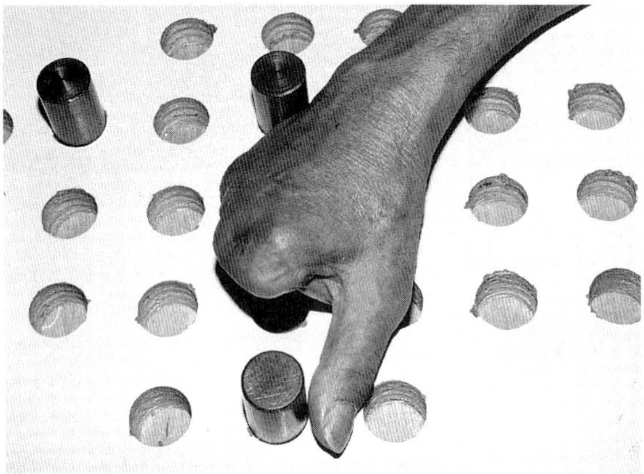

A

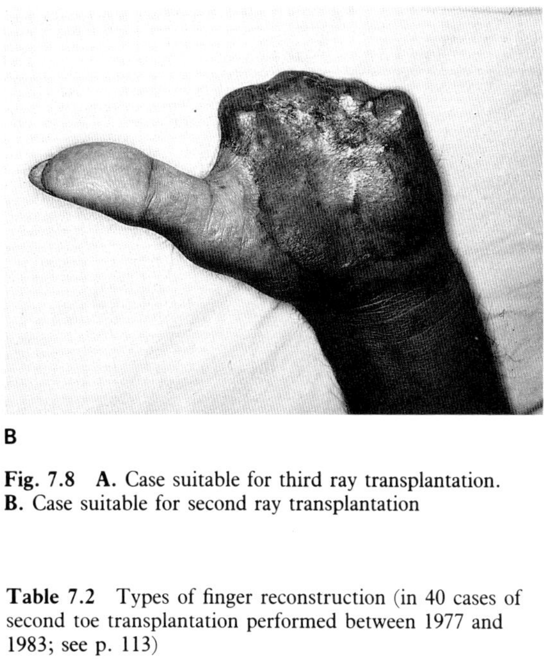

B

Fig. 7.8 **A.** Case suitable for third ray transplantation. **B.** Case suitable for second ray transplantation

Table 7.2 Types of finger reconstruction (in 40 cases of second toe transplantation performed between 1977 and 1983; see p. 113)

Finger	*Type of reconstruction*
Index	8
Middle	32

were classified as partially successful, as useful pinch function was still achieved.

Other complications included skin edge ischaemia and delayed healing, neither of which were significant. The overall hand function and individual joint movement of the transplanted toe were assessed after at least one year, with an average of four years after the surgery. The pinch function was excellent, and the strength reached that of a normal hand. In those cases where the toe was transplanted to the third ray, some gripping function would be restored, although the quality of the grip was quite poor (Fig. 7.9).

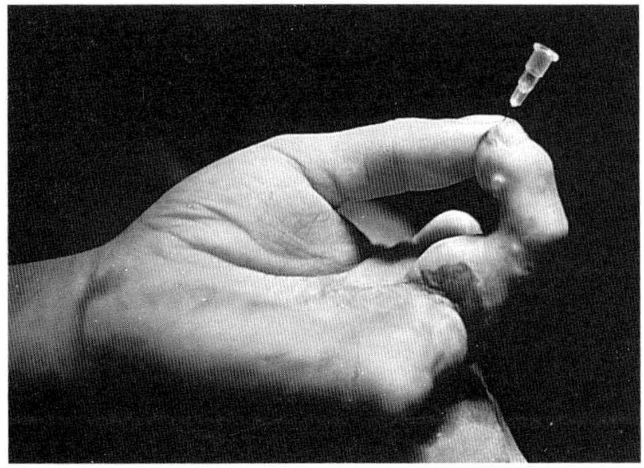

Fig. 7.9 Pinching functions of the transplanted toe.

In the assessment of individual joint motion, it was found that most of the motion of the transplanted toe occurred at the proximal interphalangeal joint, whereas the distal interphalangeal joint motion could not be properly measured because of the extremely short segments. The motion at these joints added together ranged from 80 to 100°, averaging 95°. The original metacarpophalangeal joints of the fingers had the same motion as before the surgery, whereas the transplanted metatarso-phalangeal joints of the foot moved from +100 to +135° only. In the latter case, limited motion of the toes was found in the foot before toe transplantation.

Protective sensation was always achieved, but the sensory acuity attained depended very much on the amount of scarring related to the traumatic amputation. When tested with the two-point discrimination test, the findings ranged from 3–12 mm, averaging 5.5 mm.

Osteosynthesis at the transplantation site has been straightforward. This was established 8–12 weeks after surgery, and failure of union never occurred.

Discussion

Although reconstruction of the fingers in the mutilated hand using various methods — such as elongation of the residual finger stumps, and building up of one of the stumps with a bone graft strut and encircling skin flap — have been attempted, the results of the reconstructions are usually poor, because of the weakness and frequent fracture of the bone strut, and the absence of sensation in the lengthened stump. The transplanted toe offered an attractive alternative. The new finger created is mobile, strong and sensitive; it also has an excellent tactile distal pulp with a nail to accomplish pinch function. Although the hand is still far from being normal in both functional performance and appearance, it satisfied the patient greatly. As Bunnell, in the early days, remarked, 'When there is nothing, even a little is a lot'.

In the first two cases of toe transplantation for finger reconstruction, the toe was implanted on the second ray irrespective of the length of the second ray. Later, it was found that transplanting the toe to the second ray would achieve pinch function only, whereas transplanting it to the third ray increases the span between the thumb and the reconstructed finger, thus achieving some effect of grip. Moreover, if the second ray is long enough, and there is no fibrosis in the thumb web, side pinch between the thumb and the distal part of the second metacarpal is possible. That is why, in all the subsequent transplantations, the toe was placed mostly on the third metacarpal.

In the single case of toe transplantation for cosmetic elongation of the index finger, the overall function of the hand remained the same, but the appearance did improve. However, the limited improvement might not be considered sufficient to warrant the surgery of toe transplantation.

The donor foot, as we have reported for thumb reconstruction, does not suffer functionally in long-term follow-up of up to six years. When scar formation is not hypertrophic, even the cosmetic appearance is highly acceptable.

PINCER RECONSTRUCTION

In mutilating injuries of the hand, not only are the fingers badly damaged and destroyed, but the metacarpal bones and palmar soft tissues may also be deficient. In such situations, functional reconstruction depends upon the residual tissues. Usually either a radial or ulnar component is maintained. This component may be a full digit or a residual stump of a digit. The aim of reconstruction for such mutilated hands is to restore a simple pinch function.

Clinical types

Mainly three types of cases are found. Type 1 refers to the absence of ulnar component, Type 2 to the absence of radial component, and Type 3 to the situation where both are absent and need to be replaced by transferring two toes (Fig. 7.10). The presence of either the radial or ulnar component may have been maintained by the use of a skin flap at an earlier stage.

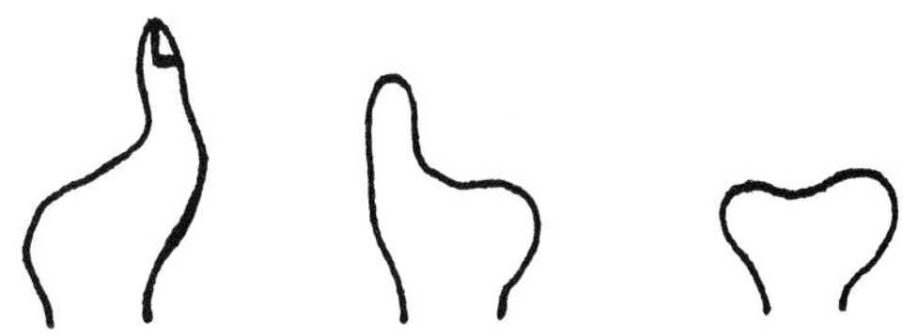

Type I Type II Type III

Fig. 7.10 Types of mutilated hand indicated for pincer reconstruction.

Technical considerations

The level of amputation resulting from trauma varies. The remaining length of metacarpal determines the length of second toe to be transplanted. The mutilating injury producing the amputation usually leaves a lot of scarring around the amputation sites and, not infrequently, a flap repair has been performed initially in order to preserve the length of residual stump. Therefore, recipient site preparation tends to be complicated. Scar tissue removal needs to be more thorough, existing flap needs to be preserved carefully and the bony stump to receive the transplant needs to be specially prepared.

A varying length of metatarsal bone might be required to build up the necessary length. This length must not be too long, otherwise the skin in the recipient hand might not be sufficient to provide adequate coverage, and excessive length is a hindrance to good pinch. Depending on the availability of this coverage, a skin flap may be raised in continuity with the second toe in order to give good closure. Apart from this consideration, the harvesting of the second toe follows exactly the some procedures as already described.

The greatest difficulty in toe transplant for pincer reconstruction lies in the selection of suitable vessels for anastomosis. The usually preferred sites, like the anatomical snuff box and dorsal area of the wrist, might not be suitable, or the vessels might have been damaged. Putting the vascular anastomoses on the same side of the wrist is always advisable, because the postoperative positioning will be made much easier. However, very often the ulnar artery or the radial artery at the proximal volar wrist level has to be utilised, and in such a situation postoperative splinting is always a problem, because the anastomosed artery and vein lie on different sides of the hand; hence, relaxing one component leaves the other tense. The ulnar artery in this type of hand may be extraordinarily tiny, and extra care needs to be taken with the anastomosis.

Not only may the vascular components of the recipient site be problematic, but the sensory nerves and tendons may also be too short for proper anastomosis, as a result of direct damage or marked fibrosis around the injury sites. To compensate for this reality, longer tendons and nerves are taken from the donor site.

Osteosynthesis is done in the same fashion as in other transplantations. The intramedullary bone peg is either introduced into the proximal metacarpal bone, or a hole is prepared in a suitable carpal bone site to accommodate the bone peg. The transplanted toe needs to be of the right length to give pulp pinch with the other residual stump. Either too much or insufficient length will affect the resulting pinch. The transplanted toe should also be correctly rotated and inclined towards the opposing stump in order to maintain a decisive pinch action.

Very often, the tendon ends are retracted proximally. It is therefore good practice to have the tendon junctions well proximal in the distal forearm, so as to avoid adhesions forming to the fibrotic scars.

Results

The survival rate is not as good as for the transplants done for thumb or finger reconstruction, since vascular complications are common in cases with fibrosis and scarring, which are always present in pincer reconstruction. Re-explorations with the intention of rescuing the circulation are common procedures. Among nine cases performed in the last six years, only five had smooth recovery and complete survival. Four cases required re-exploration to maintain vascular patency, and three of these had two re-explorations. Only two re-explorations resulted in total rescue of the transplant. One re-exploration failed totally, while one other resulted in partial rescue. The anastomosed artery was totally re-opened to allow a proper irrigation of the distal vasculature, and then re-anastomosed. In the partial restoration, gangrene of the tip of the transplanted toe resulted, probably as a consequence of intra-arterial embolisation during the irrigation.

Wound healing, again because of the presence of fibrosis and scarring, was not straightforward. Secondary skin grafting was often necessary. Sensory recovery was similarly defective. The sensitivity with the two-point discrimination test was 4–12 mm, averaging 7 mm. Fortunately, not much joint mobility is required for the pincer function; hence, although tendon gliding is usually unsatisfactory because of the scarring, effective pincer effect is gained (Fig. 7.11).

Secondary procedures are often required to improve the pincer function by widening of the

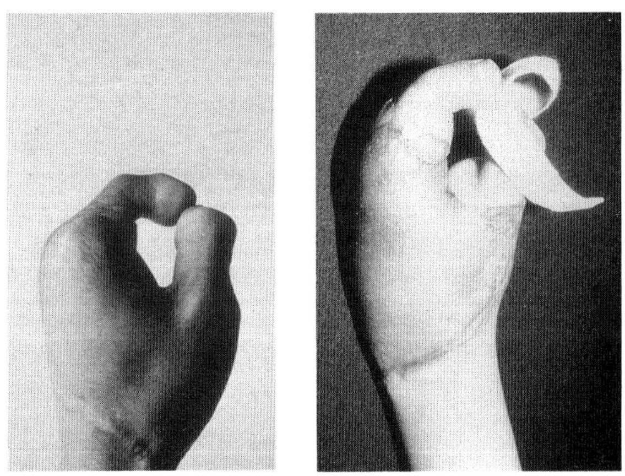

Fig. 7.11 Pinching function of reconstructed pincer.

web space between the pincer components. These simple procedures will allow bigger objects to be held.

DOUBLE-FINGER RECONSTRUCTION

Pinching with one transplanted toe gives pulp, tip and key pinch, but never chuck pinch. Therefore, it may be justified to use two toes instead of one, to achieve better functional reconstruction of chuck pinch.

The indications include total loss of fingers and special pincer reconstructions.

The second and third toes may be removed together, based upon the dorsalis pedis vascular pedicle, and then transplanted onto the recipient hand as already described (Tsai & Jupita 1981). Alternatively, the second toe from both feet may be removed at two different stages to give two neighbouring fingers, so as to achieve the chuck pinch effect. Such staged double-toe transplants may also be used to build up a pincer for metacarpal amputations, or through-wrist amputation (Fig. 7.12). The techniques for the stage one transplant are similar to those for any such procedure. During the second stage, however, techniques are more demanding. Most likely, vessels will not be readily available, and end-to-side anastomoses may have to be performed. Also, adhesions and fibrosis compromise the return of nerve and tendon function.

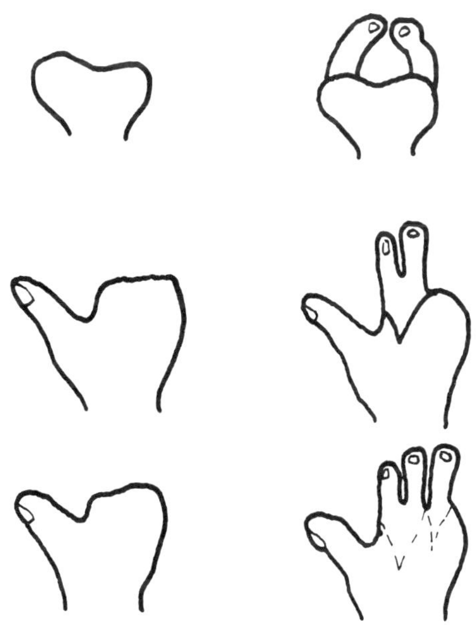

Fig. 7.12 Double toes transferred to give pinching function.

Combined second toe with 'wrap-around flap'

As an alternative, the second toe may be removed together with the lateral three-quarters of the soft tissue of the great toe (the wrap-around flap) to give two new fingers in the reconstruction of chuck pinch. The second toe forms a mobile component, whilst the wrap-around flap encircling a bone core, created either from the iliac crest or metatarsal, forms an immobile component. (Fig. 7.13).

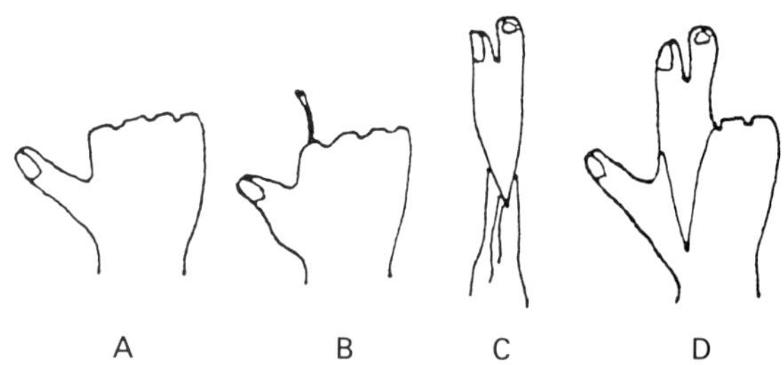

Fig. 7.13 Double-toe transplants created from the second toe and 'wrap-around flap'.

Technically, this is an easy procedure. Harvesting the second toe together with the first web and soft tissues on the lateral side of the great toe actually makes the procedure simpler and easier because the whole distal vasculature is utilised and much fewer ligations are necessary. The soft tissues on the web side of the great toe need to be taken with the toe nail. This wrap-around flap is taken from the non-weightbearing area and non-shoe contact area of the great toe, and contains the equivalent proportion of the nail of the great toe. The wide raw area of the wrap-around flap allows free oozing of blood after vascular anastomoses, and venous congestion is guaranteed not to occur. Hence, vascular problems are less likely. In fact, of the 10 such procedures performed by the author, only one required re-exploration.

Results of double-toe transplants

Survival of double-toe transplants has never been

a problem for reasons already discussed. Although staged toe transplant is technically demanding, the extra care and attention may balance the greater possibility of complication.

Functional results compare favourably with the standard thumb or finger construction. For the combined second toe and wrap-around flap, the rigid and mobile components produce excellent material for chuck pinch reconstructions (Fig. 7.14). Since the function is so satisfactory by using one toe from each foot, it makes one wonder if double-toe transfer from the same foot, which gives a mutilated donor foot, is at all justified.

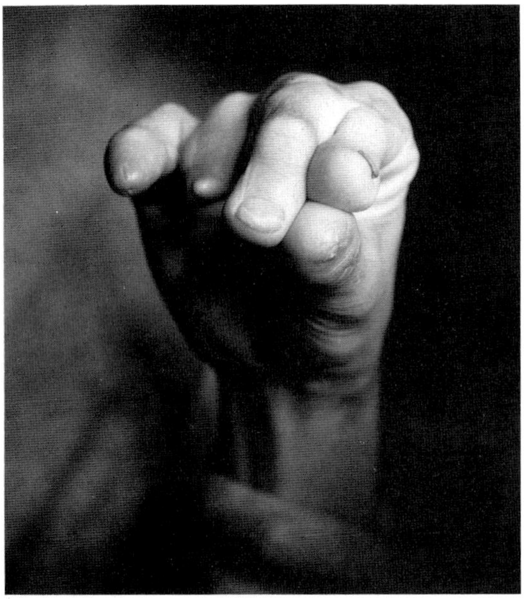

Fig. 7.14 Chuck pinch satisfactorily performed with the double digits created from second toe and wrap-around flap.

THE DONOR FOOT

The vast experience of over 120 second-toe transplant procedures have confirmed the earlier belief that the donor foot, after removal of its second toe, does not suffer from any functional loss. Should healing in the donor foot be unusually delayed, some skin grafting procedures may be necessary. Walking may be started as soon as the healing has become satisfactory. Usually, normal walking is resumed 4–6 weeks after the transplant.

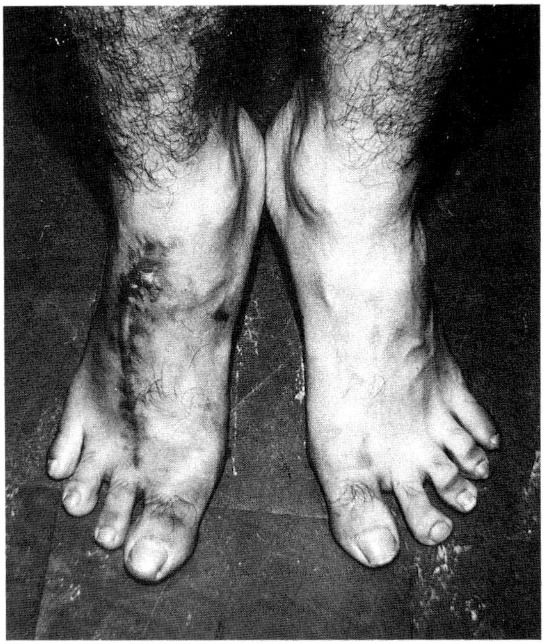

Fig. 7.15 Four-toe foot with perfect function.

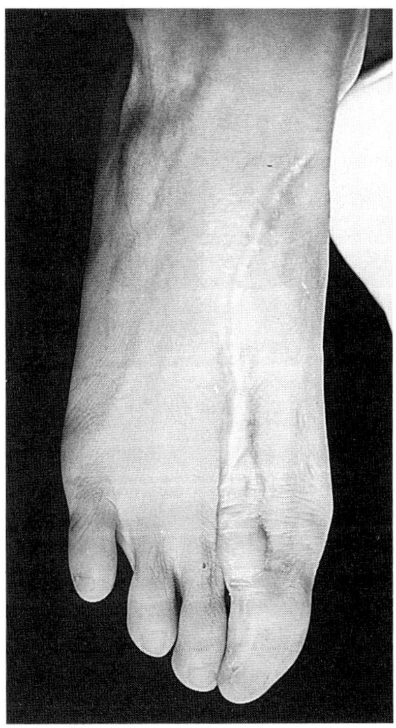

Fig. 7.16 Scar contracture resulting from removing second toe and wrap-around flap.

Cosmetically the four-toe foot suffers very little indeed (Fig. 7.15). When the wrap-around flap is used together with the second toe, scarring is marked over the first web. Some discomfort is therefore experienced on prolonged walking. Of all the cases done, only two developed first web contracture bad enough to warrant correction and skin grafting as a secondary remedial procedure (Leung 1979) (Fig. 7.16).

Pedobarographic studies on the four-toe feet have been done, using the Harris mat and a simple mechanical pressure-sensitive mat, on the static and dynamic pressure distribution of the foot. The pressure patterns of the four-toe feet, when compared with that of normal feet, show only mild differences both on level and slope walking.

Although great toe transplanters have claimed that the donor foot, without the great toe, is functionally satisfactory, with the patient walking and even running, all these observations were made with the patients being assessed on level ground. It is of great doubt whether such feet can stand the same tests on slope or stair walking. Pedobarographic studies on our patients with missing second toes repeated on slopes, however, have given the same assuring features.

The overall high survival rates, and very satisfactory functional achievements, obtained in all varieties of digital replacement using the second toe transplantation method, may have already established this method as a very useful technique in hand reconstruction.

REFERENCES

Buck-Gramcko D 1971 Pollicization of the index finger — method and results in aplasia and hypoplasia of the thumb. Journal of Bone & Joint Surgery 53A: 1605–1617

Gilbert A 1976 Composite tissue transfer from the foot: anatomic basis and surgical technique. In: Daniller A, Stranch B (eds). Symposium on microsurgery. C V Mosby, St Louis

Leung P C 1979 Early complications in toe to hand transplantation — their recognition and prevention. Annals of Academy of Medicine, Singapore 8: 419

Leung P C 1979 The 'throbbing sign' — an indication of early venous congestion in replantation surgery. Journal of Hand Surgery 4: 409–411

Leung P C 1980 Transplantation of the second-toe to the hand. Journal of Bone & Joint Surgery 62A: 990–996

Leung P C 1981 Use of an intramedullary bone peg for osteosynthesis in digital replantations, revascularisation and toe transfers. Journal of Hand Surgery 6: 281–284

Leung P C, Wong A, Wan C Y 1981 A proposed programme of physical rehabilitation for patients undergoing toe-to-hand transfer operations. British Journal of Occupational Therapy 26: 187–191

Leung P C, Ma G F Y 1982 Digital reconstruction using the toe-flap. Journal of Hand Surgery 7: 366–370

Leung P C 1983 Thumb reconstruction using second-toe transfer. Hand 15: 15–21

Leung P C, Wong W L 1983 The vessels of the first metatarsal web space — an operative and radiographic study. Journal of Bone & Joint Surgery 65A: 235–238

Leung P C 1985 Thumb reconstruction using second-toe transfer. Hand Clinic 1: 285–295

Leung P C (In press) Finger reconstruction using toe transplantation. Journal of Hand Surgery

Marter I B 1972 New thoughts on hand surgery. In: Apley A G (ed) Modern trends in orthopaedics 6. Butterworths, London

Morrison W, O'Brien McC, MacLeod A M 1980 The surgical repair of amputation of the thumb. Australia and New Zealand Journal of Surgery 50: 237

Reid D A C 1960 Reconstruction of the thumb. Journal of Bone & Joint Surgery 42B: 444

Tsai T M, Jupita J B 1981 Reconstruction of severe transmetacarpal mutilating hand injuries by combined second and third toes transfer. Journal of Hand Surgery 6: 319–328

Yang D Y, Gu Y D 1979 Thumb reconstruction utilizing second-toe transplantation by microvascular anastomosis. Chinese Medical Journal 92: 295

G. Foucher

8 Partial toe-to-hand transfers

When, in 1965, H. Buncke first transferred the great toe of a monkey to its hand, free toe transfer became potentially available for clinical application. The first successful clinical case by J. Cobbett, in 1969, opened a 15-year period of intensive refinement of indications and techniques. These include: second toe transfer (Yang 1979, Ohmori & Harii 1975); partial toe transfers — pulp (Buncke 1976), pulp and nail (Morrison et al 1980, Foucher et al 1980); and joint transfer (Buncke et al 1967, Foucher & Merle 1976, Hurwitz 1979, Foucher et al 1980, Tsai et al 1982).

TECHNIQUE OF DISSECTION

The technique of toe dissection has already been discussed in preceding chapters. Only original points will be outlined here.

The vascular anatomy at first web level has been extensively described (O'Brien et al 1975). This knowledge allows one to dissect the dorsalis pedis artery in continuity with the first dorsal or plantar metatarsal arteries. An anatomical study and clinical series of 118 toe transfers has allowed us to stress the availability of the second dorsal and/or plantar metatarsal artery. The latter is constant and is usually of good diameter. Unfortunately, it runs under the second metatarsal bone, but is easily reached after proximal osteotomy of this bone. This is only possible in case of complete sacrifice of the second toe. We frequently use an early osteotomy in such cases for several reasons. Firstly, it simplifies dissection of both first and second web vessels, avoiding a plantar incision. The flexor tendon is cut last when using the dorsal approach. Secondly, at the end of the operation, the intermetatarsal ligament is secured between first and third toes, thus improving both cosmesis and function.

Early walking is authorised. A foot surgeon (Moyen 1982) was asked to review 20 cases of second toe amputation. He reported that when the second metatarsal bone was left intact, there was a constant tendency to hallux valgus deformity. This tendency is not seen after ray resection, unless the angle between the first and second metatarsal bones was greater than 20°.

We usually favour a 'short' transfer (Yoshimura 1980) for long finger reconstruction, and a 'long' one for thumb reconstruction. The recipient artery and vein are usually approached by a short transverse incision to minimise scar on the dorsum of the hand. Various techniques for vascular anastomosis are available:

1. End-to-end suture with collateral artery, princeps pollicis or radial artery
2. End-to-side suture with palmar arch or radial artery
3. T-shaped intercalated graft in the palmar arch or the radial artery, mainly when two (or three) feeding arteries are harvested. Two end-to-end sutures are performed, one with the dorsalis pedis artery, the other with the plantar arch.

A key point in partial toe transfer remains defatting. To improve cosmesis, facilitate direct closure and avoid the need for an unsightly graft, a thorough defatting is mandatory with very distal dissections of vessels and nerves.

Special technical points will be discussed separately with each technique, dealing successively with: joint transfer; partial toe transfer for distal reconstruction — pulp, compound pulp, nail complex, compound nail complex (with bone); and partial toe transfer for thumb reconstruction (wrap-around and twisted two toes).

JOINT TRANSFER

Destruction of finger joints by trauma, infection or neoplasia, may severely impair hand function. Prosthetic replacement of finger joints is now well accepted (Swanson 1970), but there are limitations with regard to durability, stability and mobility. The problem is amplified in young patients still growing. Surgeons have long searched for means of transplanting joints (Lexer 1925, Herndon & Chase 1952, Porter & Lance 1974), but most research centred on large weight-bearing joints, such as the knee. This meant that the donor would have to be another individual, and this necessarily introduced the immunological problems of allografts. This approach has nevertheless been tried (Pritcker et al 1977, Gross et al 1983), and certainly should gain in popularity with development of immunosuppressive drugs.

The availability of toe joints for substitution of damaged finger joints by autografting, means that immunological rejection problems are eliminated, although technical problems remain (Campbell et al 1963).

The first reported transplantation of a whole toe joint to replace a finger joint was by Goebell in 1913, but despite many small series, the use of such free, non-vascularised, whole transplants did not become widespread. Free transplantation of whole toe joints to replace finger joints was reintroduced by Cuthbert in 1945, and subsequently reported by Bunnel (1948), Graham (1954), Wilson (1966) and others, showing that the results were unpredictable, but that children fared better than adults. The possibility of growth of such transfers in young patients remains controversial. Clinically, isolated successful cases have been published (Freeman 1959 and 1971, Graham 1954, Snowdy et al 1980, Vercauteren & Van Vynckt 1983, Whitesides 1977). Two short, but encouraging series (Goldberg & Watson 1982, Wilson 1966) have demonstrated that the age (around 6 months) and the technique (with preservation of periosteum) are important contributory factors, although the end result remains unpredictable.

On the other hand, experimental radiological and histological studies have demonstrated degenerative changes of cartilage and successive replacement by fibrotic tissue (Entin et al 1962 and 1968, Erdelyi 1963, Herndon & Chase 1952, Kettelkamp et al 1968, Kettelkamp & Ramsey 1971, Kettelkamp 1972).

Clinically, however, despite these cartilage changes, several authors have demonstrated that limited but useful motion can be obtained (Entin et al 1962, Erdelyi 1963, Kettelkamp & Ramsey 1971, Lexer 1908).

The major problem encountered in these autograftings was the delay of revascularisation of the subchondral bone, with secondary collapse and degenerative changes of the joint surface. Absence of living synovium and immobilisation deplete the synovial fluid, the sole means of nourishment of the articular cartilage. (Judet 1908).

A logical step was to try to revascularise bone and synovium by vascularised transfer. Slome and Reeves (1966) showed the technical feasibility of free vascularised joint transfer in a dog's knee model, and Judet and Padovani (1968) proved their long term survival.

The first island vascularised joint transfer was performed by Buncke et al in 1967, and we published the first clinical case of free vascularised compound toe joint transfer in 1976. Further cases have been reported, but all the series only comprise small numbers of patients (Watanabe et al 1978, 1980, Foucher et al 1980, Tsai et al 1982, 1985, Yoshizu et al 1984, Kuo et al 1984).

Techniques

Several techniques will be discussed:

1. Single transfer:
   - —toe proximal interphalangeal joint (PIPJ) for PIPJ or metacarpo-phalangeal joint (MCPJ) finger reconstruction
   - —toe metatarso-phalangeal joint (MTPJ) for MCPJ or trapezo-metacarpal (TMJ) reconstruction.

2. Double transfer for PIPJ or MCPJ reconstruction.

1. Toe PIPJ transfer for finger PIPJ reconstruction

A cutaneous flap is outlined on the dorsum of the toe PIPJ in continuity proximally with an extension onto the dorsum of the toe and foot. The vascular dissection is standard, the feeding vessels being plantar and dorsal with anastomotic connections (Yoshimura et al 1984). The extensor tendons are included in the transfer, and the toe is transected through the DIPJ distally and the proximal phalanx proximally. The skin on the plantar surface is reflected laterally until the vascular bundle is reached. The flexor sheath is opened medially, keeping the rims intact for later repair of the sheath at the recipient site. The flexor profundus tendon is extracted, and the flexor superficialis dissected without jeopardising the tiny vessels of the volar plate. Then, when the compound transfer remains attached to the foot only by its artery (or arteries) and vein, the tourniquet is released to allow circulation during the time of hand dissection.

At the recipient site, a longitudinal dorsal medial incision is centred on the destroyed PIPJ, and thorough debridement of scar tissue is done. The dorsal aspect of the flexor sheath is exposed, but not opened, and the remnant of the volar plate is thinned. The bone ends are trimmed, and a tenolysis of the extensor mechanism is performed if necessary.

Usually, a 'long' transfer is used, and a separate approach through a transverse incision is made at radial artery level. The dorsal skin is generously undermined to make way for the donor vessels. The different, necessary lengths of bone, tendons and vessels are carefully assessed and transected at the donor site.

The first step of the transfer is bony fixation. We have used various types of osteosynthesis (wiring, K-wire, bone peg, cemented nail or screw), but there has been no correlation with the final range of motion. Now, most frequently, wc favour inserting the ends of the toe skeleton inside the recipient bone, and stabilising with an oblique K-wire.

The remaining toe flexor sheath is fastened to the recipient flexor sheath to avoid bow-stringing. The extensor hallucis longus tendon is sutured (by overlapping) to the central part of the extensor mechanism of the finger, and the extensor brevis to the intrinsic tendon. The vascular bundle is then passed through the subcutaneous tunnel and the vascular anastomoses performed.

Various methods can be adopted at the foot donor site. We usually prefer to remove entirely the second ray, but it is possible (if the patient so wishes) to preserve the toe by bone grafting (with the finger PIPJ or an iliac crest graft) covered with a cross-toe flap from the third toe. The other technique is to syndactilise the second and third toes with two cross-toe flaps. This avoids bone grafting (and non-healing) and allows early walking.

2. Toe MTPJ transfer

The MTPJ is a more bulky joint, with a mobility mainly into hyperextension. We reserve its use for MCPJ reconstruction and TMJ reconstruction.

For MCPJ reconstruction, the graft is turned 180° around its longitudinal axis, and inserted underneath the extensor mechanism after incision of the hood (on the ulnar side in the case of the index finger). We have never tried to use the flexor mechanism as an extensor graft, but, even though not actually physiological, it could be acceptable.

One of the major shortcomings of this type of transfer was the difficulty with which a skin flap could be incorporated due to the switch of the transfer. Smith and Jones (1985) described a technique using an eccentrically placed dorsalis pedis flap. The non-dominant lateral digital artery is freed from its attachment to the skin flap. By means of this manoeuvre, after joint rotation, the flap remains dorsal.

For TMJ reconstruction in certain congenital malformations, it is also possible to use the MTPJ as this can provide bone length, mobility, stability and growth plates, as for example in mild thumb ray hypoplasia (second degree in Blauth's classification). The technique is identical except that the joint is implanted on the carpus in hyperextension, as described for pollicisation (Buck-Gramcko 1967). We prefer to transfer a skin flap at the same time to improve the thenar contour and facilitate a secondary opponensplasty (abductor digiti minimi).

3. Double transfer for PIPJ and MCPJ reconstruction

For reconstruction of adjacent PIPJs, Tsai et al (1985) used the PIPJs of the second and third toes with lateral skin and intermediate web. This results in a partial finger syndactyly which is difficult to accept. We prefer to harvest each joint on a separate pedicle: the first dorsal (or plantar) metatarsal artery for the second toe PIPJ, and the second plantar (or dorsal) metatarsal artery for the third toe PIPJ. The long arteries allow the adjacent aspects of the recipient fingers and the web to be kept intact.

For reconstruction of adjacent MCPJs, we described a technique using both joints of the second toe (which is proximally amputated). The MTPJ is lifted on the second plantar metatarsal artery (which is very close, or even attached, to this joint) and the PIPJ on the first dorsal (or plantar) metatarsal artery. As previously described, the MTPJ is turned 180° on its axis. We used this technique in a case with good extensor mechanism, and after a primary stage of skin-flap transfer. Theoretically, it is possible to have two separate skin islands for each joint (as previously described).

Indications

Our indications have been limited to very complex hand trauma and a few congenital malformations.

For congenital malformations, we have two indications:

1. TMJ reconstruction in mild thumb hypoplasia as already described;
2. Epiphyseal transfer to thumbs with aplasia of the proximal phalanx. The first step is a Matev lengthening, and the second is an epiphyseal transfer to provide stability, length and growth potential.

For post-traumatic reconstruction:

1. At MCPJ level, we restrict our indication to multiple joint involvement in young patients. The transfer is mainly devoted to radial fingers to provide good lateral stability. Our mean range of flexion has been 65° (Foucher et al 1986).
2. At PIPJ level, our results (and those of others) fall short of the normal range of motion (average 36° of flexion with an extensor lag of 35°). However, it is true that this technique provides a one-stage repair of composite loss with good lateral stability of the joint, a moderate but useful arc of motion and retains the possibility of growth in young patients. Our indications are, therefore, restricted to young patients for radial finger reconstruction where there is multiple finger involvement, and where the loss is compound, necessitating skin, bone, epiphysis, joint and extensor tendon replacement.

PULP AND COMPOUND PULP TRANSFER

Pulp and compound pulp transfer allow reconstruction of distal extensive losses of the most specialised and useful skin of the finger. The flap can be taken from the great toe or the second toe. Buncke (1976) has described a pulp flap taken from the second toe, but we prefer the great toe for several reasons:

1. The diameter of the vessel is usually larger
2. The available surface is huge
3. The diameter of the nerve matches quite perfectly the diameter of the recipient nerve
4. The two-point discrimination (2PD) is better. May and Daniel (1978) found that the big toe has 7–10 mm of 2PD, compared with 10–25 mm for the second toe.

The technique is simple, only skin, vessels and nerves being dissected free. The key point of the technique is the nerve suture, which has to be performed as distally as possible without interfering with its intrinsic vascularity. Very limited access on the deep aspect of the flap is obtained without extensive dissection.

For long finger reconstruction, the contralateral foot is selected and a 'short' transfer is performed with end-to-end suture with the palmar metacarpal artery, avoiding disturbance of the digital arteries, their nerve branches and transverse anastomoses. For thumb reconstruction, the ipsilateral foot is used and a 'long' transfer is done.

The final step of the transfer is to graft the donor site area. Following such transfers, one must insist on the necessity of a programme of sensory re-education (Dellon et al 1974), which is begun at the fifth month, to improve sensation. Many variants are based on this technique, providing the opportunity of 'tailor-made' reconstruction (Foucher et al 1980, 1985).

If part of the nail bed is missing, usually with a piece of bone, the natural tendency for the nail is to adopt a 'parrot-beak' deformity, with volar tilting impeding fine distal pinch. In such a case, it is necessary to lift, with the pulp, a small piece of vascularised bone and the distal part of the nail bed. The piece of bone is cut from the lateral aspect of the distal phalanx of the toe without modifying the length. Only one or two millimetres are removed distally, to allow good distal cover by the remaining skin.

It is important to stress that any distal bone graft has to be vascularised to avoid secondary resorption (Foucher et al 1980). The flap of nail bed is then turned 90° on the chip of bone to fit exactly the finger defect. (Fig. 8.1)

When the nail matrix has been destroyed, it is desirable to replace this also. In such cases, a longer piece of bone is taken in the same way as previously explained, but without reaching the IP joint. This bone shell protects the tiny branches feeding the nail bed and nail matrix.

A first web transfer (Gilbert et al 1975, Morrison et al 1978, Strauch & Shafiroff 1979) can be performed taking the two adjacent pulps of the great and second toe. Suture of the superficial peroneal nerve is added to that of plantar nerves. In complex amputations with short finger stumps, this technique covers both aspects of the pinch surface.

The indications for pulp and compound pulp transfers are essentially extensive traumatic or surgical loss (after tumour excision) of thumb or radial fingers in young patients, mainly where local flaps or island flaps (Littler 1952) are insufficient or impossible. In addition, it is possible to reconstruct, by this means, an insensitive radial aspect of a mitten hand primarily covered by an insensitive remote flap. This technique is also sometimes an efficient means to treat distal painful neuroma when accompanied by pulp loss.

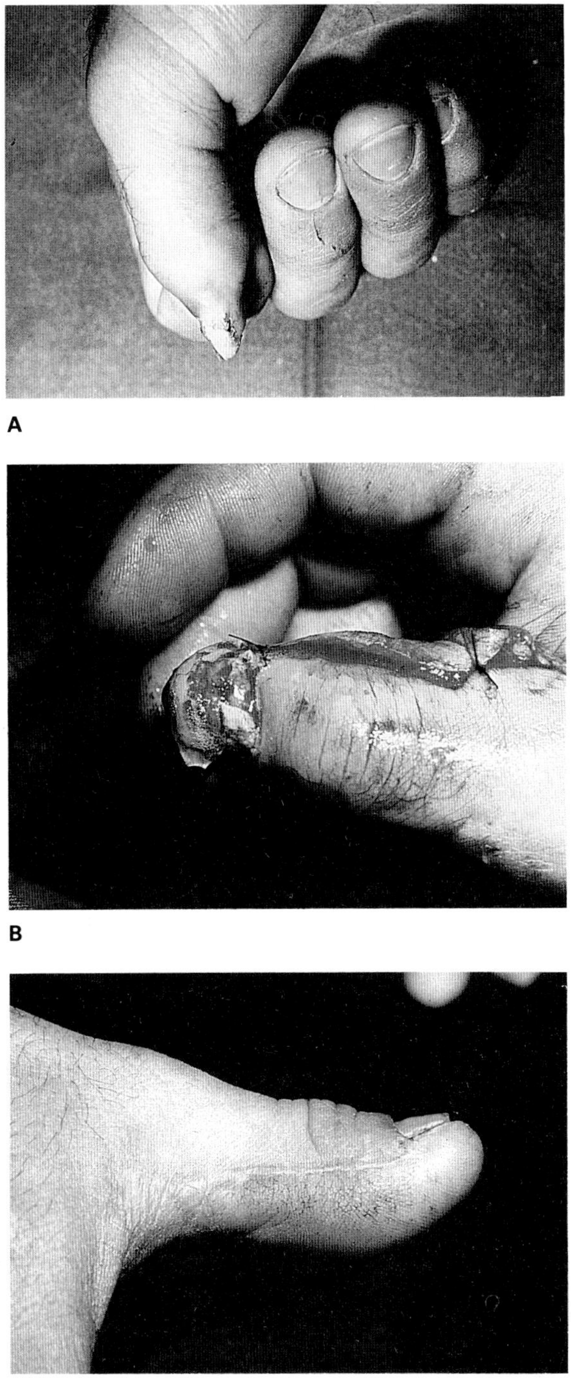

A

B

C

Fig. 8.1 **A.** Loss of pulp and nail bed in a dominant thumb of a 21-year-old male. **B.** Compound transfer of pulp, chip of bone and nail bed from the great toe. **C.** Final result 6 years later with mark of use and a 2-PD of 11 mm.

The major advantages of these techniques are that they:

1. Provide a near normal skin texture with good sensibility
2. Fit perfectly the defect (skin/bone/nail components)
3. Can be performed in only one stage
4. Entail minimal donor site morbidity.

Our results in a series of 38 cases have been encouraging, with a two-point discrimination averaging 9 mm (minimum 4.5 mm). We have found good statistical correlation between two-point discrimination, age, ischaemia time, sensory re-education programme and range of motion of the fingers.

NAIL TRANSFER

The nail complex can be transferred as a separate unit with or without bone. We only once performed a true nail transfer, in a dominant thumb of a young boy. It is well documented that the nail plays an important part in the precision of the pinch and the quality of sensory discrimination. However, we found more indications for compound transfer of nail and bone for dorsal destruction of the thumb. Usually, in such cases, the palmar skin is intact and the transfer allows a one-stage total reconstruction with quite perfect functional and aesthetic results. (Fig. 8.2)

TOTAL THUMB RECONSTRUCTION

The 'wrap-around' technique has been proposed by Morrison (Morrison et al 1980) taking a sleeve from the great toe, the skeleton being reconstructed by a bone graft taken from the iliac crest. We have used this technique only in degloving injury of thumb (or finger) with normal bone. Indeed, we stressed early the importance of distal vascularised bone to avoid the classical pitfall of osteoplastic thumb reconstruction, i.e. bone resorption (Foucher et al 1980). We were not surprised to note that many authors mentioned this complication (Leung & Ma 1982, Do et al 1983, Tomita et al 1983).

The consequence of such resorption is shortening, but also 'parrot-beak' nail deformity with impeded fine pinch. Recently, Morrison (1985) moved to techniques providing distal vascularised bone. In the same article, Morrison mentioned some problems with grafting of the donor site. Nevertheless, this technique is an improvement on classical great or second toe transfer for thumb reconstruction.

The 'twisted two toes' technique (Foucher et al 1980) is our favourite method for reconstruction of the thumb amputated at MP level in an otherwise normal hand. We stress that this technique is mainly indicated in women, and in a hand with a good aesthetic aspect. The technique seems at first glance to be more complicated, but has important advantages. Two different refinements can be used

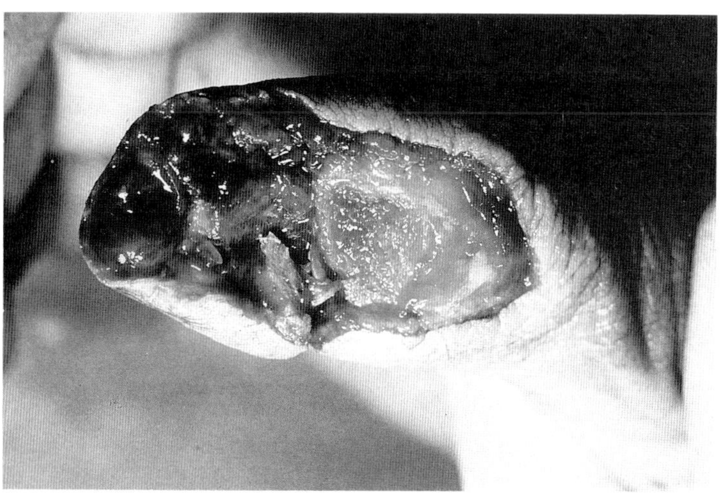

A

Fig. 8.2 **A.** Dorsal compound loss of a dominant thumb in a 25-year-old male.
B. Composite transfer from the big toe with vascularised bone and nail complex. The donor site is closed by a Tranquilli Leali flap.
C. The transfer is based on artery and vein.
D. The transfer fitting the defect and a T-shaped graft prepared to be intercalated by double end to end suture in the radial artery.
E., **F.** and **G.** Final result at the foot and the hand. The joint was reconstructed acutely, allowing a good mobility of the IP joint.

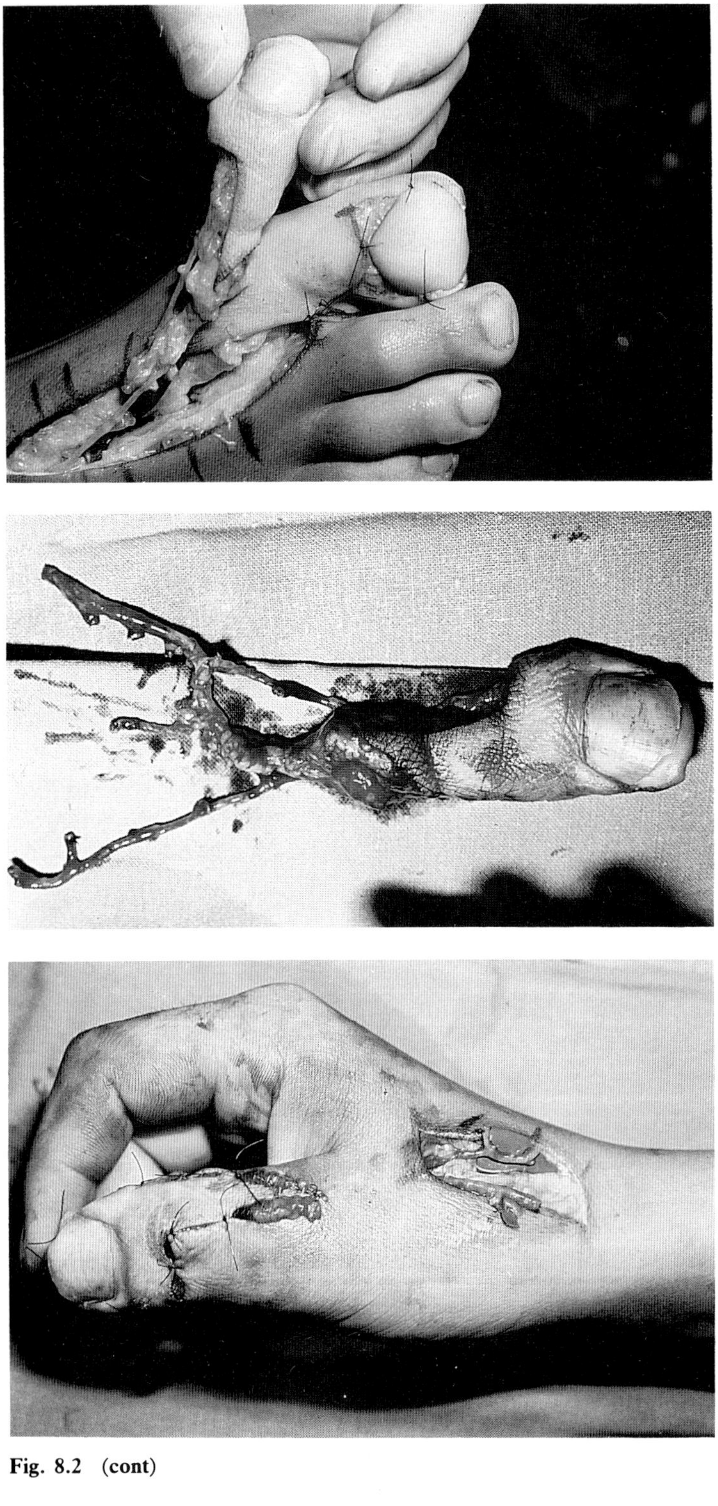

B

C

D

Fig. 8.2 (cont)

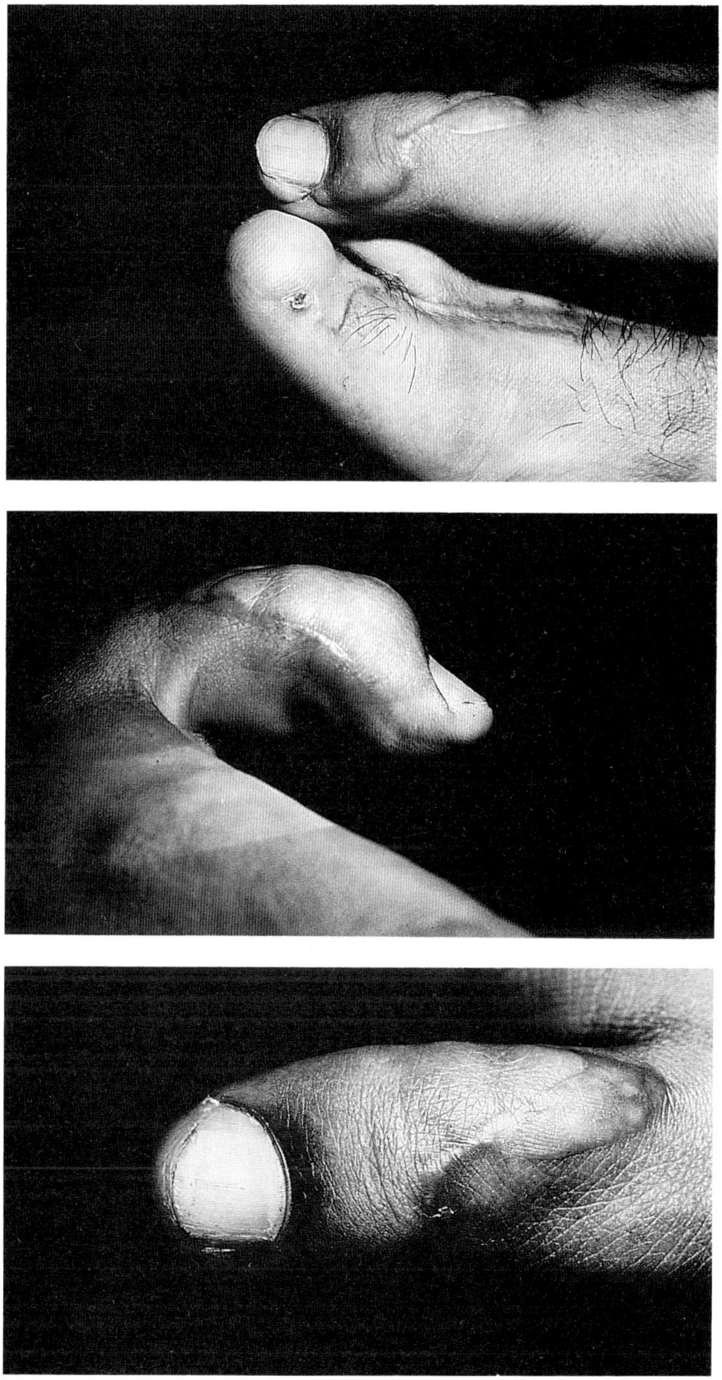

E

F

G

Fig. 8.2 (cont)

according to the size of the opposite thumb and the size of the great toe, the goal being to mimic the normal opposite thumb.

If the skin is sufficient on the big toe, it is lifted with nail complex and a piece of bone taken, as already described, longitudinally from the distal toe phalanx. Simultaneously, the PIPJ and adjacent phalanges and tendons are dissected from the second toe on the same or on a separate bundle. If needed, half of the MTPJ is preserved for MCPJ reconstruction. Then the skeleton of the second toe is shifted inside the sleeve of the great toe with distal bone stabilisation by a K-wire. The aim is for the skeleton to match the length of the two phalanges of the normal thumb. Finally, we proceed to flexor and extensor tendon suture and vessel anastomosis.

If more skin is necessary, it can be taken from the medial border of the second toe in continuity with the joint, and turned 180° to wrap it around the joint. This has never caused any problem, but it is necessary to free the vessels over a long segment to avoid interrupting the blood flow. The rest of the operation remains the same as previously described.

This technique shares the advantages of Morrison's wrap-around technique, but presents comparatively several advantages:

1. It can be useful in a child due to the transfer of epiphysis.
2. It provides a vascularised skeleton closely matching a two phalangeal thumb.
3. It provides some mobility by joint transfer (PIP and, if necessary, half the MTP).
4. The piece of bone taken en bloc with the skin of the big toe provides stability of the pulp.
5. The nerves lie between two well vascularised tissues, perhaps explaining in part the better two-point discrimination that we obtained (average 9 mm compared with 15 mm in Morrison's series (1985)).
6. Finally, the big toe is dressed by the filleted flap of the second toe, after ray amputation, affording a nail and stable cover.

CONCLUSION

Amongst the major advances provided by toe transfer for hand reconstruction, partial toe transfer is a step towards more closely reconstructing the normal appearance and function of the hand, trying at the same time to decrease the morbidity at the donor site.

REFERENCES

Buck-Gramcko D 1971 Pollicization of the index finger: methods and results in aplasia of the thumb. Journal of Bone and Joint Surgery 53A: 1605

Buncke H J 1976 Free toe to hand transfers. In: Daniller A I, Strauch B Symposium on microsurgery. C V Mosby, St Louis, p 269

Buncke H J 1980 Discussion of microsurgical free partial toe transfer in hand reconstruction by G. Foucher. Plastic Reconstructive Surgery 66: 230

Buncke H J, Rose E H 1979 Free toe to finger tip neurovascular flaps. Plastic Reconstructive Surgery 63: 607

Buncke H J Jr, McLean D H, George P T, Creech B J, Charter N L, Commons G W 1973 Thumb replacement — great toe transplantation by microvascular anastomosis. British Journal of Plastic Surgery 26: 194

Buncke H J, Buncke C M, Schulz W 1966 Immediate Nicoladoni in the rhesus monkey or hallux to hand transplantation utilizing micro miniature vascular anastomosis. British Journal of Plastic Surgery 19: 332

Buncke H J 1976 Toe digital transfer. Clinics in Plastic Surgery 3: 49

Buncke H J, Shak K G 1979 In: Serafin D, Buncke H J (eds) Microsurgical composite tissue transplantation. C V Mosby, St Louis, p 573

Buncke H J 1983 Reconstruction of the hand with free microneurovascular toe-to-hand transfer. Experience with 54 toes (Discussion). Plastic Reconstructive Surgery 71: 385

Buncke H J, Daniller A I, Schulz W P, Chase R A 1967 The fate of autogenous whole joints transplanted by microvascular anastomosis. Plastic Reconstructive Surgery 39: 331–341

Chait L A, Fleming J, Becker H 1977 Hallux-to-thumb transfer by microvascular anastomosis. South African Medical Journal 52: 429

Chang T S, Wang W S, Wu J B 1979 Free transfer of the second toe combined with dorsalis pedis flap using microvascular technique for reconstruction of the thumb and other toes. Annals of the Academy of Medicine, Singapore 8: 404

Clarkson P 1962 On making thumbs. Plastic Reconstructive Surgery 4: 325

Cobbett J R 1969 Free digital transfer. Report of a case of transfer of a great toe to replace an amputated thumb. Journal of Bone and Joint Surgery 51: 677

Comtet J J, Bertrand H G, Moyen B 1980 Free autogenous composite joint graft use in multiple finger injuries. International Journal of Microsurgery 2: 121–124

Davis J E 1964 Toe to hand transfers

(pedochyrodactyloplasty). Plastic Reconstructive Surgery 33: 422

Dellon A L 1981 Evaluation of sensibility and re-education of sensation in the hand. Williams-Wilkins

Do I K, Kotani H, Sakai K, Kuwata N 1983 Long term results of thumb reconstruction with microsurgical procedures. International Society of Reconstructive Microsurgery. Seventh Symposium, New York, abstract p 20

Donski P K, Carwell G R, Sharze L A 1979 Growth in revascularized bone grafts in young puppies. Plastic Reconstructive Surgery 64: 239–243

Donski P K, O'Brien M, Mc C 1980 Free microvascular epiphyseal transplantation. An experimental study in dogs. British Journal of Plastic Surgery 33: 169–178

Edwards E A 1960 Anatomy of the small arteries of the foot and toes. Acta Anatomica 41: 81

Elliot H R, Buncke H J 1981 Free transfer of a large sensory flap from the first web space and dorsum of the foot including the second toe for reconstruction of a mutilated hand. Journal of Hand Surgery 6: 196

Entin M A, Alger J R, Baird R M 1962 Experimental and clinical transplantation of autogenous whole joints. Journal of Bone and Joint Surgery 44A: 1518–1536

Entin M A, Daniel G, Kahn D 1968 Transplantation of autogenous half-joints. Archives of Surgery 9§: 359–368

Erdelyi R 1963 Experimental autotransplantation of small joints. Plastic Reconstructive Surgery 31: 129–139

Erdelyi R 1963 Reconstruction of ankylosed finger joints by means of transplantation of joints from the foot. Plastic Reconstructive Surgery 31: 140–150

Foucher G, Merle M, Maneaud M, Michon J 1980 Microsurgical free partial toe transfer in hand reconstruction: a report of 12 cases. Plastic Reconstructive Surgery 65: 616

Foucher G, Braun F M, Merle M, Michon J 1981 Les problèmes techniques et les indications du transfert de pulpe d'orteil. Annales de Chirurgie Plastique et Esthétique 26: 2

Foucher G, Braun F M, Merle M, Michon J 1981 Le transfert du 2ème orteil dans la chirurgie reconstructrice des doigts longs. Revue de Chirurgie Orthopédique et Réparatrice de L'Appareil Moteur 67: 235

Foucher G, Denuit p, Braun F M, Merle M, Michon J 1981 Le transfert total ou partiel du 2ème orteil dans la reconstruction digitale. A propos de 32 cas. Acta Orthopaedica Belgica 47: 854

Foucher G, Merle M 1976 Transfert articulaire au niveau d'un doigt en microchirurgie. Groupe d'avancement pour la microchirurgie. In: lettre d'information du GAM n°7

Foucher G 1982 Indication du transfert osseux vascularisé en chirurgie de la main. Revue de Chirurgie Orthopédique et Réparatrice de L'Appareil Moteur 68: 38

Foucher G, Merle M, Michon J 1984 Le traitement des mutilations traumatiques du pouce. Aspects nouveaux et apport microchirurgical. Chirurgie 110: 56

Foucher G, Van Genechten F, Morrison W A 1985 Composite tissue transfer to the hand from the foot. Recent Advances in Plastic Surgery. Jackson I T, Sommerlad B C Livingstone 65

Foucher G, Van Genechten F, Merle M, Michon J 1984 Single stage thumb reconstruction by a composite forearm island flap. Journal of Hand Surgery 9B: 245

Foucher G, Van Genechten F, Merle M, Denuit P, Braun F M, Debry R, Sur H 1984 Le transfert à partir d'orteil dans la chirurgie reconstructrice de la main. A propos de 71 cas. Annales de Chirurgie de la Main 3: 124

Foucher G (1989) Finger joint reconstruction by free vascularized transfer. In: Green D (ed) Operative hand surgery, 2nd edn. Churchill Livingstone, Edinburgh pp 1271–1293

Freeman B S 1965 Reconstruction of the thumb by toe transfer. Plastic and Reconstructive Surgery 17: 393

Freeman B S 1959 Growth studies of transplanted epiphysis. Plastic and Reconstructive Surgery 23: 584–588

Frykman G K, McC O'Brien B, Morrison W A, MacLeod A, Ciurleo A 1986 Journal of Hand Surgery 11A: 9

Furnas D W, Achauer B M 1983 Microsurgical transfer of the great toe to the radius to provide prehension after partial avulsion of the hand. Journal and Hand Surgery 8: 453

Gilbert A' 1976 Composite tissue transfers from the foot: anatomic basis and surgical technique. In: Daniller A I, Strauch B (eds) Symposium on microsurgery. C V Mosby, St Louis

Gilbert A, Morrison W A, Tubiana R 1975 Transfert sur la main d'un lambeau libre sensible. Chirurgie 101: 691

Gilbert A 1982 Toe transfers for congenital hand defects. Journal of Hand Surgery 7: 118

Goldberg N H, Watson H K 1982 Composite toe (phalanx and epiphysis) transfers in the reconstruction of the aphalangic hand. Journal of Hand Surgery 7: 454–459

Goldberg V M, Porter B P, Lance E M 1980 Transplantation of the canine knee joint on a vascular pedicle. Journal of Bone and Joint Surgery 62: 414–424

Goldberg V M, Heiple K G 1983 Experimental hemi-joint and whole-joint transplantation. Clinical Orthopaedics and Related Research 174: 43–53

Graham W C 1954 Transplantation of joints to replace diseased or damaged articulations in the hand. American Journal of Surgery 88: 136–141

Gu Y D, Wu M M 1985 Vascular variations and their treatment in toe transplantation. Journal of Reconstructive Microsurgery 1: 227–232

Gueullette R 1930 Etude critique des procédés de restauration du pouce. Journal de Chirurgie 36: 1

Haas S L 1931 Further observations on the transplantation of the epiphyseal cartilage plate. Surgery, Gynecology and Obstetrics 53: 958

Harris W R, Martin R, Tile M 1965 Transplantation of epiphyseal plates. Journal of Bone and Joint Surgery 47A: 897–914

Herndon C H, Chase S W 1952 Experimental studies in the transplantation of whole joints. Journal of Bone and Joint Surgery 34A: 564–578

Hoole J, Freilinger G, Mandl H, Frey M 1982 Grip reconstruction by double toe transplantation in cases of a fingerless hand and a handless arm. Plastic Reconstructive Surgery 69: 969

Horowitz P J 1979 Experimental transplantation of small joints by microvascular anastomosis. Plastic Reconstructive Surgery 47: 221–231

Huber J F 1941 The arterial network supplying the dorsum of the foot. Anatomical Reconstruction 80: 373

Hurwitz P J 1979 Experimental transplantation of small joints by microvascular anastomoses. Plastic Reconstructive Surgery 64: 221–231

Jacobson B H 1970 The venous drainage of the foot. Surgery, Gynecology and Obstetrics 131: 22

Jacobson H J, Suarez E L 1960 Microsurgery in anastomosis of small vessels. Surgical Forum 2: 243

Joseph J 1963 Some aspects of functional anatomy of the foot. Journal of Anatomy and Physiology in Medicine
Kettelkamp D B, Alexander H H, Dolan J 1968 A comparison of experimental arthroplasty and metacarpal head replacement. Journal of Bone and Joint Surgery 50A: 1564–1576
Kettelkamp D B, Ramsey P 1971 Experimental and clinical autogenous distal metacarpal reconstruction. Clinical Orthopaedics and Related Research 74: 129–137
Kettelkamp D B 1972 Experimental autogenous joint transplantation. Clinical Orthopaedics and Related Research 87: 138–145
Koster G 1968 Anatomy of the veins of the foot. Surgery, Gynecology and Obstetrics 127: 317
Krylov V S, Vilanov N O, Borovikow A M, Trofimov E I, Shiriaev A A 1985 Plastic Reconstructive Surgery 75: 584
Kuo E T, Ji Z L, Zheng-Lun J, Zhao Y C, Zhang M L 1984 Reconstruction of metacarpophalangeal joint by free vascularised autogenous metacarpophalangeal joint transplant. Journal of Reconstructive Microsurgery 1: 65–74
Lean M C, George P T 1973 Thumb replacement: great toe transplantation by microvascular anastomosis. British Journal of Plastic Surgery 26: 194
Le Quang C 1978 Transferts d'orteils. Revue de Chirurgie Orthopédique et Réparatrice de L'Appareil Moteur (Paris) 64: 299
Leung P C 1981 Prolonged refrigeration in toe to hand transfer — Case report. Journal of Hand Surgery 6
Leung P C 1983 Thumb reconstruction using second toe transfer. Hand 15: 15
Leung P C, Ma F Y 1982 Digital reconstruction using the toe flap — report of 10 cases. Journal of Hand Surgery 7: 366
Leung P C, Kok L C 1980 Transplantation of second toe to the hand. A preliminary report of 16 cases. Journal of Bone and Joint Surgery 62A: 990
Levame J H 1963 Les artères des orteils. Journal de Chirurgie 86: 651
Lexer E 1925 Joint transplantations and arthroplasty. Surgery, Gynecology and Obstetrics 40: 782–809
Lichtmann D, Ahbel D E, Murphy R B, Buncke H J 1982 Microvascular double toe transfer for opposable digits. Case report and rationale for treatment. Journal of Hand Surgery 7: 279
Lister G D, Kalisman M, Tsai T M 1983 Reconstruction of the hand with free microneurovascular toe to hand transfer. Experience with 54 toe transfers. Plastic Reconstructive Surgery 71: 372
Logan A, Elliot D, Foucher G 1985 Free toe pulp transfer to restore traumatic digital pulp loss. British Journal of Plastic Surgery 38: 497
Mann R A, Hagy J L 1979 The function of the toes in walking, jogging and running. Clinical Orthopaedics and Related Research 142: 24
Mateu I B 1983 Reconstructive surgery of the thumb. Pilgrims
Mathes S J, Buchannan R, Weeks P M 1980 Microvascular joint transplantation with epiphyseal growth. Journal of Hand Surgery 5: 586–589
May J W Jr, Daniel R K 1978 Great toe to hand tissue transfer. Clinical Orthopaedics and Related Research 133: 140
May J W, Smith R J, Peimer C A 1981 Toe to hand free tissue transfer for thumb reconstruction with multiple digit aplasia. Plastic Reconstructive Surgery 67: 207
May J W Jr, Chait L A, Cohen B E, O'Brien B M 1977 Free neurovascular flap from the first web of the foot in hand reconstruction. Journal of Hand Surgery 2: 387
Michon J, Merle M, Bouchon Y, Foucher G 1984 Functional comparison between pollicization and toe-to-hand transfer for thumb reconstruction. Journal of Reconstructive Microsurgery 1: 103
Mileer M R 1959 Patterns of cutaneous innervation of the human foot. Journal of Anatomy 105: 233
Morrison W A, O'Brien B, MacLeod A, Gilbert A 1978 Neurovascular free flaps from the foot for innervation of the hand. Journal of Hand Surgery 3: 235
Morrison W A, MacLeod A M, O'Brien B 1982 Digital reconstruction in the mutilated hand. Annals of Plastic Surgery 9: 392
Morrison W A, O'Brien B M, Hamilton R B 1978 Neurovascular free foot flaps in reconstruction of the mutilated hand. Clinics in Plastic Surgery 5: 265
Morrison W A, O'Brien B M, Mac Leod A M 1984 Ring finger transfer in reconstruction of transmetacarpal amputations. Journal of Hand Surgery 9A: 4
Morrison W A, O'Brien B M, Mac Leod A M 1980 Thumb reconstruction with a free neurovascular wrap around flap from the big toe. Journal of Hand Surgery 5: 575
Moyen B Toe transfers, consequences on the foot. (Unpublished)
Nicoladoni C 1897 Daumenplastik, Wien, Klinische Wochenschrift 10: 663
Nicoladoni C 1903 Weitere Erfahrungen ueber Daumenplastik, Arch Klin. Chir. 69: 697
O'Brien B M 1977 One stage toe to hand surgery. In: Microvascular reconstructive surgery. Churchill Livingstone, Edinburgh, p 183
O'Brien B M 1977 Microvascular free small joint transfer. In: Microvascular reconstructive surgery. Churchill Livingstone, Edinburgh, p 248–249
O'Brien B M, MacLeod A M, Sykes P J, Browning F S C, Threlfall G N 1978 Microvascular second toe transfer reconstruction. Journal of Hand Surgery 3: 123
O'Brien B M, MacLeod A M, Sykes P J, Donahoe S 1975 Hallux to hand transfer. Hand 7: 128
O'Brien B M, Black M J M, Morrison W A, MacLeod A M 1978 Microvascular great toe transfer for congenital absence of the thumb. Hand 10: 113
O'Brien B M, Brennen M D, MacLeod A M 1978 Simultaneous double toe transfer for severely disabled hands. Hand 10: 232
O'Brien B M, Brennen M D, MacLeod A M 1978 Microvascular free toe transfer. Clinics in Plastic Surgery 5: 223
Ohmori K, Harii K 1975 Transplantation of a toe to an amputated finger. Hand 7: 134
Ohtsuka H, Torigai K, Shioya N 1977 Two toes to finger transplants in one hand. Plastic Reconstructive Surgery 60: 561
Planas J 1969 Free transplantation of the finger joints. Plastic Reconstructive Surgery 43: 105
Reeves B 1969 Orthotopic transplantation of vascularised whole knee joints in dogs. Lancet 1: 500–502
Reeves B 1968 Studies of vascularised homotransplants of the knee joint. Journal of Bone and Joint Surgery 50B: 226–227

Roffe J L, Latil F, Chamant M, Huguet J F, Bureau H 1982 Intérêt chirurgical de l'étude radio-anatomique de la vascularisation artérielle de l'avant pied. Annales de Chirurgie de la Main 1: 84
Rose E H, Buncke H J 1980 Simultaneous transfer of the right and left second toes for reconstruction of amputated index and middle fingers in the same hand. Case report. Journal of Hand Surgery 5: 590
Schreiber A, Walker N, Nishikawa M 1976 Autologe Gelenkentransplantationen mit mikrochirurgischer gefassplastik. Helvetica Chirurgica Acta 43: 151–155
Schreiber A, Walker N, Nishikawa M, Yargarsil M G 1979 Transplantation d'articulation avec la technique de microchirurgie vasculaire. Acta Orthopaedica Belgica 45: 403–411
Smith P J, Jones B 1985 Free vascularized transfer of a metatarsophalangeal joint to the hand. A technical modification. Journal of Hand Surgery 10B: 109–112
Strauch B, Tsur H 1978 Restoration of sensation of the hand by a free neurovascular flap from the first web space of the foot. Plastic Reconstructive Surgery 62: 361
Strauch B 1977 Microsurgical approach to thumb reconstruction. Orthopedic Clinics of North America 8: 319
Tamai S, Hori Y, Tatsumi Y, Hokubo H 1977 Hallux to thumb transfer with microsurgical technique: a case report in a 45 years old woman. Hand Surgery 2: 152
Tomita Y, Kurota K, Okubo K 1983 Wrap-around flap with the tip of distal phalanx. International Society of Reconstructive Microsurgery. Seventh Symposium, New York, abstract p 20
Tsai T M, Ogden L, Jaeger S H, Okubo K 1982 Experimental vascularized total joint autografts, a primate study. Journal of Hand Surgery 7: 140–146
Tsai T M, Jupiter J B, Kutz J E, Kleinert H E 1982 Vascularized autogenous whole joint transfer in the hand, a clinical study. Journal of Hand Surgery 7: 335–342
Tsai T M, Singer R, Elliott E, Klein H 1985 Immediate free vascularized joint transfer from second toe to index finger proximal interphalangeal joint. A case report. Journal of Hand Surgery 10B: 85–89
Tsai T M 1979 Second and third toe transplantation to a transmetacarpal amputated hand. Annals of the Academy of Medicine, Singapore 8: 413
Tsai T M, Jupiter J B, Wolff T W, Asatoy E 1981 Reconstruction of severe transmetacarpal mutilating hand injuries by combined second and third toe transfer. Journal of Hand Surgery 6: 319
Vercauteren M E, Van Vynckt C 1983 A free total toe phalanx transplant to a finger. A case report. Journal of Hand Surgery 8: 336–339
Vilky S Personal communication
Wei C Z, Meyer V E, Beasley R W 1981 The versatile second toe microvascular transfer. Symposium on management of upper limb amputations. Orthopedic Clinics of North America 12: 827
Wei C Z 1981 Reconstruction by autogenous toe transplantations for total hand amputation. Symposium on management of upper limb amputations. Orthopedic Clinics of North America 12: 835
Whitesides E S 1977 Normal growth in a transplanted epiphysis, case report with 13 year follow up. Journal of Bone and Joint Surgery 59A: 546–547
Wilson J N 1966 Epiphyseal transplantation. Journal of Bone and Joint Surgery 48A: 245–256
Wray R C, Mathes S M, Young V L, Weeks P M 1981 Free vascularized whole joint transplants with ununited epiphyses. Plastic Reconstructive Surgery 67: 519–525
Yang D, Yudoing G 1979 Thumb reconstruction utilizing second toe transplantations by microvascular anastomosis. Report of 78 cases. Chinese Medical Journal 92: 295
Yoshimura M 1980 Toe to hand transfer. Plastic Reconstructive Surgery 66: 74
Yoshimura M 1984 Toe to hand transfer. Plastic Reconstructive Surgery 73: 851
Zaleske D J, Ehrlich M G, Piliero C, May J W, Mankin H J 1982 Growth plate behavior in whole joint replantation in the rabbit. Journal of Bone and Joint Surgery 64A: 249–258

A. Gilbert and R. Brockman

9 Flap coverage for the upper extremity

Techniques for covering large areas of tissue loss in the upper extremity have progressed tremendously in the last twenty years.

During the 1970s, the development of microsurgery and the appearance of free flaps with vascular anastomoses completely changed the surgical options. Previously, when thin skin grafts were not possible, one had to resort to thick, unreliable abdominal or contralateral arm flaps, requiring undesirable immobilisation, and carrying significant risk of maceration or infection. The description of axial pattern flaps, in particular the groin flap of McGregor, represented real progress.

From the beginning of reconstructive microsurgery, free flaps, initially deltopectoral and groin, have been applied to upper extremity problems. However, these particular flaps have numerous disadvantages: thickness, hair-bearing, donor site problems, etc. During the last fifteen years, many anatomical studies have been done which have placed a great variety of flaps at our disposal, each having its own particular characteristic advantages and specific indications.

Nearly one hundred free flap donor sites have been described, but barely more than half-a-dozen remain widely used. The specialised pulp flaps from the toes are described elsewhere. Here, we will address only the principal donor sites used for covering areas of tissue loss:

1. Dorsal foot flap
2. Lateral arm flap
3. Scapular flap
4. Latissimus dorsi flap.

DORSAL FOOT FLAP

The dorsal foot free flap was originally proposed to provide cover with sensibility over a large anaesthetic area in the hand (Daniel et al 1976), but the results for restoration of sensation were poor, and its use for this indication has been all but abandoned. Currently, its use in upper extremity surgery is mostly limited to those situations where an extremely thin free flap is required for the hand.

The flap is centred over the dorsalis pedis artery and its venae comitantes. In maximum dimension, it can extend from the extensor retinaculum at the ankle to the interdigital web spaces of the foot, and from the extensor hallucis longus to the fifth metatarsal, giving a flap measuring 9 cm by 12 cm. Smaller flaps should be centralised over the dorsalis pedis vessels, and include some part of the dorsal venous arch. The flap may include skin, tendons and the second metatarsal bone if required.

The dorsalis pedis artery is the continuation of the anterior tibial artery. Proximally, it is between the extensor hallucis longus (EHL) and the tibialis anterior tendons, and then passes under the EHL and the extensor retinaculum. It then lies in close proximity to the tarsal bones, and here gives off numerous fine cutaneous branches. At the level of the extensor hallucis brevis (EHB), it gives off two tarsal arteries — the medial one going directly to the skin, and the larger lateral one going to the skin and then continuing to the short toe extensors. The dorsalis pedis artery ends over the base of the second metatarsal by dividing into the arcuate artery, which passes laterally, and the plantar communicating artery, which then passes between the heads of origin of the first interosseous muscle to join the deep plantar arch.

The first dorsal metatarsal artery arises usually from the dorsalis pedis artery, but sometimes from the plantar communicating artery, and travels distally, usually superficially, between the heads of the first and second metatarsals. This first dorsal metatarsal artery is the only arterial supply to the distal 3 cm of the flap.

Venous drainage from the flap is through the dorsal venous arch, long saphenous vein and the venae comitantes.

The sensation of the majority of the flap is via the superficial peroneal nerve, a purely sensory nerve, which enters the flap proximally just lateral to the midline. The sensory input for the first web space is supplied by the deep peroneal nerve, which follows the first dorsal metatarsal artery.

The second metatarsal is supplied through its periosteum from proximal and distal cortical branches of the first dorsal metatarsal artery. In 12–18% of cases, there is inadequate vascular supply for distal skin flap survival, due to absence of the dorsalis pedis or first dorsal metatarsal arteries (Hollingshead 1982, Man & Acland 1980, May et al 1977). Therefore, a preoperative Doppler examination should be performed to assess flow in the posterior tibial and dorsalis pedis arteries at the ankle, and to ensure that there is a clear signal in the region of the proximal web space, indicating communication between the dorsalis pedis artery and the first dorsal metatarsal artery.

Elevation of the flap is performed under tourniquet control. The flap should be designed on the foot, and the position of the pedicle marked.

The initial incision is made medially on the foot. The flap is elevated, keeping nerves and veins with the flap but leaving the paratenon with the tendons. Elevation continues just to the lateral border of the long extensor of the second toe. The distal incision is then made, and the neurovascular bundle located in the first intermetatarsal space and ligated distally. The flap is then elevated deep to the first dorsal metatarsal artery. The plantar communicating artery is ligated. The tendon of extensor hallucis brevis lies superficial to the artery and must be divided. Dissection of the dorsalis pedis artery and superficial peroneal nerve proximal to the flap is performed via a zig-zag incision over the pedicle.

Meticulous technique must be used for donor site closure to avoid complications. Haemostasis must be complete, any rents in the paratenon must be closed, the dorsal retinaculum should be repaired and a split-thickness skin graft applied.

Donor site complications, notably poor healing, and the tedious nature of the dissection have reduced the use in recent times of the dorsal foot flap. However, its long, large-diameter pedicle, the possibility for re-innervation, the thin skin and relatively inconspicuous donor site make it a useful tool in appropriate circumstances.

LATERAL ARM FLAP

The lateral arm flap is a fasciocutaneous flap on the lateral arm centred on a line joining the lateral epicondyle to the deltoid tubercle. It is based on the posterior radial collateral artery, the terminal branch of the profunda brachii artery. The artery travels in the lateral intermuscular septum. It should not be confused with the anterior radial collateral artery, which is deeper and travels with the radial nerve between brachioradialis and brachialis. The length of the pedicle is 7–8 cm, and the vessel diameter is 1.5 mm (0.9–2.4 mm) proximally and 1 mm (0.6–1.7 mm) distally. Venous drainage is through venae comitantes, which are approximately 2.5 mm in diameter.

Cutaneous innervation of the flap can be achieved using the posterior cutaneous nerve of the arm, which runs through the flap. The posterior cutaneous nerve of the forearm also traverses the flap, and its sacrifice during harvesting of the flap creates anaesthesia on the posterior forearm.

Surgery can be performed with a high sterile tourniquet. The flap dissection begins with the posterior incision, which is carried down through the fascia over the triceps. Subfascial dissection continues to the septum, where the artery will be seen. The anterior incision is then made, and carried subfascially over the biceps and the brachialis to the intermuscular septum. The septum is liberated from the bone beginning distally at the lateral epicondyle. At the superior margin of brachioradialis, the radial nerve and the anterior radial collateral artery will be seen. This artery should be divided to allow the profunda brachii artery to be taken with the flap.

If the width of the flap is less than 6 cm, the defect can be closed primarily. However, the flap may be as wide as 15 cm if the donor site is skin grafted (Urbaniak 1987). The maximum recommended length is 12 cm, beginning distally at the lateral epicondyle (Song et al 1982).

The lateral arm flap is useful for hand reconstruction as it has thin elastic skin. Other advantages include a constant vessel, its sensory potential, the possibility of taking bone and part of triceps tendon with the flap or, conversely, of harvesting the well-vascularized fascia alone. The vessel at both ends of the flap may be anastomosed to create flow through the flap. The main disadvantages of the flap are the obvious donor site scar and the anaesthesia of the forearm.

SCAPULAR FLAP

The scapular flap is a cutaneous flap based on the cutaneous branch of the circumflex scapular artery. It was described in an anatomical study in 1980 (Dos Santos 1980) and has gained wide clinical use since its first application.

Most commonly, the subscapular artery arises from the third part of the axillary artery. It travels inferiorly and then divides into the thoracodorsal artery and the scapular circumflex artery. The latter then curves around the lower border of the subscapularis, gives off its muscular branches and emerges posteriorly through the triangular space; this is bordered by teres minor superiorly, teres major inferiorly, and the long head of the triceps laterally. It then divides into two terminal cutaneous branches. One, which travels horizontally to supply the skin over the scapula, is the basis of the scapular flap. The other, a descending branch, is the artery of the parascapular flap. The pedicle is 3–6 cm long, but can be lengthened up to 5–10 cm if dissection is carried to its origin from the subscapular artery. The diameter of the transverse cutaneous branch is 1.5–2.5 mm, and that of the circumflex scapular 2.5–3.5 mm in the adult. There are two venae comitantes, usually with diameters similar to the arterial diameter.

The flap is designed centred over the artery on the inferior two-thirds of the scapula. With the patient's arm at his side, the border limits are as follows: medially, 2 cm lateral to the spinous process; laterally, 2 cm superior to the posterior axillary crease; superiorly, 2 cm inferior to the spine of the scapula; and inferiorly, 2 cm superior to the inferior margin of the scapula. A flap of 10 cm by 20 cm can be developed. The width should not be over 10 cm, to allow primary closure of the donor site.

Dissection of the flap is relatively easy. The flap should be elevated from medial to lateral just superficial to the muscle fascia. The pedicle is found exiting from the triangular space. It is advantageous to include the circumflex scapular artery with the pedicle, in order to have an adequate diameter vessel for anastomosis, and to lengthen the pedicle. This requires deep, careful dissection in the triangular space.

The scapular flap is good for covering medium-sized defects (Fig. 9.1). It is relatively thin, hairless and has a long, large, constant pedicle. There is no functional donor site morbidity, although the scars do spread. The flap does not have cutaneous innervation. It can be combined with the parascapular flap or the latissimus dorsi flap, if necessary, to cover very large defects.

LATISSIMUS DORSI FLAP

The latissimus dorsi flap can provide musculocutaneous coverage for defects extending from the shoulder to the middle third of the forearm. First described as a pedicled flap by Tanzini in 1896 (Lassen et al 1985), and first used as a free flap by Maxwell (Lassen et al 1985) in 1978, it has been modified and widely used for back, chest wall, breast, and head and neck reconstruction, as well as its upper extremity applications.

The latissimus dorsi (LD) muscle takes its

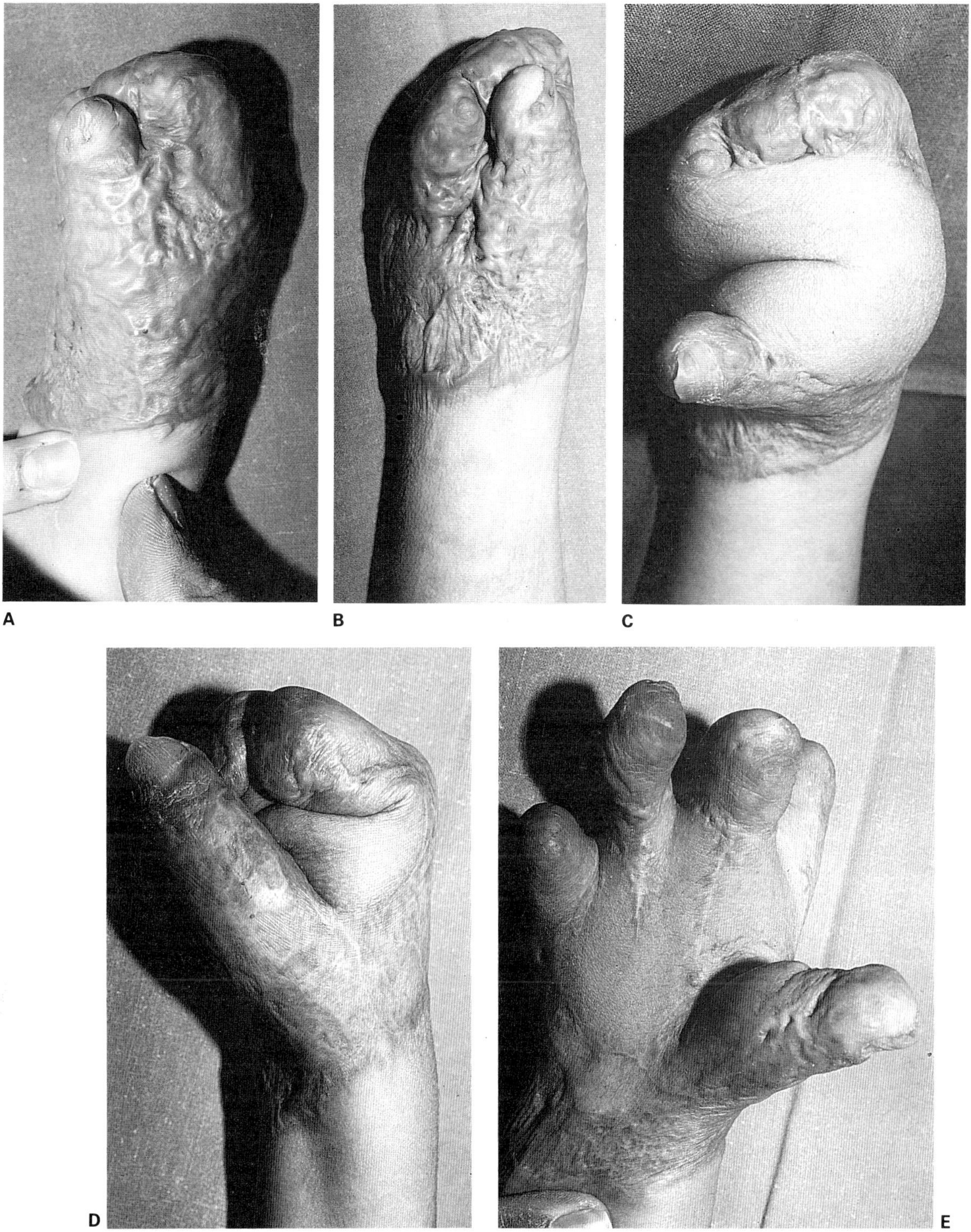

Fig. 9.1 Three-year-old girl victim of a severe burn to both hands. A. and B. Right hand: hypertrophic scar completely enveloping the hand. C. Transfer of an inguinal free flap freeing the commissure and bringing a large amount of skin. D. and E. After separation of the fingers and defatting of the flap.

origin from the lower six thoracic, the lumbar and the upper sacral spinous processes, by an aponeurosis from the iliac crest, and the inferior angle of the scapula. It inserts into the intertubercular groove of the humerus. Its dual blood supply is provided by a dominant pedicle; the thoracodorsal artery, and the posterior paraspinal perforators. The thoracodorsal artery is a branch of the subscapular artery, and enters the deep surface of the muscle with the thoracodorsal nerve 8–9 cm medial to the lateral border of the muscle. In the muscle, it divides into two branches at 45° to one another, allowing independently vascularised, smaller flaps when needed (Urbaniak 1987).

The neurovascular pedicle is long, 9–15 cm, and the artery measures approximately 2.5 mm in diameter. A muscular flap with maximum dimensions of 30 cm by 20 cm can be taken.

Skin directly overlying the muscle can be taken with the flap, although it is not recommended. The skin will not have sensation, as the thoracodorsal nerve is purely motor and its sensory innervation comes from the dorsal cutaneous rami of T6–T12. The patient should be in the lateral position or slightly tilted dorsally or ventrally, with the arm draped free. The incision is made in the posterior axillary line and the pedicle is identified. The muscle is then dissected from distal to proximal. The donor site can be closed primarily.

The usefulness of the flap outweighs most of its disadvantages. Seroma and pain are frequent donor site complications. Functional disability is minimal if the rest of the musculature in the shoulder and back is intact, although loss of the latissimus dorsi does compromise posterior push-off (essential for snow skiing and for some polio patients).

As well as its uses for soft tissue coverage, the latissimus dorsi muscle flap can be transposed with a preserved neurovascular pedicle to restore elbow flexion (Zancolli & Mitre 1973) or extension along with soft tissue cover (Fig. 9.2).

ISLAND FLAPS

Parallel to the clinical development of microsurgical flaps, anatomical work completely altered our understanding of the vascular anatomy of the integument of the limbs, and research directed at discovering new free flaps defined arterial pedicle flaps that might be locally transposed as island flaps. More progress was made when it was discovered that, in certain circumstances, a flap could survive perfectly well with retrograde flow. The radial 'Chinese' flap provided the proof for this idea, and opened the door to a series of anatomical discoveries that were once again to alter the surgical indications for free flaps, introducing simpler procedures and removing the necessity for vascular anastomoses.

In the upper extremity, the following flaps have such great importance that their description is indispensable:

1. 'Chinese' or radial forearm flap
2. Posterior interosseous flap
3. Becker's flap
4. Brachioradialis flap.

Radial forearm or Chinese flap

The radial forearm flap was first described by Chinese authors (Yang Guofan & Gao Yuzhi 1981), and introduced to the west by western surgeons who visited China in the early 1980s (Foucher et al 1984, Muhlbauer et al 1982). Initially designed as a free flap, it was later used as an island flap supported by retrograde blood flow.

In the proximal one-third of the forearm, the radial artery is medial to the brachioradialis muscle belly. Distally, the artery is more superficial, lying between the brachioradialis and flexor carpi radialis with only fascia and skin above. Proximally, it gives off the radial recurrent artery, and more distally in the forearm gives off several muscular branches. The cutaneous branches are contained in an areolar septum, containing the radial artery, which becomes better defined as one progresses distally in the forearm.

The flap should be centred anterolaterally overlying the radial arterial axis. Its largest recommended dimensions extend from the ulnar margin of the forearm medially to the middle of the posterior aspect of the forearm, and from 3 cm proximal to the wrist flexion crease to 3 cm distal to the elbow flexion crease (Masquelet 1984). The

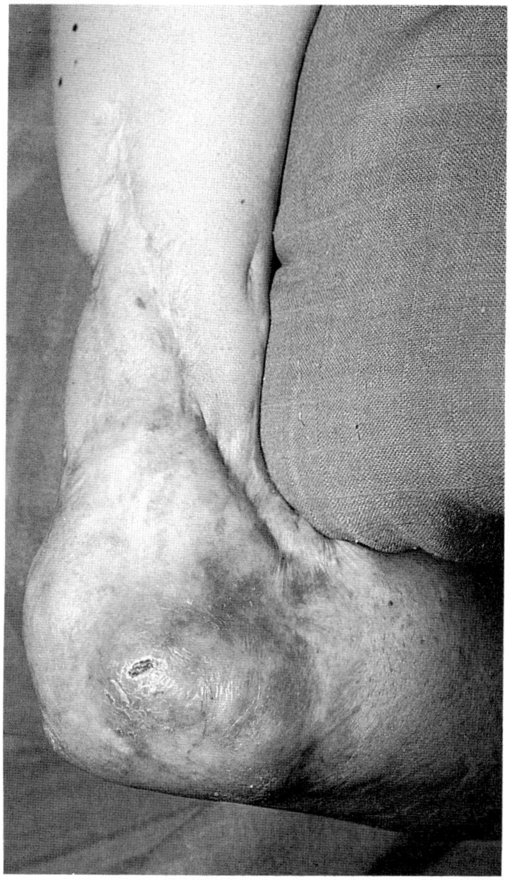

A

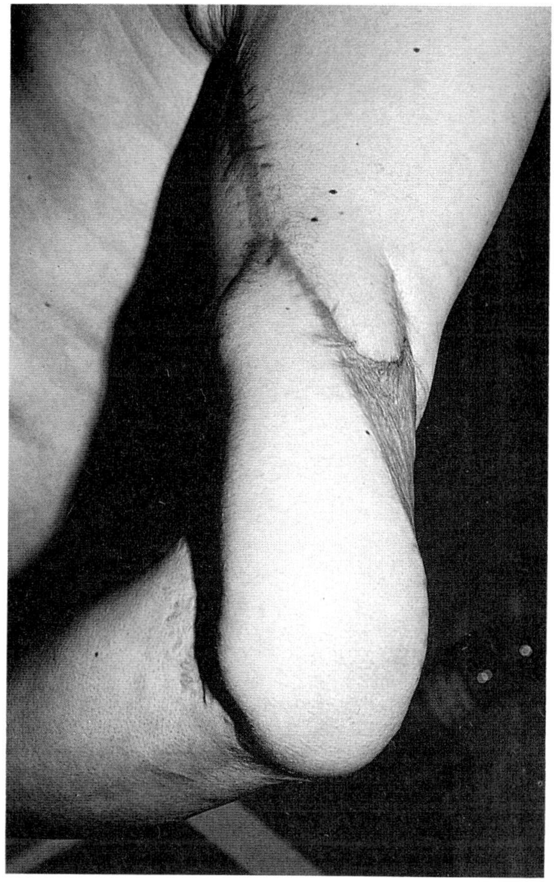

B

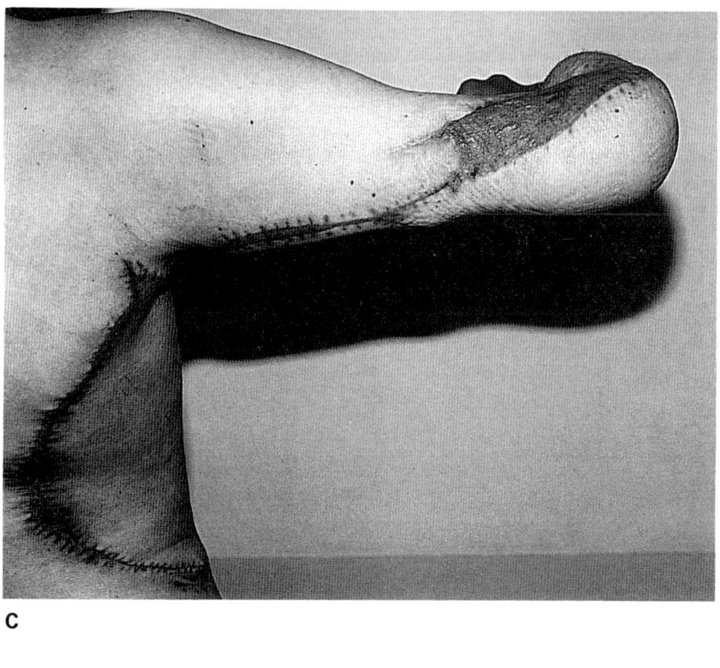

C

Fig. 9.2 Tissue loss from the posterior aspect of the elbow with destruction of the triceps. **A.** Posterior aspect of the elbow and the ulcerated zone. **B.** and **C.** After transfer of latissimus dorsi as an island flap.

lateral and medial cutaneous nerves of the forearm may be included with the flap to innervate it. When used as a pedicled flap, the venae comitantes provide sufficient drainage, and the cephalic vein should not be taken as this can provoke venous congestion in the flap. However, when used as a free flap, the cephalic vein should be included. Preoperatively, the Allen test and a Doppler examination should be performed to confirm the presence of a functioning ulnar artery.

Flap dissection should begin by finding the radial artery proximal and distal to the flap. The flap is then dissected from the ulnar side, taking care to elevate the deep fascia with the flap. At the radial border of the FCR, the dissection must go deep to the radial artery. Similar subfascial dissection is performed from the radial side, plunging deep at the ulnar border of brachioradialis. The superficial branch of the radial nerve must be identified and preserved. A clamp can be put on the radial artery, and the tourniquet released to assess the vascularity of the hand before the artery is divided. The donor site is skin grafted. The Chinese flap is very versatile. It may be used as a pedicled or a free flap, and may include nerve, tendon and bone as well as skin and fascia. Donor site morbidity may include failure of the skin graft, and hand swelling or stiffness. Ligation of the radial artery carries the risk of ischaemic complications, but these have not been reported.

Posterior interosseous flap

After the first description by the Chinese of a successful flap based on retrograde flow through anastomotic channels, other authors exploited this idea in the development of other flaps. One such flap is the posterior interosseous flap, a fasciocutaneous flap on the posterolateral aspect of the arm based on the posterior interosseous artery (Zancolli & Angrigianni 1986, Masquelet 1987).

The posterior interosseous artery is a branch of the interosseous arterial trunk, which is a branch of the ulnar artery. As it enters the posterior compartment of the forearm, it divides into two branches — an ascending one supplying the elbow joint and forearm musculature, and a descending one which travels in the septum between the extensor carpi ulnaris (ECU) and extensor digiti quinti (EDQ) giving off small branches which travel through the fascial septum to the skin. The largest of these is the first branch, which is constant and leaves the posterior interosseous artery near its origin. Near the ulnar head, the posterior interosseous artery anastomoses with the perforating branch of the anterior interosseous artery and the dorsal carpal arch. In his cadaver study, Masquelet (1984) found that the posterior interosseous artery did not reach the wrist in 4 of 70 forearms, and that in 1 of 70 forearms, although the artery reached the wrist, there was no distal anastomosis. Venous drainage is through venae comitantes.

The posterior interosseous nerve and the posterior interosseous artery leave the deep surface of the supinator in the proximal forearm, and travel throughout the posterior compartment together. All of the branches of this motor nerve are lateral to the artery.

Because of its vascular anatomy, the posterior interosseous flap can be used as a proximally based, anterograde-flow pedicle flap, or as a distally based pedicle dependent on retrograde flow.

Because the distal arterial anastomoses are not constant, it is recommended that preoperative Doppler examination be performed and that the distal pedicle be explored surgically before elevating a distally based flap.

The flap is centred on a line which follows the course of the artery, i.e. a line drawn between the lateral epicondyle and the ulnar head. The limits of the skin territory that can be elevated extend medial to the ulnar crest, lateral to the midline posteriorly, distal to the wrist and proximal to 3 cm proximal to the point of emergence of the artery at the junction of the middle and proximal third of the line described above. Small flaps must be centred distal to the point of arterial emergence.

Flaps using a proximally based pedicle should be elevated from the lower third of the forearm, and those with a distally based pedicle designed over the site of emergence of the artery.

The elbow should be flexed and the forearm pronated to facilitate dissection, which should proceed from radial to ulnar and then from ulnar to radial, taking care to preserve the septum between the ECU and EDQ which contains the vessels. The nerve must be separated from the artery and left unharmed. For the proximally based flap, the pedicle is raised to the level of the fibrous band deep to EDQ, and for the distally based flap this band must be divided to release the pedicle. The motor nerve to ECU, which is near the origin of the pedicle, must be preserved.

The donor site can usually be closed directly.

The flap is useful for covering the dorsum of the hand, the first web space, the wrist and the elbow. It does not require sacrifice of a major artery to the hand. It is, however, a difficult dissection and the arteries are small. Thus, there is the possibility of ischaemic loss which has not been reported with the radial forearm flap.

Becker's flap

Becker's flap is a fasciocutaneous flap located on the anteromedial side of the distal forearm. It was originally described to provide coverage for the median nerve in cases of revision carpal tunnel surgery where skin and subcutaneous tissue were inadequate for closure (Becker & Gilbert 1988).

The flap is based on the fasciocutaneous branch of the dorsal branch of the ulnar artery. The dorsal branch divides from the ulnar artery 2.5 cm proximal to the proximal wrist crease. This artery, which is 1–1.3 mm in diameter, passes under the flexor carpi ulnaris (FCU) and then divides into three branches. The first and second go to the pisiform and the FCU respectively. The third branch is the fasciocutaneous branch, which itself divides into an ascending branch supplying the ulnar two-thirds of the skin of the forearm and the fascia of the FCU, and a descending branch which supplies the palmar skin over the fourth and fifth metacarpals.

The flap is designed with maximum dimensions of 10 cm in width and 20 cm in length on the ulnar part of the hand and forearm. Dissection begins with a longitudinal anteromedial incision at the anterior border of FCU. The fascia over the FCU is divided longitudinally and perpendicularly. The dissection continues in the subfascial plane until the origin of the dorsal branch of the ulnar artery is found.

The flap can be used to cover defects on the hypothenar eminence and the dorsal aspect of the hand to the MCP joints, as well as for revision carpal tunnel surgery. It can, in the latter case, be wrapped around the median nerve.

Advantages of the flap include: the relative ease of dissection; large flap with minimal donor site morbidity; good blood supply; and the fact that no major arterial axes are sacrificed. Its disadvantages are its short pedicle and the non-innervated skin.

Brachioradialis flap

The use of the brachioradialis muscle has been described by one of the authors (Gilbert & Restrepo 1980) for covering soft tissue defects around the elbow joint when skin grafts are insufficient.

The muscle measures approximately 30 cm (range 24–33 cm) from its origin on the lateral supracondylar ridge of the humerus to its insertion on the lateral side of the distal radius. Of that length, 22 cm is muscle belly and the remaining 8 cm is tendon.

The blood supply of the muscle is through a principal and one or two accessory pedicles. The principal pedicle usually originates from the radial recurrent artery, but may branch from the brachial, radial or recurrent ulnar arteries. The pedicle penetrates the muscle belly approximately 10 cm from its humeral origin (range 6–16 cm). As the pedicle is 3.8 cm long, and its diameter ranges from 0.9–1.6 mm, the flap can be used also as a free flap.

The radial nerve branch which innervates brachioradialis enters the muscle approximately 6 cm from its origin, i.e. proximal to and distinct from its vascular pedicle.

The muscle is dissected in the forearm to its pedicle from distal to proximal after it has been divided at the musculotendinous junction. This provides a flap 10–12 cm long and 3–4 cm wide, which can be swung to cover anterior or posterior defects about the elbow. The width can be increased by stretching the muscle after removing the perimysium (Fig. 9.3).

SURGICAL INDICATIONS

The surgical choices for flaps to the upper limb

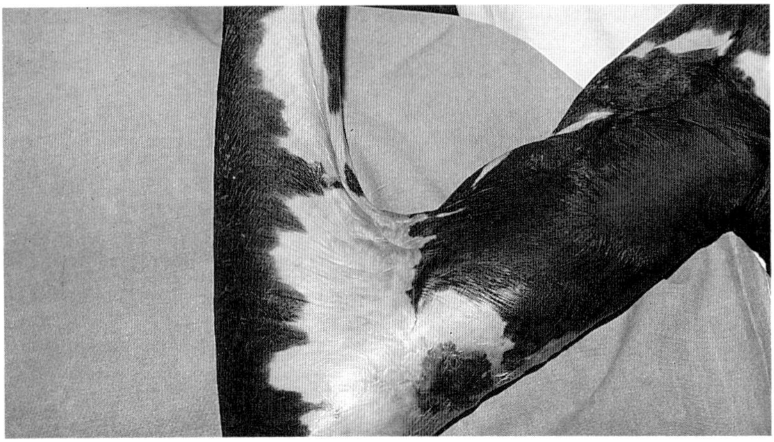

A

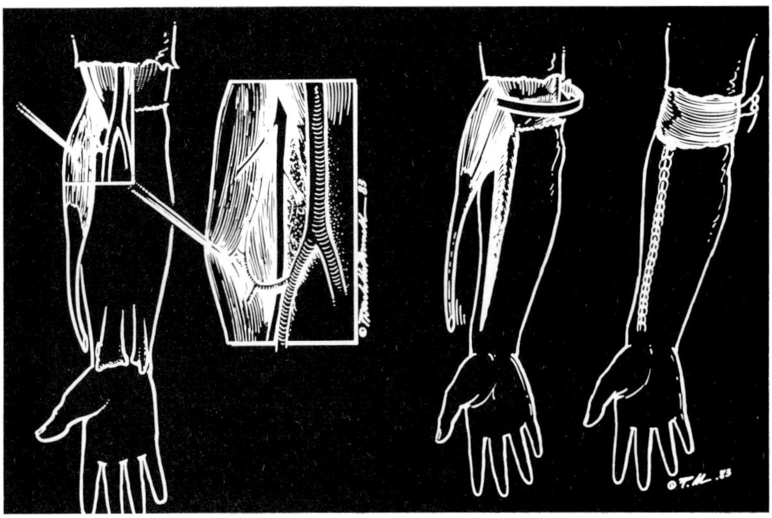

B

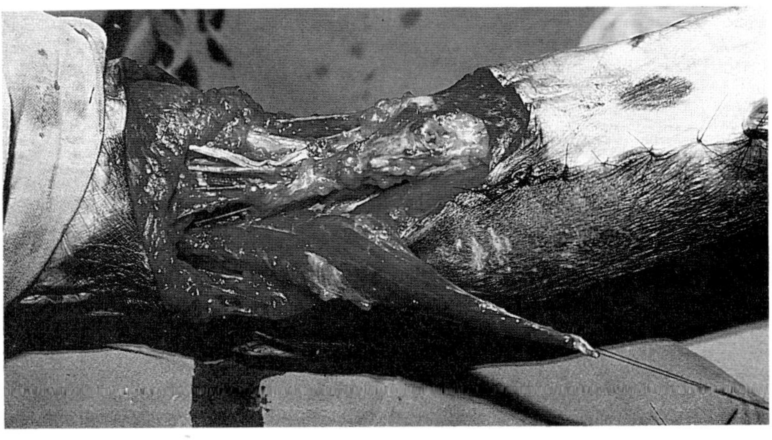

C

Fig. 9.3 Significant elbow contraction after a burn in a ten-year-old child. **A.** Anterior elbow scar. **B.** Design of the brachioradialis flap. **C.** The elbow has been extended, the biceps elongated and the flap sectioned distally. **D.** The flap is spread out over the anterior aspect of the elbow and will be covered by a skin graft. **E.** and **F.** Results after one year.

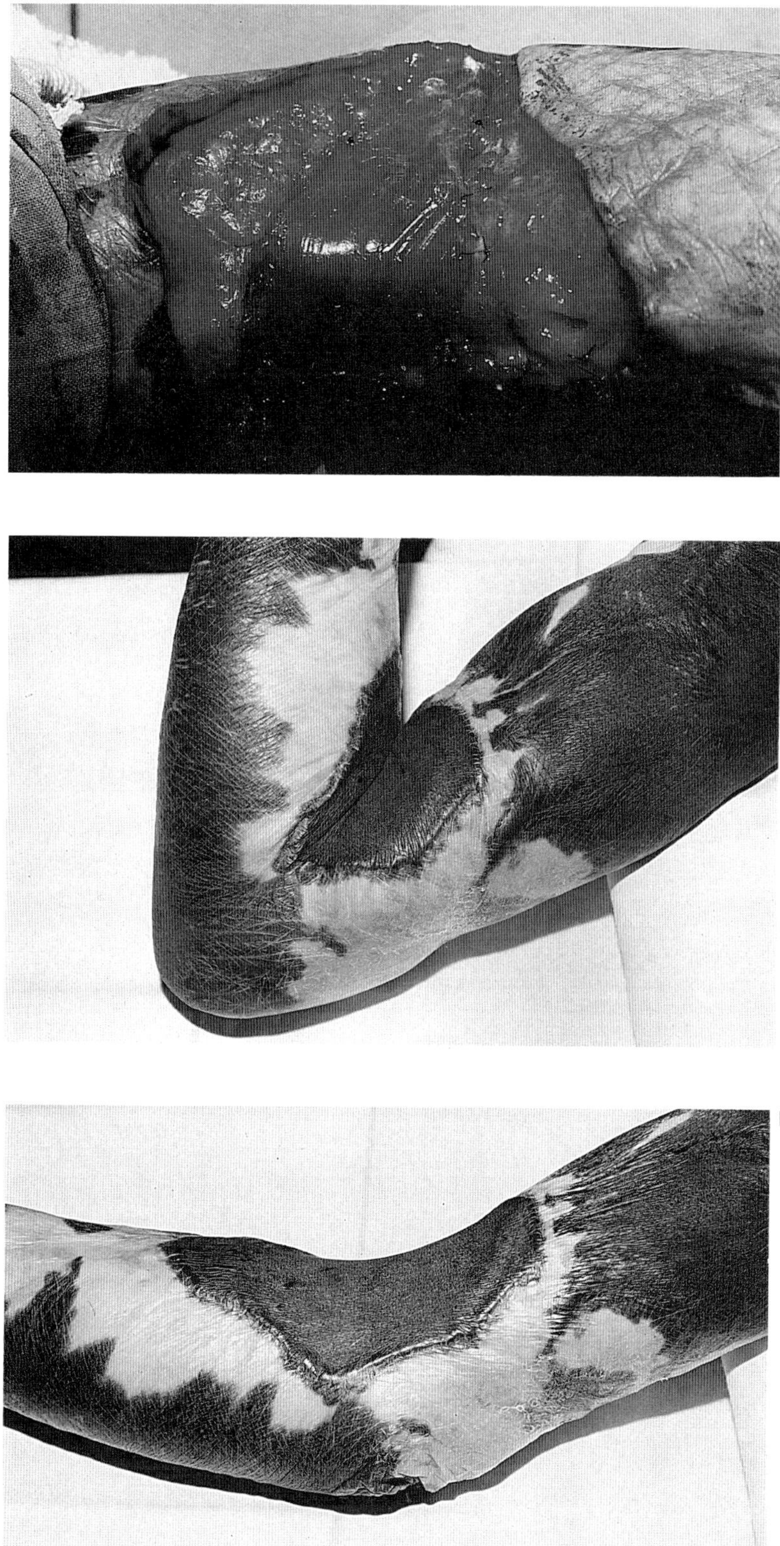

Fig. 9.3 (cont)

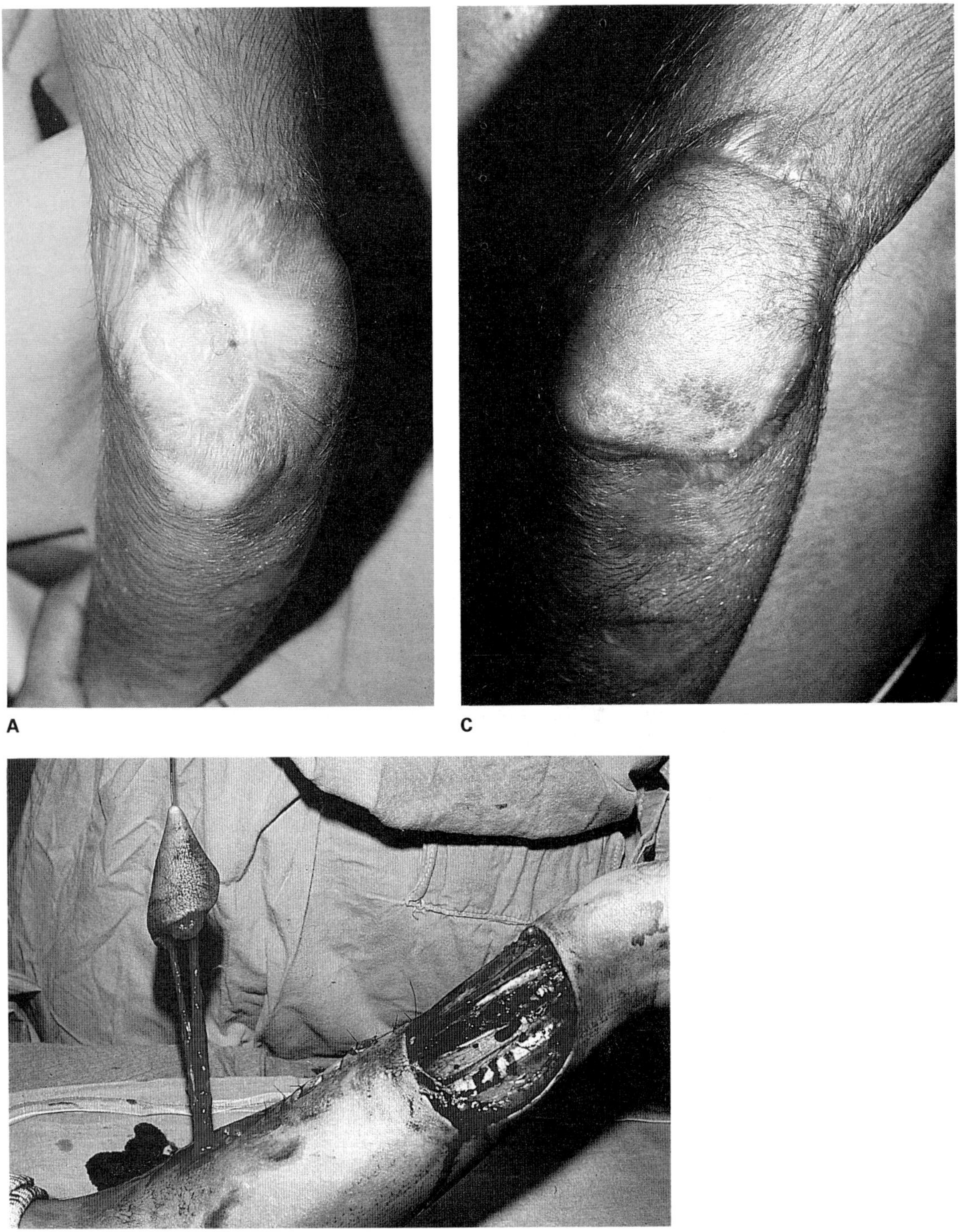

A C B

Fig. 9.4 Post-traumatic scarring on the posterior surface of the elbow. **A.** The scar is adherent to bone. **B.** Radial forearm flap with a proximal pedicle. **C.** The posterior tissue loss is covered by the flap.

A

B

C

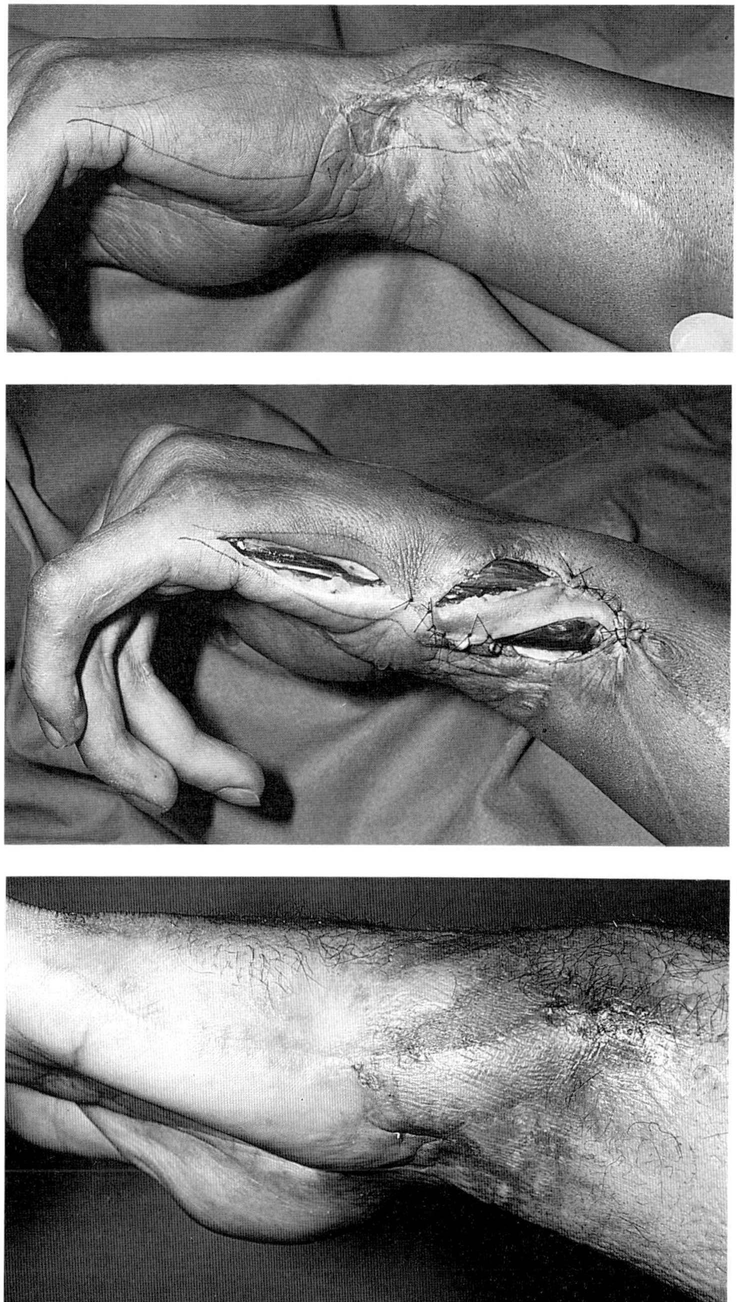

Fig. 9.5 Osteitis with adherent scar on the ulnar border of the wrist. **A.** The adherent zone is excised; sketch of the abductor digit minimi. **B.** The abductor digiti minimi has been rotated 180° with a small cutaneous flap. Skin grafts will be added. **C.** After healing.

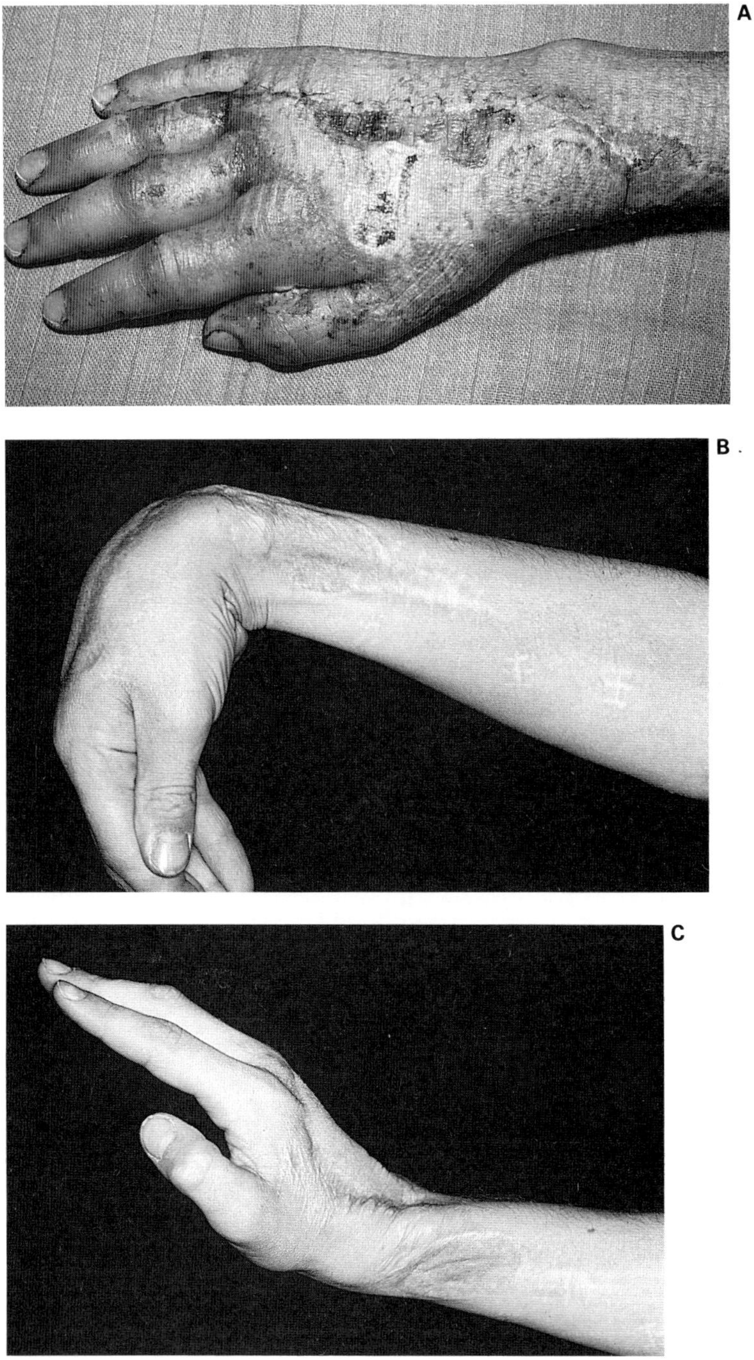

Fig. 9.6 Crush injury to the dorsum of the hand with destruction of the extensor tendons. **A.** The dorsal necrosis. **B., C., D.** and **E.** The 'Chinese' flap and extensor tendon grafts two years after surgery.

D

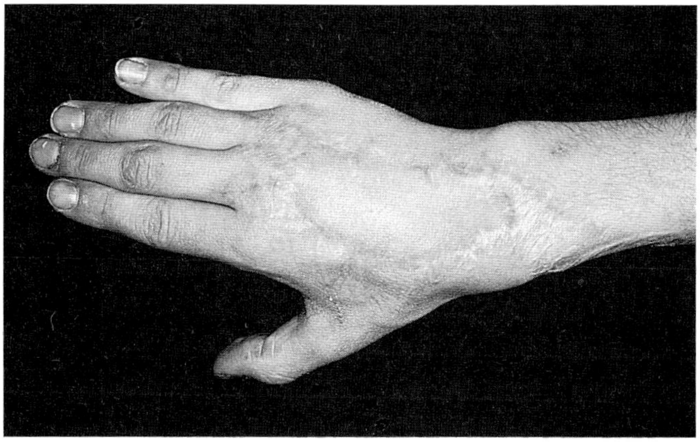

E

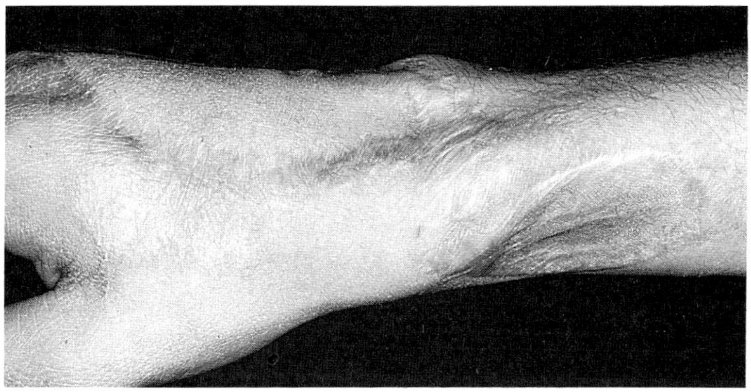

Fig. 9.6 (cont)

have varied enormously over the years, and have passed through successive phases. These have been: the classic pedicled flaps (abdominal, groin, tube); the microsurgical phase, a technique sometimes used in excess; and, finally, the phase of local or regional island flaps that have reduced the indications for microsurgical procedures.

Many factors enter into the operative plan; one of the principal ones is the position of the defect.

Tissue loss at the shoulder and arm

Tissue loss at the shoulder and arm is incontestably the domain of the latissimus dorsi flap. This flap can be used with or without attached skin, and allows coverage of a large surface to the level of the elbow. It can also be used as a functional transfer for reconstruction of the biceps or the triceps. If this transfer is impossible for vascular reasons, or if the area to be covered is smaller, it is possible to use the scapular or parascapular flaps. These cutaneous flaps can cover the shoulder or axilla.

Tissue loss at the elbow

The elbow region has always been difficult to cover, and there are few local possibilities. Two local flaps can be used:

1. The brachioradialis muscle flap which, when turned on its vascular axis, can cover a small loss of tissue on the anterior aspect of the elbow or above the medial epicondyle (Fig. 9.3).
2. The lateral arm flap, which can be brought to the anterior or posterior aspects of the elbow.

The most difficult area to cover is the medial aspect of the elbow and the epitrochlear area, but

A B

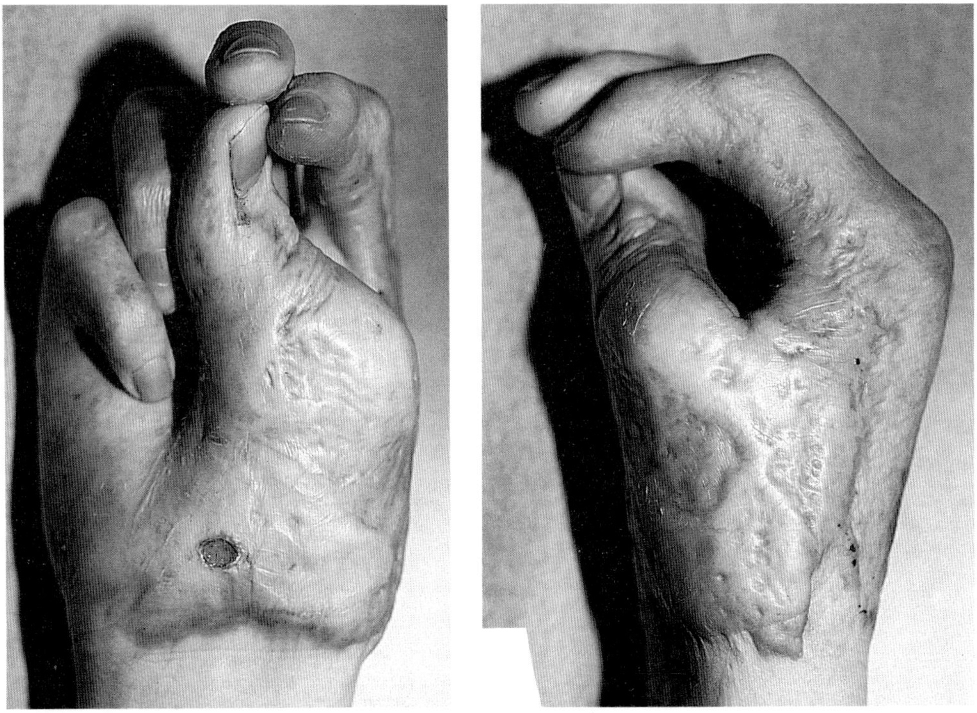

C

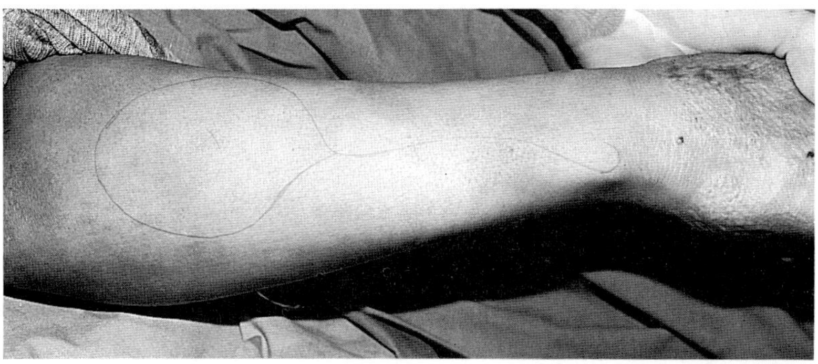

D

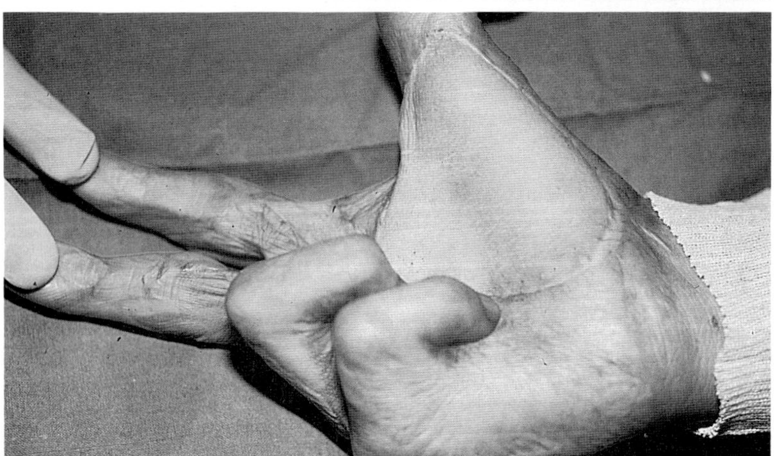

Fig. 9.7 First web space contracture after a severe hand burn. **A.** and **B.** Severe scarring on anterior aspect of the thumb, dorsum and first web space. **C.** Sketch of posterior interosseous flap. **D.** The flap has been placed on the palm and in the first web space allowing a wide separation of the thumb from the hand.

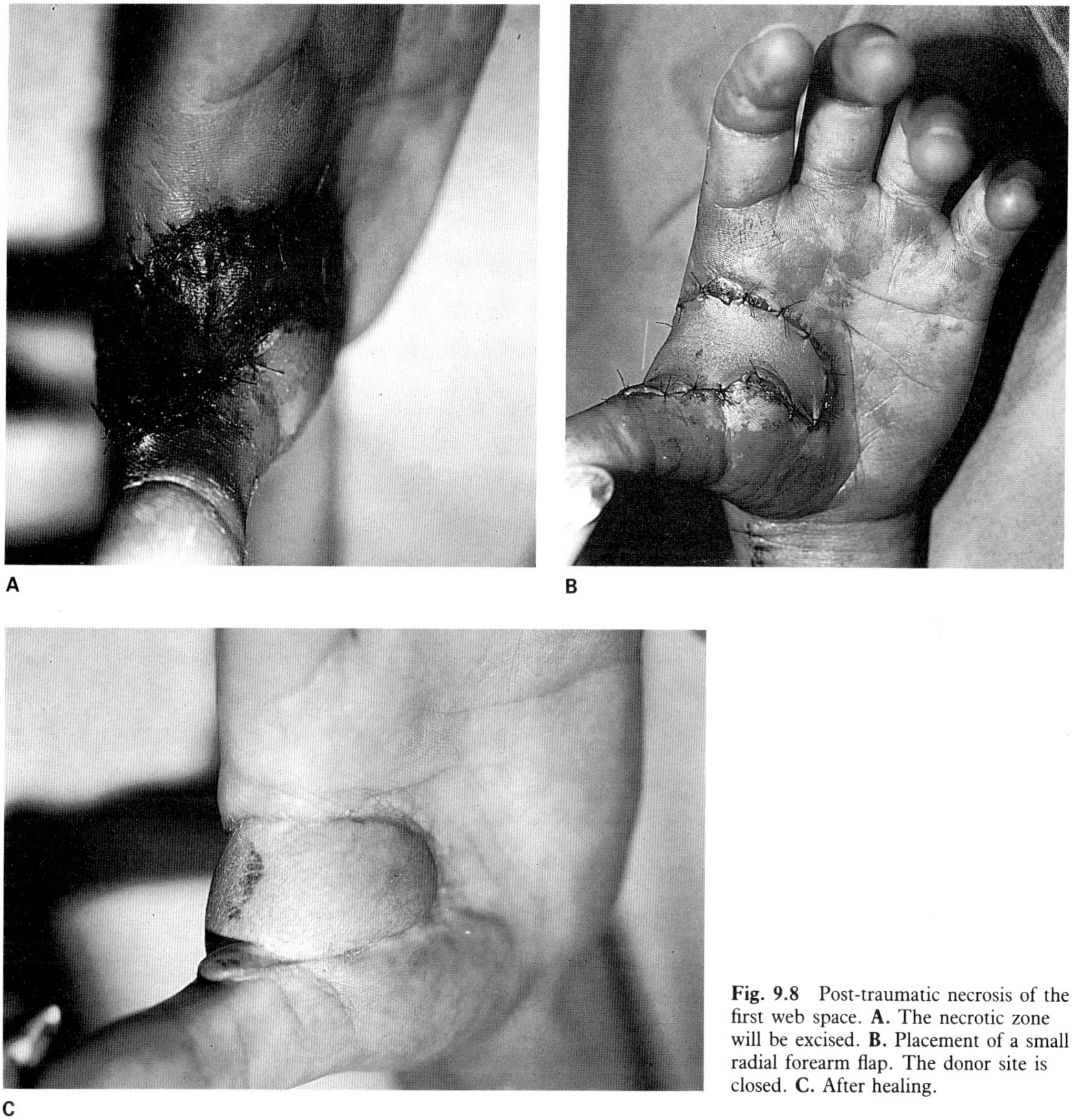

Fig. 9.8 Post-traumatic necrosis of the first web space. **A.** The necrotic zone will be excised. **B.** Placement of a small radial forearm flap. The donor site is closed. **C.** After healing.

this can be reached by a long lateral arm flap or by an anterograde radial forearm island flap (Fig. 9.4).

The use of microsurgical free flaps has become limited to those cases where local or regional flaps are contraindicated or not available.

Anterior aspect of wrist and palm (Fig. 9.5)

Many flaps can reach the anterior aspect of the wrist and palm: the radial flap, the ulnar flap, Becker's flap and the posterior interosseous flap. Their respective uses are dictated by the aetiology and the size of the defect.

To cover a small zone or to replace a dystrophic scar, the flap of choice is Becker's flap, which can be used with the skin or simply as a fat flap.

When the deficit is in the palm, it is better to use the radial forearm flap, which is large and well vascularised.

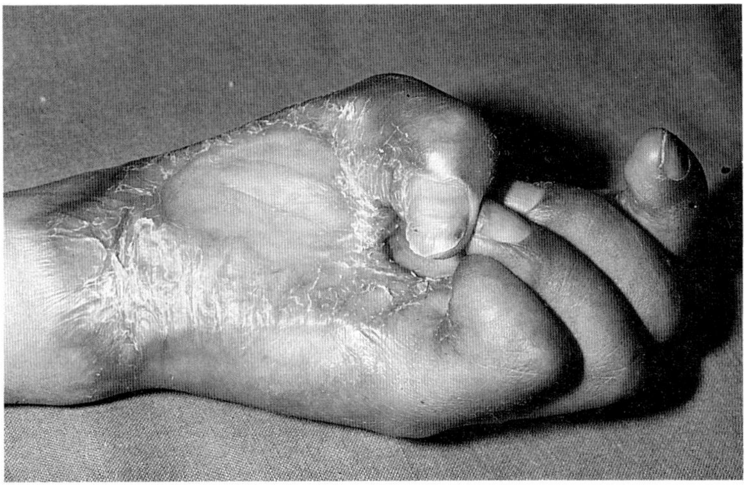

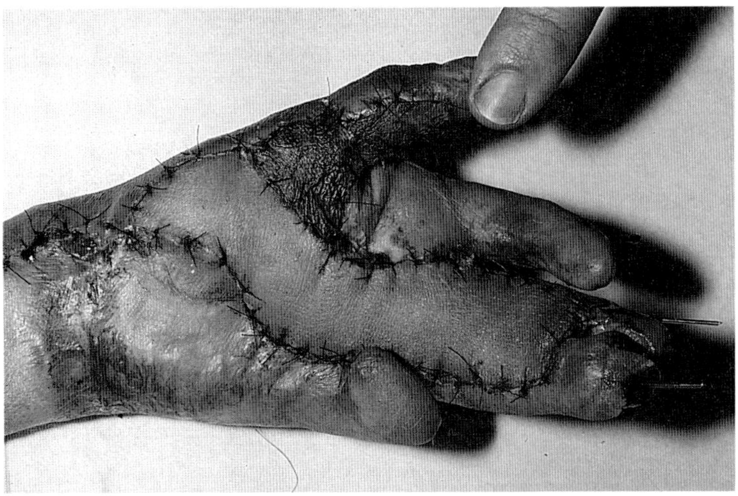

Fig. 9.9 Scar contracture of a burned hand. **A.** There is severe contracture of the fingers and thumb. **B.** The thumb contracture has been treated by full thickness skin grafts, and the finger contractures by a long radial forearm flap to be divided at a second stage.

Free flaps are sometimes necessary if there is extensive scarring of the forearm. The scapular flap or the lateral arm flap are the ones most often used.

Dorsum of the wrist and hand

The flap of choice is the radial forearm flap (Fig. 9.9) because it is thin and because its arc of rotation allows coverage of the entire dorsal surface without difficulty (Fig. 9.6). If this is not available, the posterior interosseous flap can be used. Distant pedicle flaps and free flaps are avoided, because they are thick and leave a significant aesthetic problem.

First web space

Although first web space contractures are better treated by a local flap, it is sometimes necessary to use a regional flap, and in this case it is the posterior interosseous flap (Fig. 9.7) that is best suited. Microsurgical free flaps are rarely necessary, and they must be very thin (e.g. the dorsal foot flap) (Figs. 9.8 and 9.9).

Other factors influencing the choice for flap coverage include:

1. Age: elderly patients should have the simplest possible reconstruction, without microvascular anastomosis whenever possible

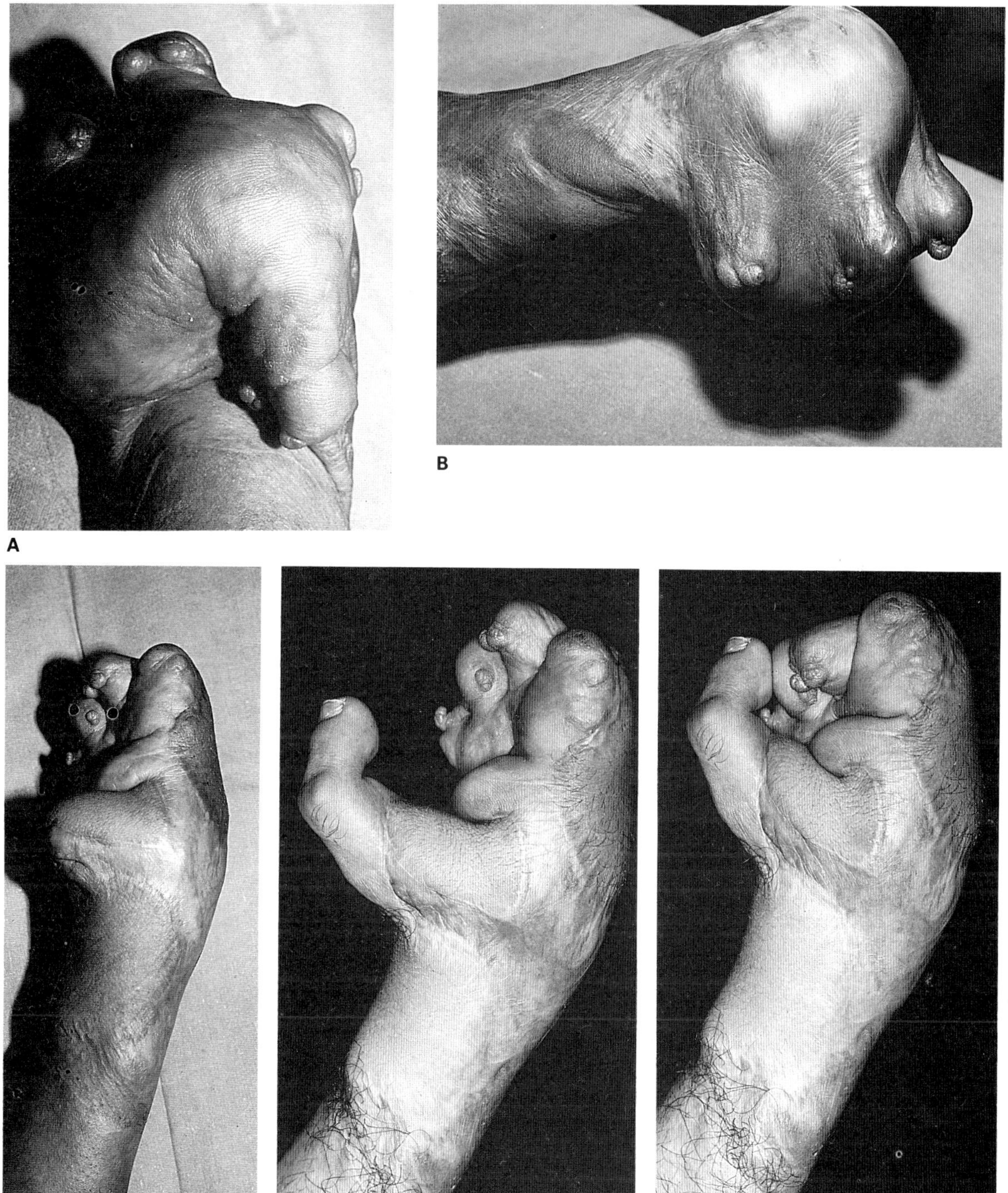

A B C D E

Fig. 9.10 Combined reconstruction for treatment of a severe burn contracture of the hand. **A.** and **B.** There are severe flexion contractures of the wrist and the first metacarpal, the metacarpals are turned completely dorsally and the skin is of very poor quality. The fingers have been amputated. **C.** Reconstruction by several techniques. A free scapular flap was used to treat the palmar wrist contracture, a pedicle inguinal flap for the dorsal finger contracture, and a radial free flap from the opposite forearm for the first web space. **D.** and **E.** The reconstruction is completed by a toe transfer to the first metacarpal, which creates a pinch.

2. Smoking: microvascular suture should be avoided in smokers
3. Sex: conspicuous scars on the arm and forearm should be avoided in women
4. Obesity.

CONCLUSION

For the upper extremity, it is no longer possible to discuss the indications for free flaps with microvascular anastomosis without also referring to pedicle flaps.

The indications for the use of free flaps result from contraindications for other flaps, e.g. extensive burns, distal vascular lesions precluding retrograde circulation, and excessive surface area.

In spite of the large number of available flaps, only a few of them are suitable for coverage in the upper extremity and hand (Fig. 9.10).

REFERENCES

Bartlett S P, May J W Jr, Yaremchuc M J 1981 The latissimus dorsi muscle: a fresh cadaver study of the primary neurovascular pedicle. Plastic and Reconstructive Surgery 67: 631

Barwick W J, Goodkind D J, Serafin D 1985 The free scapular flap. Plastic and Reconstructive Surgery 55: 177

Becker C, Gilbert A 1988 Der Ulnaris-Lappen Handchirurgie 20: 180–183

Bostwick J III, Nahai F, Wallac J G and Vasconez L O 1979 Sixty latissimus dorsi flaps. Plastic and Reconstructive Surgery 63: 31

Cormack G C, Lamberty B G H 1984 Fasciocutaneous vessels in the upper arm: application to the design of new fasciocutaneous flaps. Plastic and Reconstructive Surgery 74: 244

Daniel R K, Terzis J, Midgley R D 1976 Restoration of sensation to an anaesthetic hand by a free neurovascular flap from the foot. Plastic and Reconstructive Surgery 57: 275

Dos Santos L F 1980 Le lambeau scapulaire et l'artère cutanée scapulaire. Mem. Lab. Anat. Paris

Foucher G, Van Genechten F, Merle M, Michon J 1984 A compound radial artery forearm flap in hand surgery: An originial modification of the Chinese forearm flap. British Journal of Plastic Surgery 37: 139–148

Gilbert A, Morrison W, Tubiana R, Lisfranc R, Firmin F 1975 Transfert sur la main d'un lambeau libre sensible provenant du pied. Chirurgie 101: 621

Gilbert A, Teot L 1982 The free scapular flap. Plastic and Reconstructive Surgery 69: 601

Gilbert A, Restrepo J 1980 Le long supinateur: anatomie et utilisation comme lambeau de rotation musculaire. Annales de Chirurgie Plastique et Esthetique 25: 72–175

Katsaros J, Schustermann M, Beppu M, Banis J C, Acland R D 1984 The lateral upper arm flap: anatomy and clinical applications Annales de Chirurgie Plastique et Esthetique 12: 489

Lassen M, Krag C, Nielsen I M 1985 The latissimus dorsi flap. Scandinavian Journal of Plastic and Reconstructive Surgery 19: 41

Man D, Acland R C 1980 The micro-arterial anatomy of the dorsalis pedis flap and its clinical applications. Plastic and Reconstructive Surgery 65: 419

Masquelet A C 1984 Anatomy of the radial forearm flap. Anatomia Clinica 6: 171

Masquelet A C 1987 Le lambeau interosseux postérieur. Annales de Chirurgie de la Main 6 (2): 132

May J W, Chait L A, Cohen B E, O'Brien B McC 1977 Free neurovascular flap from the foot in hand reconstruction. Journal of Hand Surgery 5: 387

Mayou B J, Whitby D, Jones B M 1982 The scapular free flap: an anatomical and clinical study. British Journal of Plastic Surgery 35: 8

McGraw J B, Furlow L T 1975 The dorsalis pedis arterialized flap. A clinical study. Plastic and Reconstructive Surgery 55: 177

McGraw J B, Arnold P G McGraw and Arnold's atlas of muscle and musculocutaneous flaps. Hampton Press Publishing Company, Norfolk.

Muhlbauer W, Herndl E, Stock W 1982 The forearm flap. Plastic and Reconstructive Surgery 70: 336

Robinson D W 1976 Microsurgical transfer of dorsalis pedis neurovascular island flap. British Journal of Plastic Surgery 29: 209

Song R Y, Gao Y Z, Song Y G, Yu Y S, Song Y L 1982 The forearm flap. Clinics in Plastic Surgery 9.1: 21

Timmons M J, Missoten F E M, Poole M D, Davies D M 1986 Complications of radial forearm flap donor sites. British Journal of Plastic Surgery 39: 176

Tobin G R et al 1981 The intramuscular neurovascular anatomy of the latissimus dorsi muscle: the basis for splitting the flap. Plastic and Reconstructive Surgery 67 (5): 637

Urbaniak J R (ed) 1987 Microsurgery of major limb reconstruction. C V Mosby, St Louis

Urbaniak J R, Koman L A, Goldner R D, Armstrong N B, Nunley J A 1982 The vascularized cutaneous scapular flap. Plastic and Reconstructive Surgery 69: 772

Yang Guofan, Gao Yuzhi 1981, 1982 Forearm free skin transplantation. National Medical Journal of China (Journal of the Chinese Medical Association) 61: 139 (In Chinese). Abstracted in Plastic and Reconstructive Surgery 69: 1041

Zancolli E, Mitre H 1973 Latissimus dorsi transfer to restore elbow flexion. Journal of Bone and Joint Surgery 55 A (6): 1265

Zancolli E, Angrigiani C 1986 Colgajo dorsal de antebrazo (en islo) Rev. Ass. Argentina de Ortop. y Traumat. 51: 161–168

R. T. Manktelow

10 Functioning muscle transfer

Functioning microvascular muscle transfer is the transfer of a skeletal muscle from one location to another. Survival depends on microvascular anastomoses between the muscle and the recipient bed, and active contraction is produced by suturing the muscle's motor nerve to a recipient motor nerve.

INTRODUCTION

Functioning muscle transfer was first reported by Tamai (Tamai et al 1970) in the experimental animal. This work was a stimulus to surgeons to apply the technique to patients with major muscle defects.

The initial clinical experience occurred in the upper extremity to replace long finger flexor musculature. Surgeons at the Sixth Peoples Hospital, in Shanghai, reported in 1976 a successful transplantation of the lateral portion of the pectoralis major to the forearm for replacement of long finger flexor musculature. Subsequent experience was reported by Ikuta et al (1976), O'Brien (1977), Manktelow and McKee (1978) and Manktelow, Zuker and McKee (1984). Extremity muscle transfer has remained a strong area of activity. However, the use of functioning muscle transfer for facial paralysis reconstruction, which was introduced by Harii et al (1976) brought a powerful new technique to the problems of facial paralysis reconstruction.

MUSCLE PHYSIOLOGY

The purpose of skeletal muscle is to produce a controlled force. This force can be exerted while the muscle is in a static state or while it is shortening or lengthening. The basic functioning unit is the myofibril. Many myofibrils composed of actin and myosin form a cellular muscle fibre unit. Contraction is produced by the dynamic process of the adjacent actin and myosin fibres sliding over each other into an overlapped position. At maximum extension, there is very little overlap. With muscle contraction, overlap increases until it is complete. The strongest contraction of the muscle represents the point at which there is total overlap of actin and myosin fibres. With further contraction, there is crumpling of myosin fibres, less area of overlap and correspondingly less force of contraction. The surgeon who wishes to use a muscle for a functioning transfer and obtain the maximum force of contraction should transfer the muscle so that it functions within the peak portion of the length–tension curve. In our laboratory, Kuzon and McKee (Kuzon et al 1984) demonstrated that the experimental microneurovascular muscle transplantation in dogs produced muscle transfers which had a maximum force of contraction 35–125% that of the control muscle in the opposite limb. They were impressed with the potential of obtaining a normally functioning muscle after transfer in some of their animals.

The response of an individual muscle fibre is an 'all-or-none' phenomenon. The force of contraction of a muscle depends upon the number of individual muscle fibres that contract, as well the length which the muscle is required to contract. With a weak muscle contraction, only a few muscle fibres are functioning, whereas with a strong contraction, most of the fibres respond. In a strap muscle with parallel muscle fibres, the maximum strength of contraction varies directly with the cross-sectional area of the muscle. In a pennate muscle, which has shorter muscle fibres arranged in a feather-type configuration, the maximum force of contraction varies with the aggregate of all muscle fibres over the overall length of the muscle. For this reason, pennate muscles are stronger for a given total muscle mass, but have a shorter range of excursion. The maximum tension developed experimentally on tetanic stimulation in mammals is 4 kg/cm^2 (Carlson & Wilkie 1974). The surgeon's objective should be to select a muscle which has a range of excursion and a muscle strength which adequately replace the functional deficit in the extremity.

MUSCLE SELECTION

Muscle selection is based upon:

1. The anatomical requirements — neurovascular anatomy and gross anatomy which allows the muscle to fit the defect
2. Functional potential — strength, range of excursion and lack of fatigue
3. Donor site deficit — the ability of the muscle to be removed without leaving a significant cosmetic or functional deficit.

Many muscles have been used for transfer, including the gracilis, latissimus dorsi, tensor fascia lata, rectus femoris, one head of the gastrocnemius, the serratus anterior and the pectoralis major and minor. Undoubtedly many other muscles will be used as their functional anatomy becomes more clearly understood. The most commonly used muscle has been the gracilis. Its functional anatomy and the detailed technique of elevating this muscle are described by Manktelow (1986).

This muscle has a potential of shortening 12–16 cm. The muscle has a reliable neurovascular pedicle, and a good length for insertion into the upper and lower arm. There is a useful tendon of origin and a long tendon of insertion which facilitate its attachment to distal tendons. When removed, the muscle has no functional loss, and the cosmetic defect, a scar on the medial aspect of the upper thigh, is well accepted.

INDICATIONS

Functioning muscle transfer is reserved for those patients for whom no suitable simpler procedures are available, such as tendon transfers, tenodeses or fusions. The suitable patient has sustained a major loss of a functional group of skeletal muscle which has resulted in a significant deficit, such as loss of finger flexion, finger extension, elbow flexion or shoulder flexion (Fig. 10.1A). The most common causes of muscle loss have been direct trauma, including Volkmann's ischaemic paralysis, electrical burns, gas gangrene and tumour resection.

Patient selection is important. A suitable patient is one who has sustained a limited injury for which the transfer of a single functioning muscle will provide a useful functional improvement. In the most common situation of finger flexor muscle replacement, the patient will have an adequate mechanism for finger extension and wrist stabilisation, adequate finger sensibility, and sufficient intrinsic function to provide a stable balanced flexion of the fingers (Fig. 10.1B). There must be a good passive range of motion of the joints, and flexor tendons must be available with a good gliding bed. In addition, there should be skin coverage available for the distal half of the muscle transfer to allow good muscle tendon gliding.

SURGICAL TECHNIQUE (Fig. 10.1C–G)

In order to decrease the operating time, the recipient site and the muscle are usually prepared simultaneously by two teams.

Recipient site preparation involves the identification and preparation for repair of 5 structures:

1. Site of muscle origin
2. Site of muscle insertion
3. Skin flap to house the muscle
4. Vessels for revascularisation
5. A nerve for re-innervation.

The surgeon can anticipate the location of most of

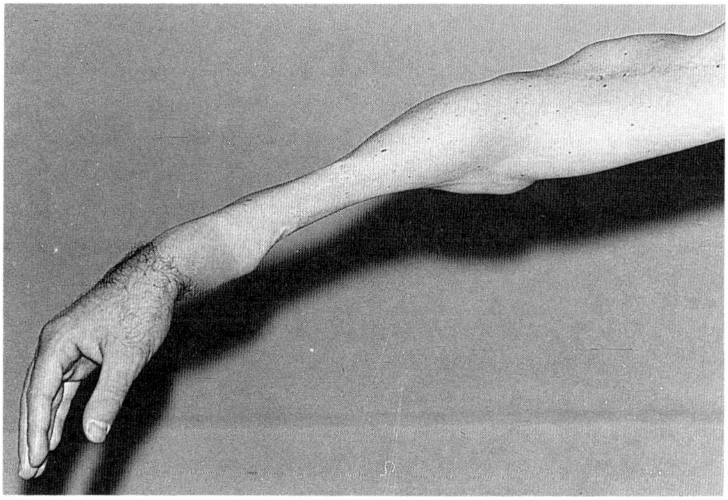

A

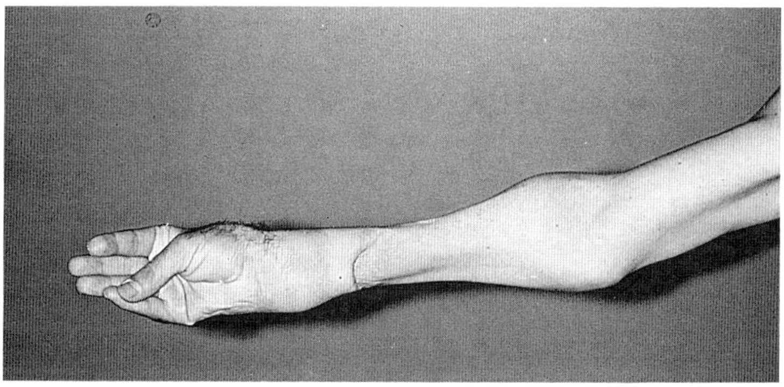

B

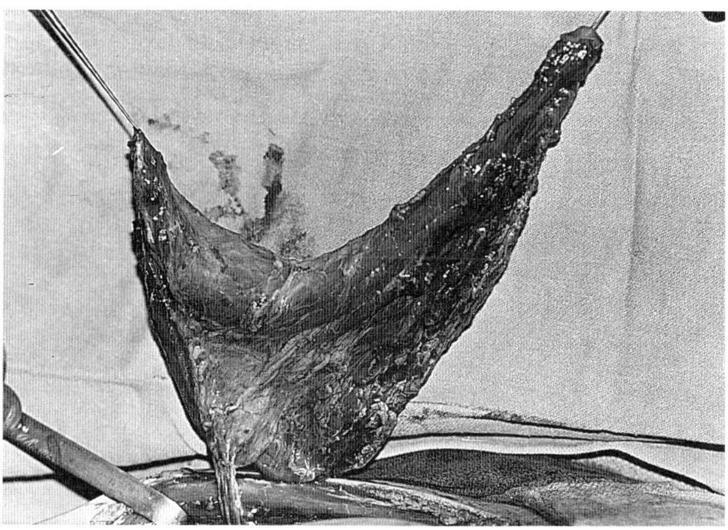

C

Fig. 10.1 **A.** Preoperative appearance of patient with a traumatic loss of flexor and extensor musculature. The only forearm muscles remaining are the extensor carpi radialis and brachioradialis. **B.** Normal hand sensation and intrinsic function are present, allowing thumb opposition and MP flexion. Patient's functional deficit is long finger flexion and extension. **C.** The right pectoralis major muscle has been separated from the chest and is viewed from below while still attached to the thoraco-acromial vascular pedicle. The curved upper surface of the muscle represents the lateral free margin.

D

E

F

G

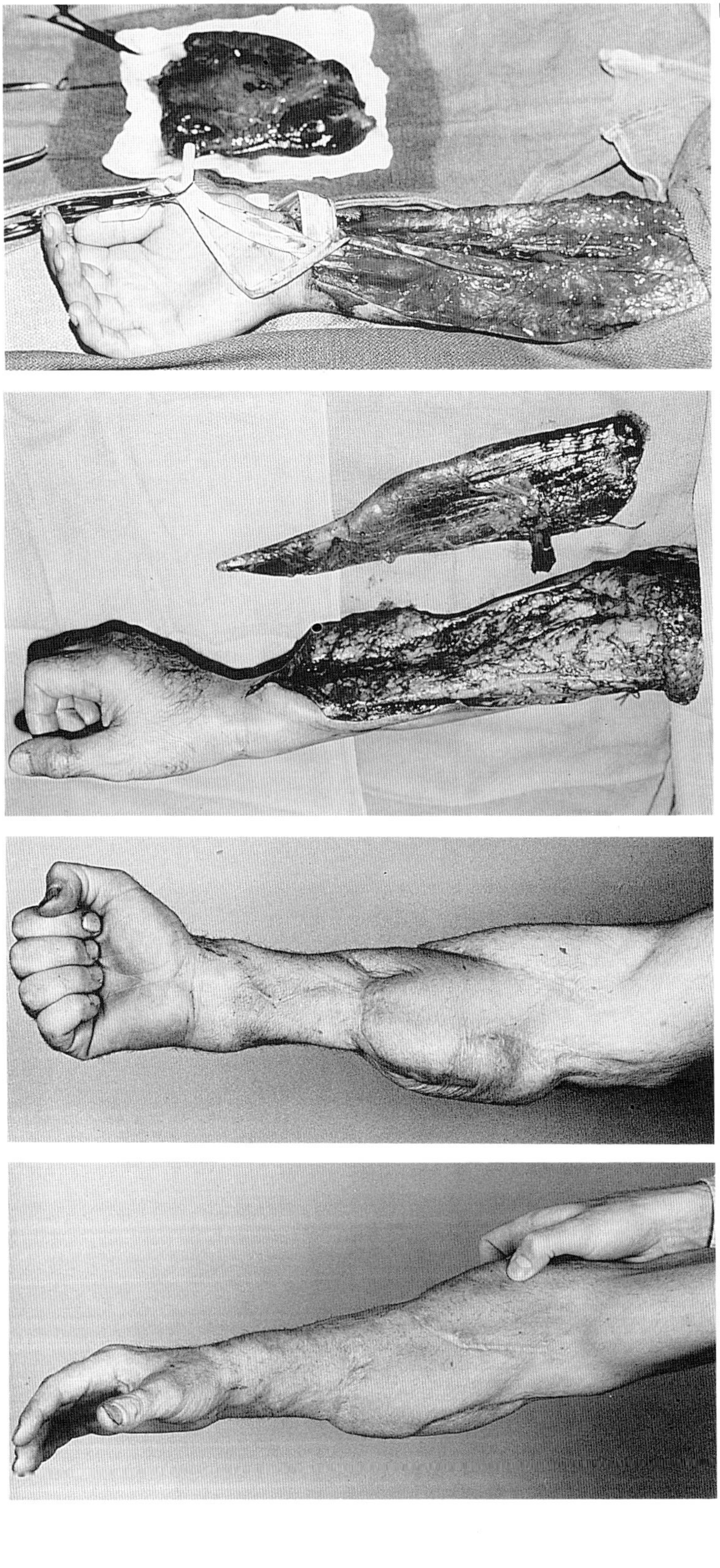

Fig. 10.1 (cont) **D.** Forearm has been prepared. Long finger flexor tendons and flexor carpi radialis are held by penrose drain. Musculature is absent. The muscle can be seen in the upper portion of the picture, lying on white sponges. The sternal origin was attached to the profundus and flexor pollicis longus tendons. Innervation was with the branches of the anterior interosseus nerve. **E.** One year later at second operation gracilis muscle is seen lying above the prepared dorsum of the forearm. Muscle was inserted into the extensor digitorum communis and extensor pollicis longus tendons. Innervation was through the posterior interosseous nerve. **F.** Pectoralis major muscle provides a full fist and thumb flexion. Grip strength is 28 kg. The bulge in the proximal half of the forearm represents the contracting pectoralis major muscle. **G.** Gracilis muscle provides good finger and thumb extension. The examiner's hand is seen palpating the contracting muscle. An extensor tenolysis could produce fuller extension (From: Manktelow 1986)

these structures from knowledge of the extent of the pathology. An arteriogram is frequently required to assess the presence and condition of recipient arteries.

Selecting a nerve for re-innervation may be difficult. In a badly damaged arm, it is often difficult to anticipate what will be available before surgical exploration. The preferred nerves in the upper extremity are: the anterior interosseous for finger flexion; the posterior interosseous for finger extension; and the motor branches of the musculocutaneous and axillary for elbow flexion and shoulder flexion. A preliminary operative procedure to explore and biopsy the nerve may be required. This is a crucial part of the operative planning, as without a normal nerve for re-innervation, useful muscle function cannot be expected.

Preparation of the muscle

Of the various muscles that are available, the most suitable one can be selected based on the anatomical and functional needs of the recipient site. A pattern taken from the arm and outlining the size and shape of the anticipated muscle and the location of the expected recipient nerve and vessels will allow the surgeon to select the most useful muscle.

The technique for removing these muscles has been described, and is based on an understanding of the gross and microneurovascular anatomy (Manktelow 1986). When the muscle is still attached by its pedicle, but has been separated from its surrounding tissues and the origin and insertion divided, its circulation should be assessed by observing the muscle's colour. Contractility, bleeding and colour are the usual signs of muscle viability. If any part of the distal portion of the muscle is not viable, it should be removed, and the cut ends re-attached to the intramuscular portion of the tendon.

Muscle transplantation

When the bed has been prepared, the muscle is transferred and immediate revascularisation carried out to minimise the ischaemia time. However, experimental evidence by Kuzon and McKee indicates that a warm ischaemia time of 3 hours is not detrimental to the function of muscle transfer (Kuzon et al 1984). When the muscle has been placed in the recipient area, the desired location is determined by its origin and insertion, and the location of the neurovascular pedicle.

Revascularisation

A technically perfect arterial and venous repair should be done. The selected point of the anastomosis is important, as with excursion of the muscle, traction can be placed on the muscle's pedicle if the intraoperative planning is incorrect.

Re-innervation

A fascicular repair, placed as close as possible to the neuromuscular hilum, is done. As there is considerable fatty connective tissue in the motor nerve of some muscles, such as the gracilis, a fascicular repair is likely to produce better apposition of axons.

Balanced tendon fixation

If the muscle is used to produce movement of more than one tendon, as in flexor or extensor finger reconstruction, it is important that the individual profundus tendons move in such a way as to provide synchronous finger flexion. This can be accomplished by initially sewing the profundus tendons side-to-side in a balanced position. If the muscle is used to provide thumb flexion as well, it is desirable to have the fingers flex first and the thumb come down afterwards to provide a key pinch type of contact with the radial aspect of the index finger. After side-to-side fixation of the tendons, the transferred muscle is then attached to the tendons by a strong interweaving technique.

Optimum tension

Using a marking technique, as shown by Manktelow (Manktelow & McKee 1978), the muscle can be transferred in such a manner that the optimum portion of the length–tension curve will be used by the patient (Fig. 10.2 A and B).

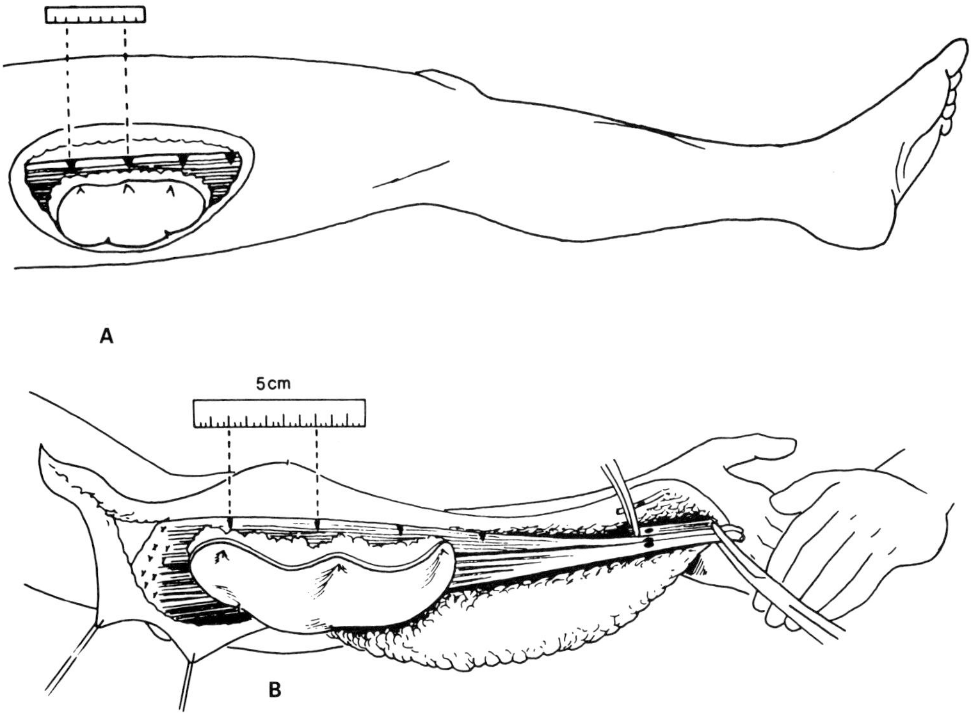

Fig. 10.2 **A.** The technique of stretching the gracilis muscle preoperatively, and application of markers at 5 cm intervals is outlined. This is done with the muscle at its physiological extended maximum length which is produced by abducting the thigh and extending the knee. **B.** The gracilis muscle is shown transferred to the forearm. The origin is attached to the medial epicondyle and common flexor fascial origin. The correct tension is determined by pulling on the gracilis tendon until the previously placed marks on the surface are at 5 cm intervals. This represents the maximum physiological stretched length of the muscle, which is the length which is desired when the wrist and fingers are fully extended, and can be used in the forearm when the wrist and fingers are fully extended. With the wrist and fingers fully extended, the position of the tendons relative to each other is the position at which the suture repair between the transferred gracilis tendon and the flexor digitorum profundus tendon is done. (Reproduced with permission from Manktelow R T 1986 Microvascular Reconstruction: Anatomy, Applications and Surgical Technique, Springer–Verlag, Heidelberg).

Skin flap coverage

There must be good skin flap cover for the neurovascular repairs and for the distal half of the muscle and tendon-to-tendon repair (Fig. 10.3). In an injured extremity, there may be insufficient skin cover for this portion of the muscle, and a preliminary flap or tissue expansion procedure may be necessary to develop flap coverage. The proximal half of the muscle can be covered with a split-thickness skin graft, and this will not impede functional excursion.

POSTOPERATIVE CARE

The extremity is splinted in such a way as to relax the muscle attachments. It is unlikely that the tendon repairs will be pulled apart, as there is no active function within the muscle for some time. After a three week period for tendon healing, the muscle is stretched by extending or flexing the extremity to develop a good tendon gliding bed at the tendon–muscle junction. When innervation has occurred, the patient is encouraged to use the extremity actively, and increase the range of excursion of the functioning muscle. When reasonable excursion has been obtained, the patient is placed on an exercise program designed to produce maximum strength in the muscle.

Muscle transplantation can provide successful restoration of function for finger flexion, finger extension, elbow flexion or shoulder flexion. However, this operative procedure is complex, and maximum functional results are not obtained for

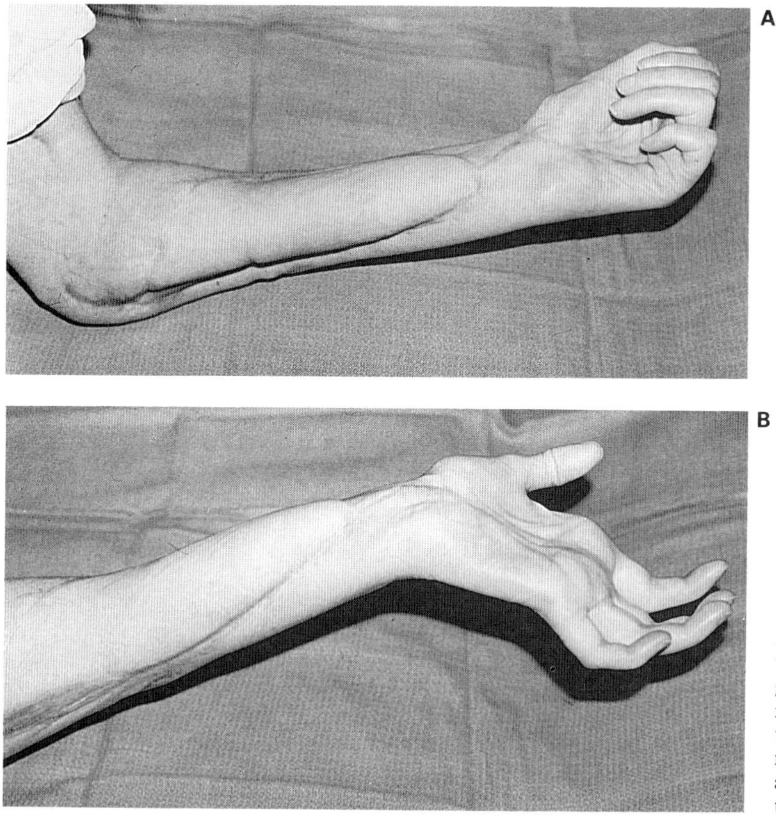

Fig. 10.3 **A.** Patient who sustained a loss of all flexor musculature and injury to the extensors with a gunshot wound to the forearm. An abdominal skin flap has been applied to the flexor aspect of the forearm. One year following gracilis muscle transplantation, the muscle provides almost full flexion of the fingers. **B.** With relaxation of the muscle, nearly full finger extension is allowed. Note slight clawing from the ulnar nerve paralysis.

1–2 years following surgery. If simpler techniques of tendon transfer are available, they should be used. Careful preoperative planning, meticulous surgical technique and a thorough program of postoperative exercises are required for a successful result.

REFERENCES

Carlson F D, Wilkie D R 1974 Muscle physiology. Prentice-Hall, Englewood, New Jersey

Harii K, Ohmori K, Sekiguchi J 1976 The free musculocutaneous flap. Plastic and Reconstructive Surgery 57: 294

Ikuta Y, Kubo T, Tsuge K 1976 Free muscle transplantation by microsurgical technique to treat severe Volkmann's contracture. Plastic and Reconstructive Surgery 58: 407

Kuzon W M, Fish J S, Pynn B R, McKee N H 1984 Determinants of contractile function in free muscle transfers. Surgical Forum 35: 610

Manktelow R T, McKee N H 1978 Free muscle transplantation to provide active finger flexion. Journal of Hand Surgery 3: 416

Manktelow R T, Zuker R M, McKee N H 1984 Functional free muscle transplantation. Journal of Hand Surgery 9A: 32

Manktelow R T 1986 Microsurgical reconstruction: anatomy, applications and surgical technique. Springer Verlag, Heidelberg

O'Brien B McC 1977 Microvascular and reconstructive surgery. Churchill Livingstone, Edinburgh, p 29

Shanghai Sixth Peoples Hospital 1976 Free muscle transplantation by microsurgical neurovascular anastomoses. Chinese Medical Journal 2: 47

Tamai S, Komatsu S, Sakamoto H et al 1970 Free muscle transplants in dogs with microsurgical neurovascular anastomoses. Plastic and Reconstructive Surgery 46: 219

R. W. H. Pho

11 Vascularised bone grafts in upper extremity reconstruction

INTRODUCTION

Vascularised bone graft was first described by Huntington in 1905. He transferred the diaphysis of a fibula based on a muscular pedicle to bridge a large bony defect in the tibia. The transfer of free vascularised bone grafts was first initiated by Ostrup and Fredrickson's experimental work in 1975. The first documented clinical case of free living fibular graft, based on a peroneal vascular pedicle, was reported by Taylor, Miller and Ham in 1975. Weiland and others reported the use of free vascularised bone grafts in upper extremity reconstruction in 1979, and Pho reported the use of vascularised fibular grafts in replacement of the radius, as a vascularised hemi-joint transfer in 1979. This technique has clearly demonstrated its value in difficult reconstructions of the upper extremity. The vascularised bone graft not only acts as a space filler and strut support to bridge the bony defect, but also introduces new vascular supply at the recipient site.

INDICATIONS FOR VASCULARISED BONE GRAFTS IN UPPER EXTREMITY RECONSTRUCTION

Indications for vascularised bone grafts in upper extremity reconstruction are no different from lower extremity reconstruction. They are mainly used for:

1. Bridging a large bony defect in congenital conditions, such pseudo-arthrosis of radius, ulna, humerus or in radial club hand
2. Reconstruction following bone tumour resection
3. Management of osteomyelitis
4. Post-traumatic bone loss
5. Revascularisation of avascular scaphoid or lunate
6. Complicated arthrodesis of joints.

I want to emphasise that vascularised bone grafts are indicated mainly to solve difficult problems in upper extremity reconstruction, when conventional techniques could lead to unpredictable results and protracted rehabilitation with multiple surgical procedures.

In severe injuries of the extremities, very often we encounter the associated problems of soft tissue and bony loss, infection, poor vascularity and loss of segments of bone, leading to secondary deformities. There is only one technique that can overcome all these problems as a one-stage reconstruction, that is, the use of vascularised composite tissue transfer. There are many types of transfer available:

1. Composite skin, nail, pulp, tendon, nerves, toe phalanx and joint for reconstructing thumb or digits
2. Composite bone and tendon to replace metacarpals in hand reconstruction
3. Composite skin, bone and muscle in forearm reconstruction
4. Proximal fibula and its fibrocartilaginous head for vascularised hemi-joint transfer, or its epiphysis for replacement of radius or humerus in growing children.

SOURCES OF VASCULARISED BONE GRAFTS

1. Local pediculed transfer of bone graft from neighbouring parts of the body

1. Rib graft and sternum for proximal humeral replacement (Fig. 11.1A and B), distal radius or ulna for replacement of distal humerus (Fig. 11.2)
2. Proximal radius or ulna for replacement of metacarpals in thumb and hand reconstruction
3. Pisiform branch of ulnar artery; pronator quadratus transfer (Braun); dorsal metacarpal or volar digital vascular pedicle transfer in revascularisation of the avascular scaphoid or lunate.

2. Free vascularised bone graft

1. Iliac crest based on superficial or deep circumflex iliac vessels
2. Fibula and its epiphysis based on peroneal or anterior tibial vessels
3. Second metatarsals based on the dorsalis pedis vessels
4. Radius or ulnar osteocutaneous transfer based on radial, ulnar, or anterior or posterior interosseous vessels.

All the local pedicled transfers from adjacent bones in the same limb, may also be used as free vascularised bone grafts for opposite limb reconstruction.

REVASCULARISATION OF AVASCULAR CARPAL BONES (Fig. 11.3)

The following techniques have been used in revascularisation of Kienböck's disease and avascular necrosis of scaphoid:

1. Transfer of the second dorsal metacarpal vessels as reported by Harii and Tamai. It is believed that revascularisation with this technique arises from proliferation of capillaries around the transferred bundle, which gradually extend to vascularise the entire avascular bone. The revascularisation process would help in the resorption of the necrotic bone, and the stimulation of new bone formation and remoulding.

A

B

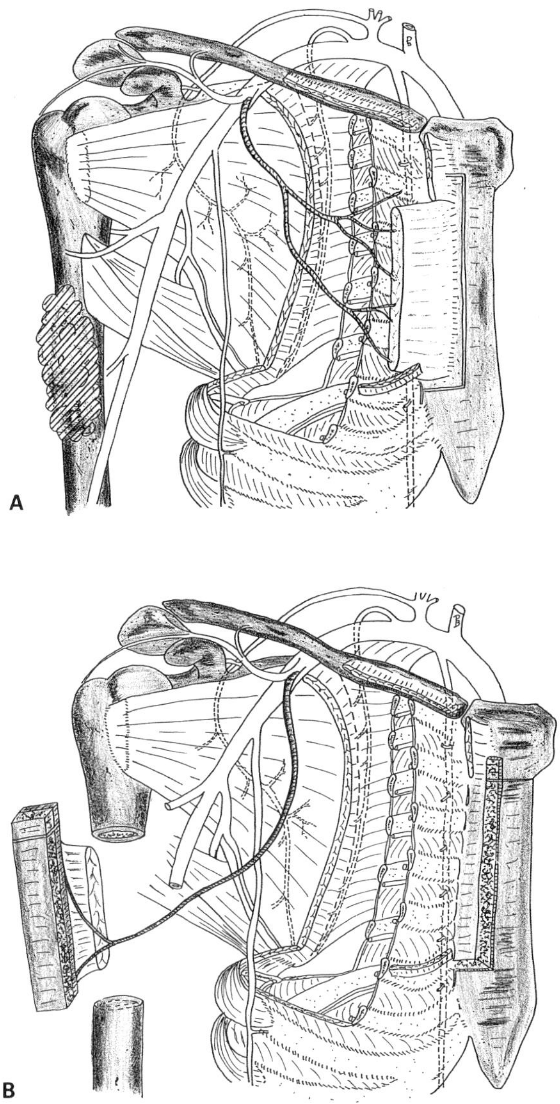

Fig. 11.1A. and **B.** Sternal bone graft based on pectoral vessel for replacement of proximal humerus.

2. Muscular pedicle bone grafts as reported by Braun, where part of the radius was elevated based on pronator quadratus muscle.
3. Use of the pisiform branch or second dorsal metacarpal vessels in revascularisation in Kienböck's disease.

The method I have used is based on the second dorsal metacarpal artery with part of the cancel-

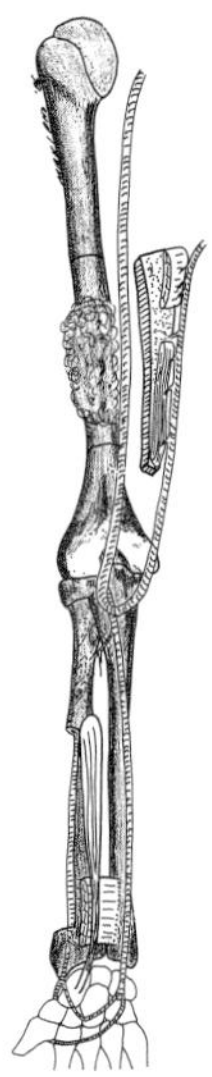

Fig. 11.2 Radial artery osteo flap for replacement of humerus.

lous bone of second metacarpal head (Fig. 11.4). The second metacarpal vessels vary in size but in most cases they are present. They can be raised together with the epipmysium of the dorsal interosseous muscles in order that the bundle can be harvested safely. One has to include the periostium, and take the bone graft at the second metacarpal head. This will ensure that the cortical and cancellous bone are connected to the vascular pedicle. It is important to preserve the periostium to ensure a good attachment of the vascular pedicle to the bone. I have used this technique for revascularisation of avascular necrosis of the scaphoid, and in those cases of non-union of the scaphoid with the avascular necrosis of the proximal pole. This technique could also be indicated for revascularisation of Kienböck's disease, and in neglected dislocation of the lunate where complete release of surrounding soft tissue is required before the lunate can be reduced. The lunate, very often, is completely avascular, and therefore will require revascularisation. Although the revascularisation concept is excellent, my own experience is that it is difficult to achieve complete revascularisation and prevent collapse of the carpal bones. This could be related to the size of the bone to be revascularised and, possibly, mechanical factors which lead to the collapse of the avascular bone.

The insertion of the vascularised bone graft into the recipient carpal bone is often difficult. Cortical strips provide strut support but it is not easy to slot them in, as most of the carpal bones tend to have large articular surfaces, thus making the seating of the graft and its pedicle very difficult. For non-union of the scaphoid, bony union is often achieved by using this technique. Symptomatically, improvements are often obtained following this procedure. This could be due to improved wrist movements and also grip strength, resulting from relief of pain.

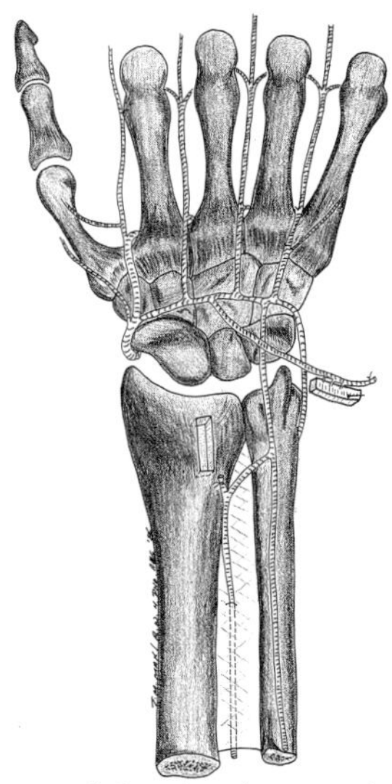

Fig. 11.3 Bone graft based on intercarpal vessel for revascularisation of carpal bone

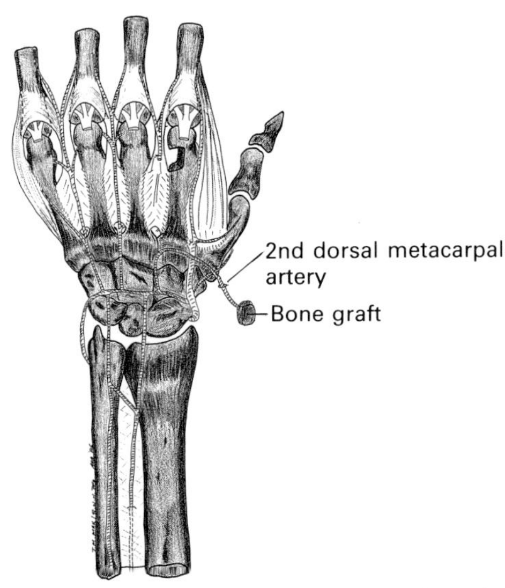

Fig. 11.4 Bone graft based on 2nd dorsal metacarpal vessel.

FREE VASCULARISED FIBULAR BONE GRAFTS IN UPPER EXTREMITY RECONSTRUCTION

Free vascularised fibular bone grafts have been our main workhorse for reconstruction of large bone defects in the upper extremity.

The vascularised fibular bone graft has the following advantages:

1. It is readily available, with length reaching about 30 cm
2. The fibula is a straight and relatively strong cortical bone
3. The vascular pedicle consists of the peroneal artery and its two venae comitantes which, although short, are large
4. The proximal part and its fibrocartilage can be harvested as a vascularised hemi-joint transfer, especially for shoulder and wrist reconstruction
5. In growing children, the proximal fibular epiphysis can also be transplanted to replace the upper humerus and the lower radius
6. The overlying skin, measuring up to 20 cm by 10 cm, can be included as an osteocutaneous transfer to provide soft tissue padding and skin cover.

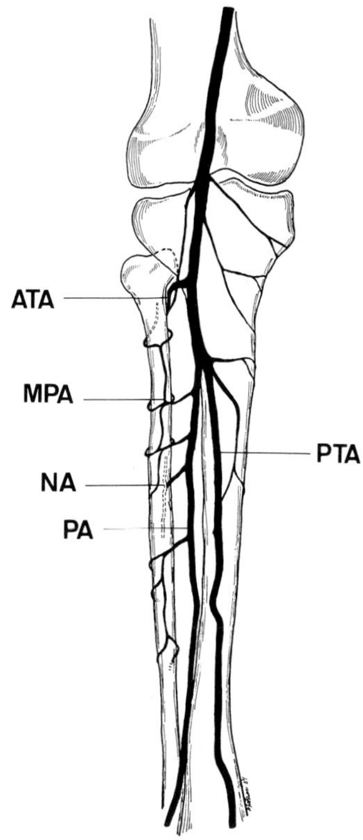

Fig. 11.5 Blood supply to fibula. PTA = posterior tibial artery. ATA = anterior tibial artery. MPA = musculoperiosteal artery. NA = nutrient artery. PA = peroneal artery.

Blood supply of the fibula (Fig. 11.5)

The diaphyseal part of the fibula receives its blood supply from the peroneal artery through the musculoperiosteal vessels and the main nutrient artery.

The peroneal artery arises from the posterior tibial artery or the popliteal artery at varying levels, and can replace the posterior tibial artery as dominant blood supply to the posterior compartment of the leg. Two venae comitantes run parallel to the peroneal artery, and provide for venous drainage from the fibula.

As intercommunicating branches, multiple longitudinal vessels run parallel to the long axis of the fibula, within and superficial to the periosteum. My own studies have shown that, in adults, the fibular head receives adequate blood supply from the peroneal artery, via the musculoperiosteal vessels. In children, the contribution of epiphyseal branches from the descending genicular vessel and anterior tibial vessel may be significant in supplying the proximal fibular epiphysis.

The skin on the lateral aspect of the leg along the whole length of the fibula receives multiple fasciocutaneous branches from the peroneal vessel, which runs along the intermuscular septum between the soleus and the peroneal compartment. These branches are each accompanied by two venae comitantes. A large piece of skin can safely be raised together with the fibula, based on its peroneal vascular pedicle. When the skin flap is incorporated, the vascular pedicle should be lengthened using the short saphenous vein as a loop, to facilitate vessel anastomosis. (Fig. 11.6A and B).

Indications for vascularised fibular bone grafts

I have used free vascularised fibular bone grafts

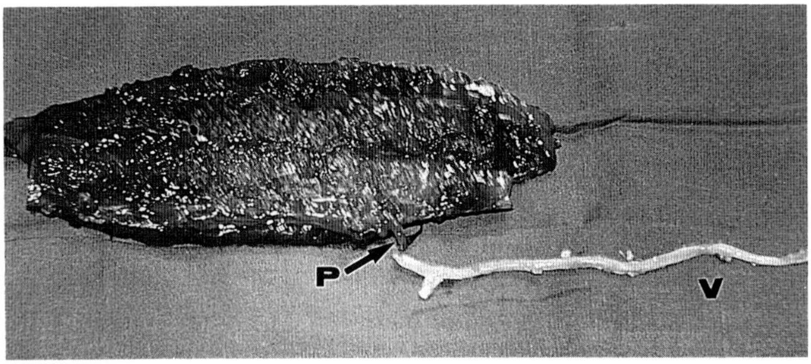

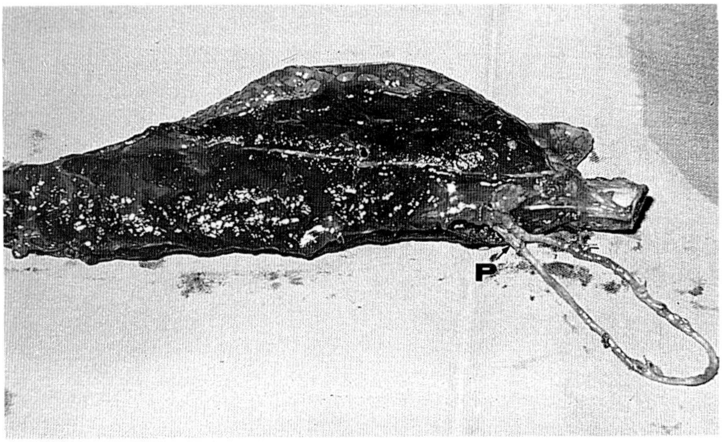

Fig. 11.6 A. Osteocutaneous fibular graft with short vascular pedicle (P) to be lengthened by vein graft (V)
B. Osteocutaneous fibular graft closed loop lengthening of vascular pedicle (P)

for upper extremity reconstruction in the following situations:

1. As an epiphyseal transplant for replacement of the lower end of the radius after tumour resection, for radial club hand, and for replacement of missing proximal humerus following osteomyelitis in children.
2. In management of problematic post-traumatic non-union of radius and ulna associated with bone gaps or soft tissue loss
3. For reconstruction of large bony defects following bone tumour resection from radius, ulna and humerus. The fibula acts as a tissue spacer to provide internal strut support for stability, and soft tissue cover. (Fig. 11.7A and B).

BONE HEALING IN FREE VASCULARISED BONE GRAFTS

Free vascularised bone grafts should be regarded as similar to a segmental fracture, with preservation of the vascular supply to the middle segment. The healing process, therefore, should be comparable to this type of fracture, with the exception that during transfer the initial ischaemic time may range from 2 to 6 hours. The time taken for bone union is therefore comparable to normal segmental fracture healing.

Although free vascularised bone grafts can be regarded as being similar to segmental fractures, they are completely denervated. Therefore, when stress fracture develops, it may be painless, unless there is extraperiosteal compression of the surrounding tissues. This is a very important point to remember when using free vascularised bone grafts for reconstruction after tumour excision. The undisplaced stress fracture site may show swelling and increased temperature, but no pain, and may be mistaken for local tumour recurrence.

The clinical observation of bone healing in free vascularised bone grafts indicates that the periosteum plays a major role in external callus

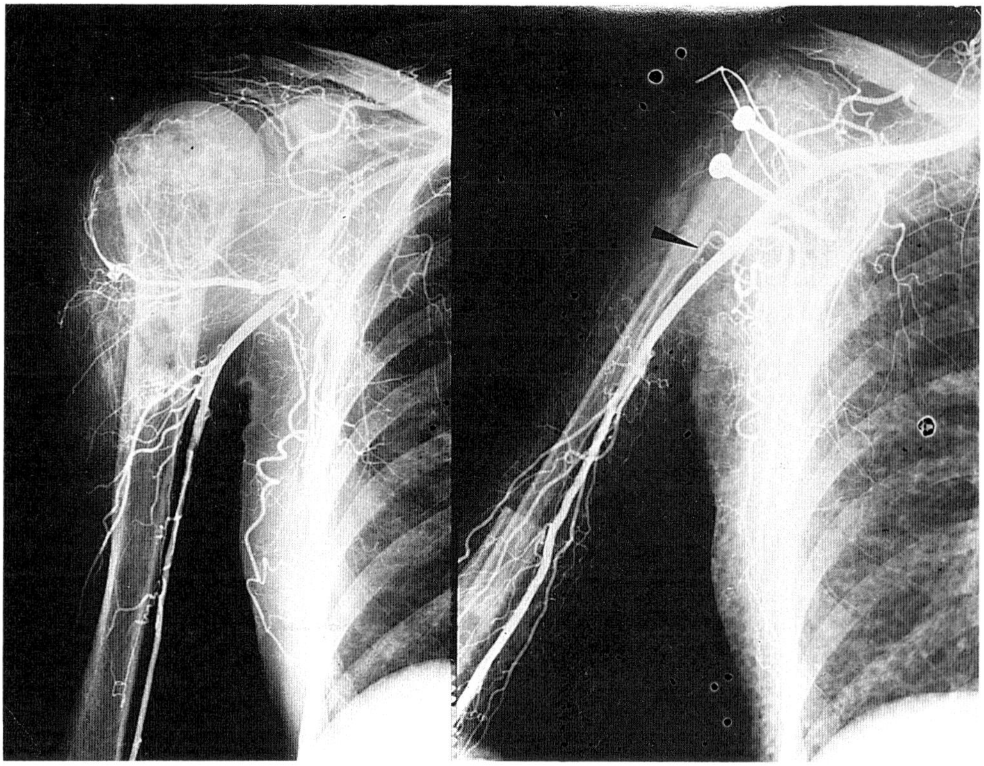

A

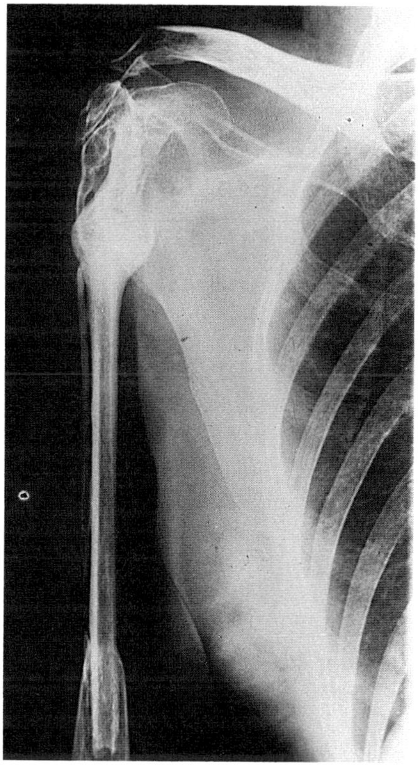

B

Fig. 11.7 A. Chondrosarcoma proximal humerus replaced with proximal fibula. Recipient circumflex vessels were sutured to peroneal vascular pedicle **B.** Successful transfer of proximal fibula in replacement of proximal humerus. The shoulder is fused with healed stress fracture at screw site.

formation. This may be related to preservation of musculoperiosteal blood vessels, as sometimes the harvested segment may not include the nutrient vessels of the bone.

BONE FIXATION

The following four different techniques of bone fixation are all used in free vascularised bone transplantation.

1. Direct plating with compression
2. Step-cut osteotomy with screw or plate fixation
3. Intramedullary type of fixation
4. Periosteocortical flap.

In most cases, I have used minimal implants and small screws, to avoid splitting the fibula, damage to the periosteal vessels and the possibility of developing stress fracture. To increase immediate stability, one should reinforce with an external fixator if indicated.

VASCULARISED FIBULA FOR REPLACEMENT OF RADIUS OR ULNA (Fig. 11.8)

Our experimental work on the torsional strength and stiffness of the fibula has shown that the radius is a stronger bone than the fibula.

We have noted the concept of Vitale, that the ulna makes the elbow joint and the radius makes the wrist joint. The stability we observed tends to depend on the extent of the residual forearm bone. Substantial defects of the proximal radius, especially after tumour resection, may result in instability of the proximal radio-ulnar joint.

If the fibula is fixed to the radius in this type of case, although one may theoretically get subluxation of the proximal radio-ulnar joint, this may be related to the demands made upon the reconstructed limb. The other factor may be the length of remaining proximal ulna. If it is too short, stability depends upon the short length of interosseous membrane, and this may be inadequate. Therefore, the choice depends on the patient. If the patient needs strength more than pronation and supination, it would be best to fix the fibular graft to the ulna proximally. If, on the other hand, rotation of the forearm is needed more than strength, and there is an adequate length of proximal radius, it is possible to fix the graft to the proximal radius. We use plates to stabilise the host graft juncture.

When proximal fibula is used as a vascularised hemi-joint transfer, the palmaris longus is used to reconstruct the wrist joint. (Figs 11.9 and 11.10)

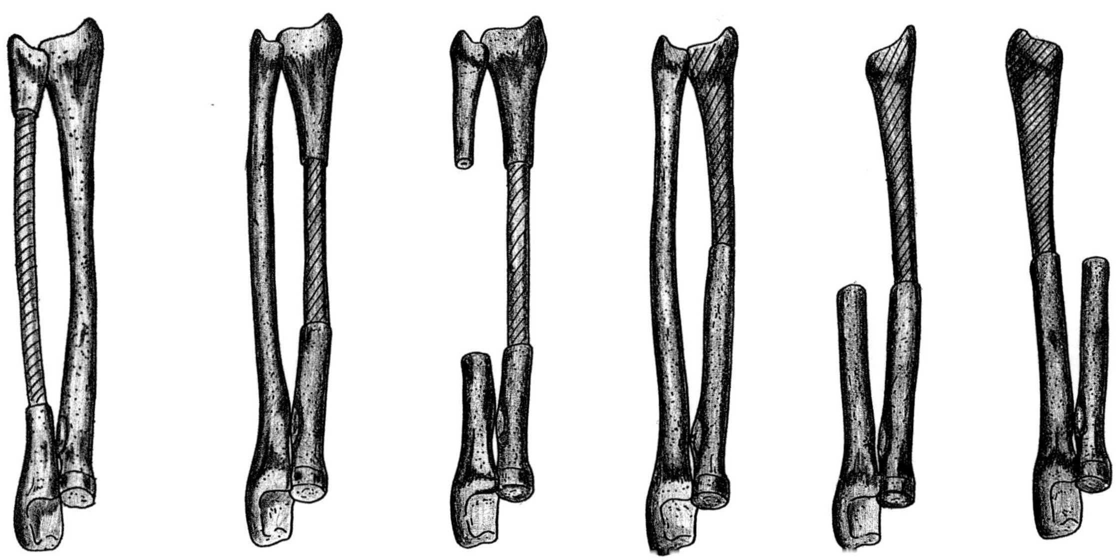

Fig. 11.8 Free vascularised fibula for replacement of radius and ulna.

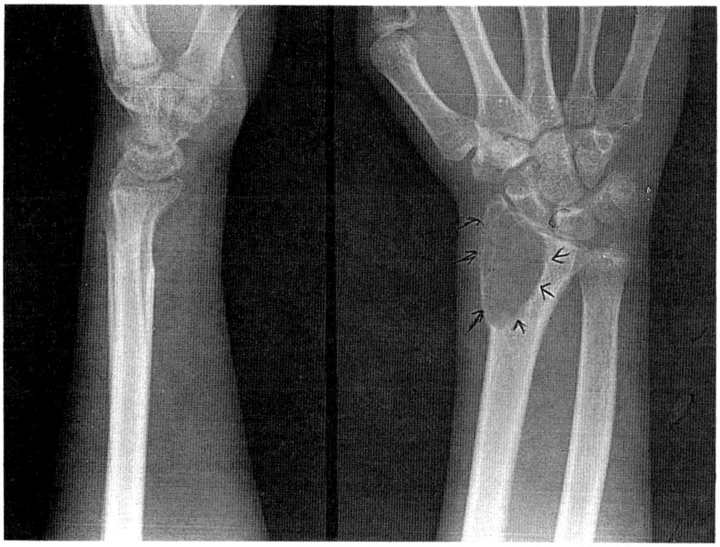

Fig. 11.9 Giant cell tumour of lower end of radius.

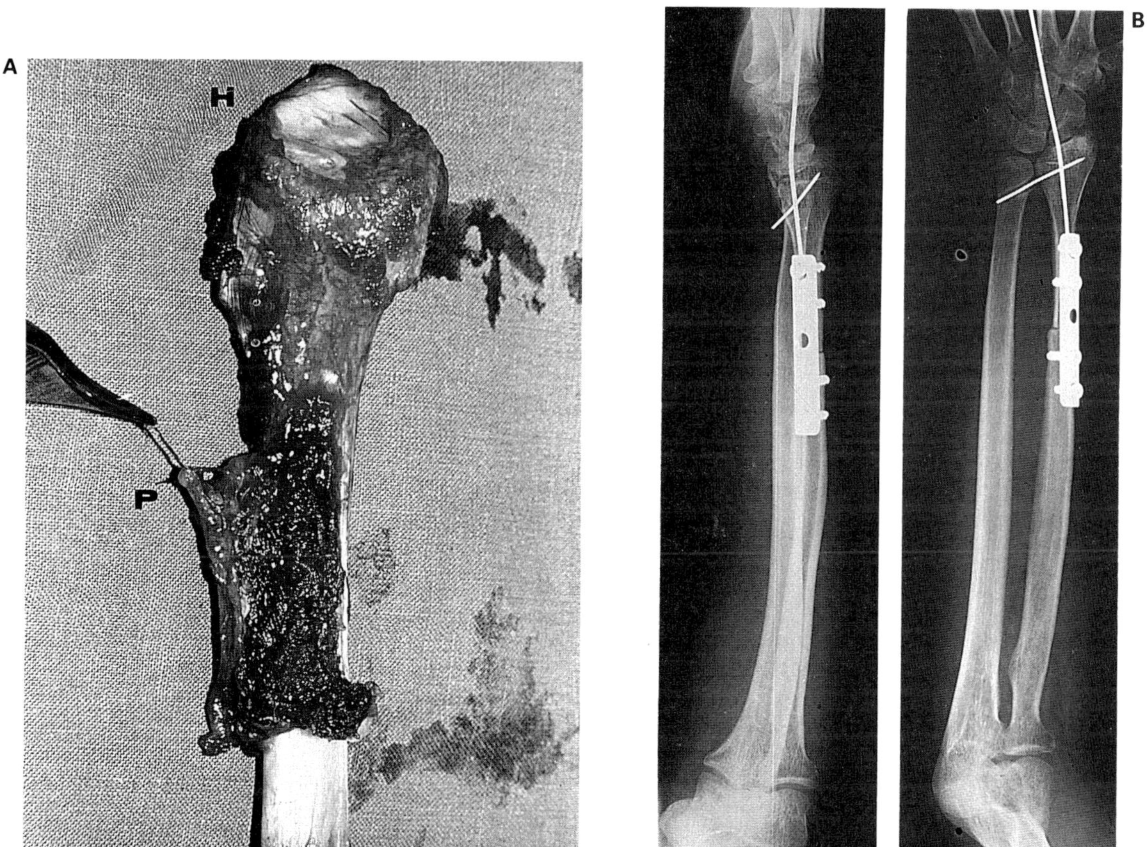

Fig. 11.10 A. and **B.** Proximal fibula as hemi-vascularised joint transfer to replace lower end of radius. Joint stability was achieved by: (1) Palmaris tendon reconstruction; (2) Kirschner wire fixation for three months.

A B C D

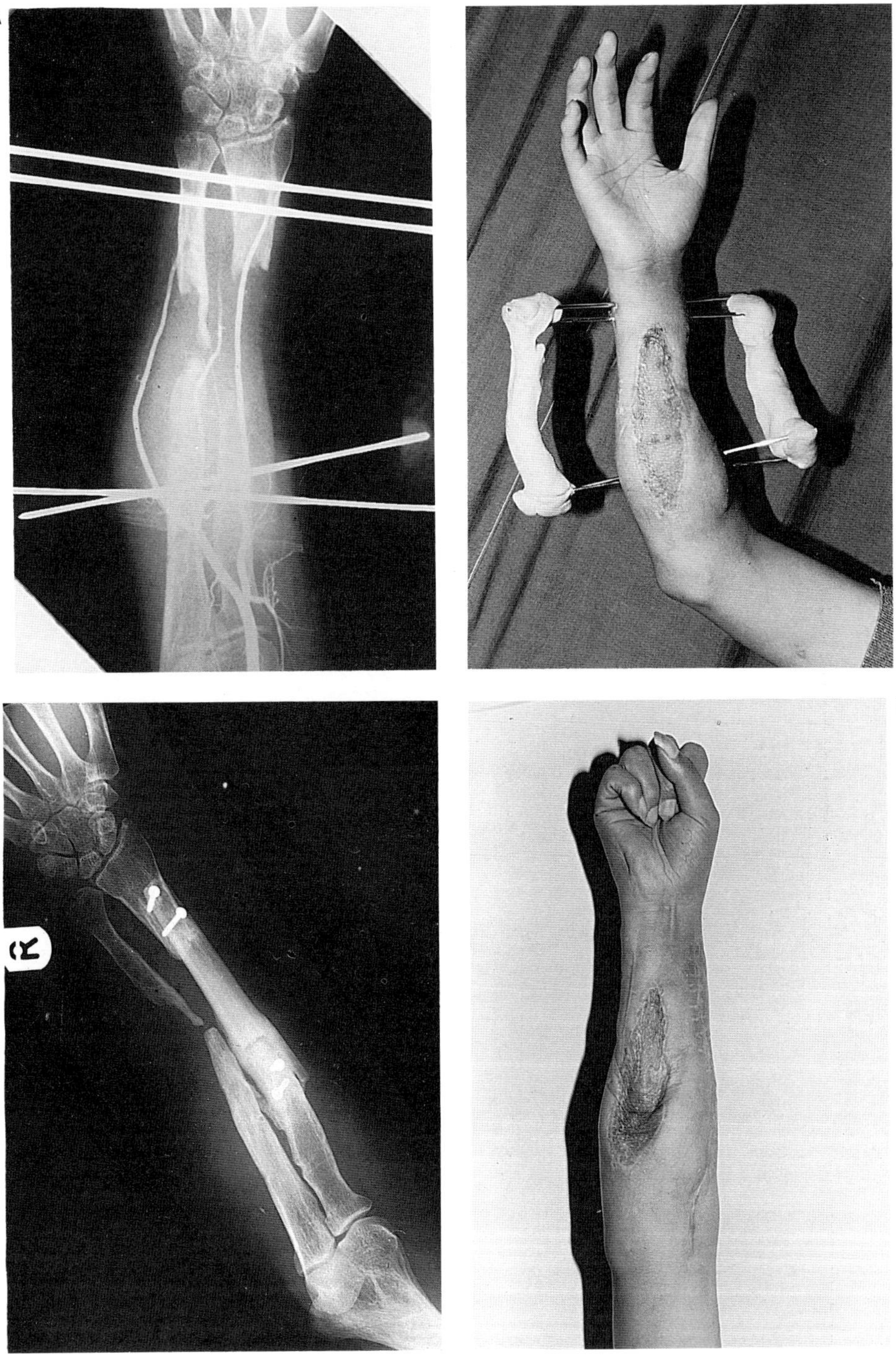

Fig. 11.11 A. Chronic osteomyelitis with large bony defect in radius and ulna with persistent discharge. **B.** External stabilisation with Steinmann's pin and cement to control infection. **C.** Successful transfer of free vascularised fibular graft to bridge bony defect in radius. Note marked hypertrophy of fibula with healed stress fracture at proximal juncture. **D.** Excellent functional results after surgery.

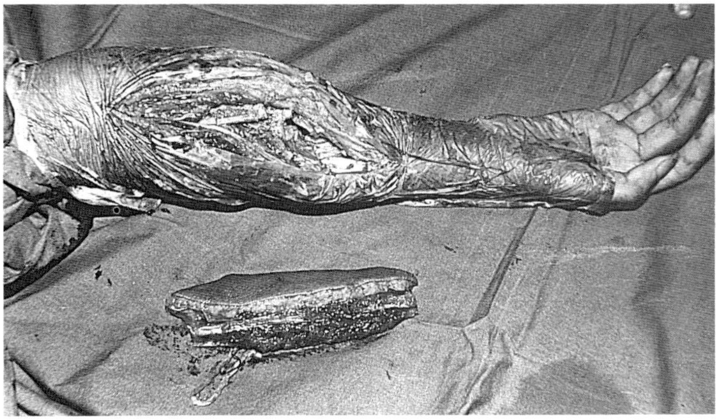

A

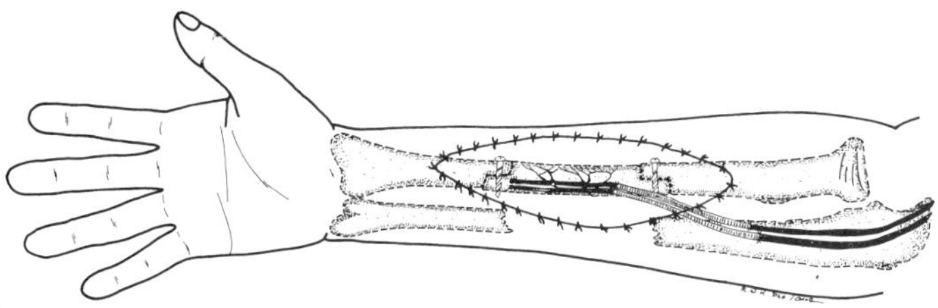

B

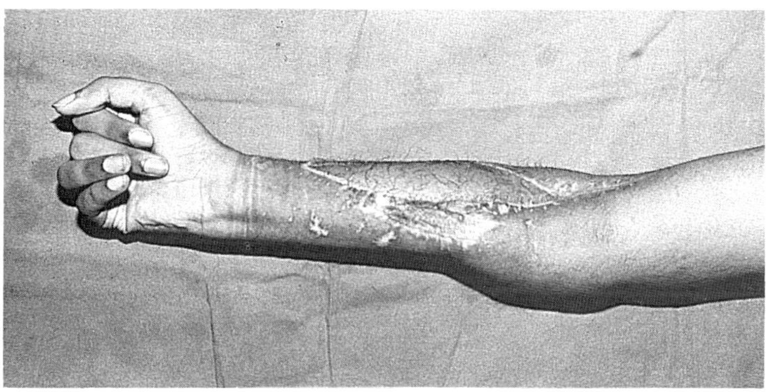

C

Fig. 11.12 A. Combined skin, muscle and bone loss in the forearm associated with infection. Radical resection of infected necrotic bone and soft tissue before replacement with osteocutaneous fibular graft **B.** Schematic representation of fixing the bone graft and vessel anastomosis using long vein grafts. **C.** Functional results after transfer. This technique provides:
(a) introduction of new vascular bed;
(b) soft tissue padding to restore contour;
(c) bony strut for stability; (d) skin flap for resurfacing.

Our results after using the fibula to replace the radius have been rewarding. We noticed that four cases developed stress fracture. This occurred when the fibula was used to replace the radius and ulna, as the fibula took over the load of both radius and ulna (Fig. 11.11A, B, C and D). The fracture was due to the high stress load on the single bone forearm, as compared with the normal forearm where two bones share the load. We also noticed that three of the four fractures occurred in patients who actively used their arms. Three of these cases had their wrists fused, and this may be associated with increased stress load at the bone graft. All the fractures united with external immobilisation and plaster fixation, except in two patients where bone graft was needed.

In infected non-union, we advocated aggressive resection of infected necrotic bone. Very often, the recipient area is badly scarred with poor skin cover. The use of osteocutaneous flaps, with the pedicle lengthened as a closed loop, would enable the surgeon to choose healthy recipient vessels far away from the scarred area, so as to facilitate vessel anastomosis (Fig. 11.12A, B and C).

Functional results

The long-term follow-up of functional results has

shown that the wrist joint, after using the proximal fibula as a vascularised hemi-joint transfer, retains more than half of its normal flexion, extension, supination and pronation (Fig. 11.13). Late volar subluxation of the wrist may occur if the wrist ligaments are not reconstructed. However, the longest follow-up, of more than 10 years, showed that there was no pain in this area. This could be related to the resection of both anterior and posterior interosseous nerves during resection of the tumour.

In those cases where the wrist is fused and the fibula is fixed to the radius, the patient retains very good pronation and supination of the hand, with a stabilised, arthrodesed wrist.

EPIPHYSEAL TRANSPLANT IN THE UPPER EXTREMITY

In a growing child, where limb length discrepancy is likely to develop following loss of an epiphysis, epiphyseal transplant may be indicated.

The selection of donor epiphysis should not interfere with the function and growth at the donor site. Similarly, the growth rate of the transferred epiphysis should, if possible, be similar to the growth rate of the replaced epiphysis, at the recipient site.

We have observed that the transfer of the proximal epiphysis of the fibula and the epiphysis of a toe phalanx are least likely to result in donor site morbidity.

The proximal epiphysis of the fibula has intercommunicating branches through musculoperiosteal vessels from the peroneal vessels. Injection studies have shown that the lateral inferior genicular artery and anterior tibial artery also supply the epiphysis. However, the lateral inferior genicular artery is relatively small, especially when transfer is done in the very young, making harvesting of this vessel for anastomosis very difficult. Therefore, either the anterior tibial vessels or the peroneal vascular pedicle have been used in the transfer of the proximal epiphysis of fibula.

The indications for epiphyseal transfer to the upper extremity are:

1. Congenital deficiency of bone and joint, such as in radial club hand
2. Epiphyseal arrest, secondary to injury or infection
3. Loss of epiphysis and diaphysis following injury, infection or tumour resection.

1. Radial club hand

I have used proximal fibula and its epiphysis, based on its peroneal vascular pedicle, together with its surrounding soft tissue to ensure preservation of intercommunicating branches supplying the proximal epiphysis, for reconstruction of radial club hand as a replacement for missing radius. The fibular epiphysis is large, but shows little ossification if transfer is done in the young, especially those under one year of age, but the articular cartilage is always of large size to support the carpal bones.

Seating of the fibula at the recipient site is often very difficult. It is not easy to place it close to the ulnar border, because the ulna also has a large cartilagenous head, and on X-ray the distal ulnar and fibular head are seen to be widely separated. It is best that one should attempt to create a groove on the ulnar head into which the fibular head can be placed.

The proximal fibula should be placed under the extensor tendons as proximaly as possible. The more proximal the junction, the more difficult is the seating of the proximal fibula within the surrounding muscles.

I have attempted to fix the proximal and distal fibula by transfixing with Kirschner wires to provide stability.

From a study based on the growth of the proximal radius and ulna, we have estimated that the proximal fibula can provide 90% of the growth rate of the radius, with the understanding that, in radial club hand, the growth of the radius and ulna may be retarded and unpredictable as compared with the normal hand. At the present stage, free vascularised fibular graft, with its epiphysis, has helped in achieving initial centralisation of the wrist in radial club hand. The procedure is still empirical. Long term follow-up is required to assess whether the transferred fibula will grow

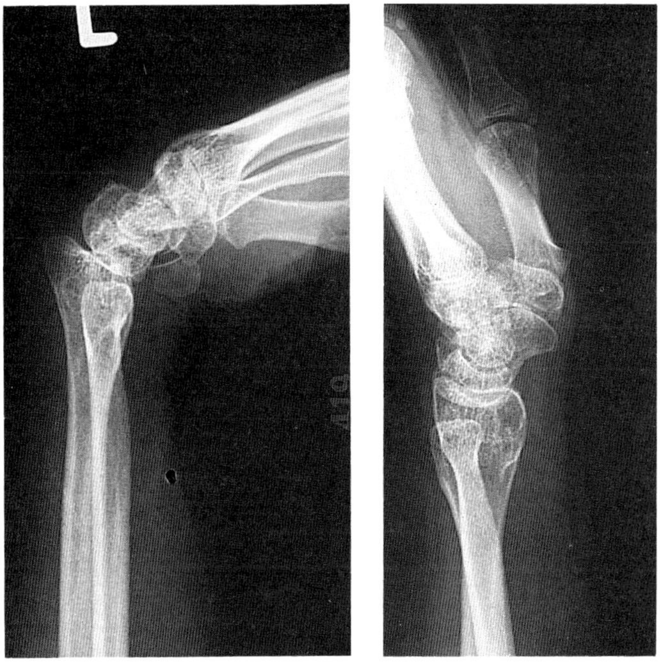

Fig. 11.13 Late results (6 years) of successful transfer of proximal fibula as hemi-vascularised joint transfer to replace lower end of radius in wrist reconstruction.

like a 'normal' radius, preventing deformity of the wrist.

2. Tumour resection of distal radius

I have used proximal fibula to replace both the radius and ulna after resection of osteogenic sarcoma involving both the ends of the radius and ulna in an 8-year-old child. In this type of case, carpal joint stabilisation is very important if one wants to preserve the wrist. The transferred epiphysis will provide growth, but carpal stability will require prolonged Kirschner wire stabilisation. For vessel anastomosis, I have joined the peroneal artery to the radial artery, and peroneal venae comitantes to the cephalic vein. Six years follow-up showed continued growth of fibula to support carpal bone.

3. Osteomyelitis of proximal humerus

I have used proximal fibula and its epiphysis to replace the proximal half of the humerus, lost as a result of osteomyelitis, as a vascularised hemi-joint transfer in a child of 4 years of age (Fig. 11.14A and B). Bony union occurs at six weeks, with normal uptake at the proximal fibular epiphysis on bone scan, using ^{99}Tc (Fig. 11.15). However, after two years follow-up, the X-rays showed that the fibular epiphysis had increased in size by hypertrophy, but irregularly. The fibular epiphysis had simulated the humeral head. The patient had obtained stability with restoration of contour of the shoulder joint; however, movements were restricted.

The follow-up of my experience of free vascularised epiphyseal transfer has, so far, been relatively short. I consider that this technique is still empirical surgery. It can only be assessed after the child has reached maturity. However, at the present stage, transfer of free vascularised epiphyses seems to offer the only solution in treating this very difficult situation.

ACKNOWLEDGEMENTS
I would like to thank Dr Philippe Bayon and Miss Mak Tsui Mei for the illustrations, Mr S. H. Tow and Mr S. S. Moorthy for the photographs, and Mrs Janet Han for typing the manuscript.

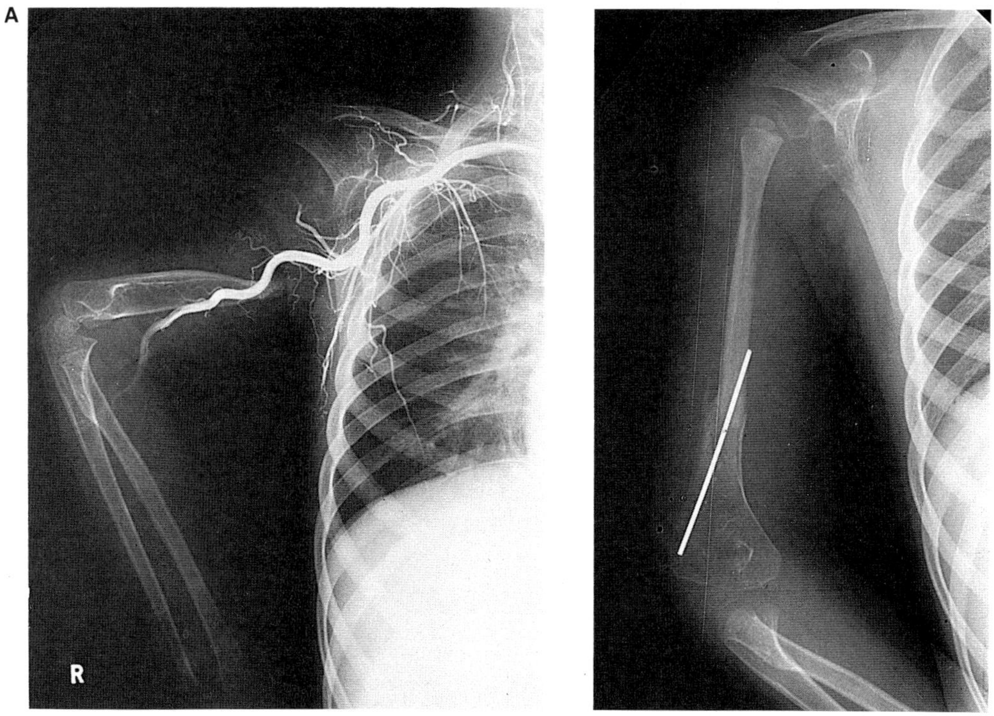

Fig. 11.14 A. Absent proximal humerus and its epiphysis following osteomyelitis in a four-year-old. **B.** Successful transfer of proximal fibula and its epiphysis based on peroneal vascular pedicle.

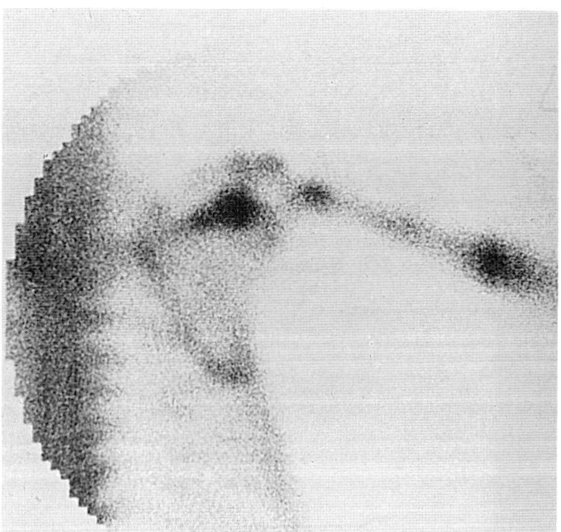

Fig. 11.15 Bone scan (^{99}Tc) showed normal uptake of proximal fibula epiphysis (FE).

REFERENCES

Abbott L C, Schottstaedt E R, Saunders J B, Bost F C 1947 The evaluation of cortical and cancellous bone as grafting material. A clinical and experimental study. Journal of Bone and Joint Surgery 29: 381–414

Albee F H 1923 Fundamentals in bone transplantation. Experience in 3000 bone graft operations. Journal of the American Medical Association 81: 1429–1432

Allieu A, Gomis R, Yoshimura M, Dimeguo A, Bonnel F 1981 Congenital pseudoarthrosis of the forearm. Two cases treated by free vascularised fibular graft. Journal of Hand Surgery 6: 475–481

Bonfiglio M 1958 Repair of bone transplant fracture. Journal of Bone and Joint Surgery 40A: 446–456

Bonfiglio M, Jeter W 1972 Immunological response to bone. Clinical Orthopaedics and Related Research 87: 19–27

Chase S N, Herndon C H 1955 The fate of autogenesis and homogenesis bone grafts. A historical review. Journal of Bone and Joint Surgery 37A: 809–841

Chen Z W, Yu Z J, Wang Y 1979 A new method of treatment of congenital tibial pseudoarthrosis using free vascularised fibular graft. A preliminary report. Annals of the Academy of Medicine, Singapore 8: 465–473

Enneking W F, Burchardt H, Puhl J J 1975 Physical and

biological aspect of repair in cortical bone transplant. Journal of Bone and Joint Surgery 57A: 232–251

Enneking W F, Eady J L, Burchardt H 1980 Autogenous cortical bone graft in the reconstruction of segmental skeletal defects. Journal of Bone and Joint Surgery 62A: 1039–1058

Gilbert A 1979 Vascularised transfer of the fibular shaft. International Journal of Microsurgery 1: 100–109

Gregory C F 1972 The current status of bone and joint transplant. Clinical Orthopaedics and Related Research 87: 165–166

Hammack B L, Enneking W F 1960 Comparative vascularisation of autogenous and homogenous bone transplantation. Journal of Bone and Joint Surgery 42A: 811–817

Huntington T W 1905 Case of bone transference. Annals of Surgery 41: 249–256

Kumar V P, Pho R W H 1986 Tikhoff procedure in recurrent chondrosarcoma following free vascularised fibular graft. The Hand. The British Society for Surgery of the Hand. In press.

Mankin S J, Fogelson F S, Trasher S Z, Zaffer F 1976 Massive resection and allograft transplantation in the treatment of malignant bone tumour. New England Journal of Medicine 294: 1247–1255

Nisbet N W 1966 Immunology of bone transplantation. Clinical Orthopaedics and Related Research 47: 199–228

Ostrup L T, Frederickson J M 1975 Reconstruction of mandibular defects after radiation using a free living bone graft transferred by microvascular anastomoses. An experimental study. Plastic and Reconstructive Surgery 55: 563–572

Parrish F F 1973 Allograft replacement of all or parts of the end of the long bone following excision of a tumour. Journal of Bone and Joint Surgery 55A: 1–22

Pho R W H 1979 Free vascularised fibular transplant for replacement of the lower radius. Journal of Bone and Joint Surgery 61B: 362–365

Pho R W H 1981 Malignant giant cell tumour of the distal end of the radius treated by a free vascularised fibular transplant. Journal of Bone and Joint Surgery, 63A: 877–884

Pho R W H 1983 Free vascularised bone and joint transplant in bone tumour resection. In: The design and application of tumour prostheses for bone and joint reconstruction. Thieme-Stratton Inc., New York, p 93–97

Pho R W H, Levack B, Satku K, Patradul A 1985 Free vascularised fibular graft in the treatment of congenital pseudarthrosis of the tibia. Journal of Bone and Joint Surgery 67A: 64–70

Pho R W H, Levack B 1986 Preliminary observations on epiphyseal growth rate after vascularised fibular graft in congenital pseudarthrosis of tibia. Clinical Orthopaedics and Related Research 206: 104–108

Ray R D, Holloway J A 1957 Bone implants. Journal of Bone and Joint Surgery 39A: 1119–1128

Ray R D 1972 Vascularisation of bone graft and implants. Clinical Orthopaedics and Related Research 87: 43–48

Restrepo J, Katz D, Gilbert A 1980 Anterior vascularisation of the proximal epiphysis and the diaphysis of the fibula. International Journal of Microsurgery 2: 49–54

Sim F H, Chao E Y S 1979 Prosthetic replacement of the knee and large segment of the femur or tibia. Journal of Bone and Joint Surgery 61A: 887–892

Taylor G I, Miller G D H, Ham F J 1975 The free vascularised bone grafts, clinical extension of microvascular techniques. Plastic and Reconstructive Surgery 55: 533–544

Taylor G I, Watson N 1978 One stage repair of compound leg defects with free vascularised flaps of groin skin and iliac bone. Plastic and Reconstructive Surgery 61: 494–506

Urist M R 1976 Practical applications of basic research on bone graft physiology. In: Instructional Lecture, The American Academy of Orthopaedic Surgeons, Vol 25. C V Mosby, St Louis, p 1–26

Weiland A J, Daniel R K 1979 Microvascular anastomosis of bone graft in the treatment of muscle defect. Journal of Bone and Joint Surgery 61A: 98

P. R. Ellis, Tsu-Min Tsai and J. E. Kutz

12 Joint transplantation with microvascular anastomosis

Treatment of severely traumatised joints in the hand has long been a significant challenge to the hand surgeon. The reconstruction of congenital joint deformities of the hand presents a difficult problem as well. Numerous techniques have been used to meet this challenge, including amputation, arthrodesis, resection arthroplasty, silastic interposition arthroplasty, distraction arthroplasty, perichondrial arthroplasty, non-vascularised joint transfer and allografts. Unfortunately, none of these have been universally successful.

The concept of autogenous joint replacement as an alternative form of treatment in these difficult cases is not new. Bachman (Wray et al 1981), in 1907, reported the first free whole joint transfer to the upper limb when he described a transfer of the metatarso-phalangeal (MTP) joint to the elbow. In 1909, Wolffe (Wray et al 1981) performed the first autogenous half-joint replacement, by removing a tuberculous proximal phalanx of the fourth finger and replacing it with the proximal phalanx from the second toe. Rudolf Goebell reported in 1913 (O'Brien et al 1984) the first free whole autogenous toe-joint-to-finger transfer. He replaced a musician's painful arthritic distal interphalangeal joint of the left small finger with the PIP joint of the second toe. Following Goebell's publication, little was written on the topic until 1945, when Cuthbert (Erdelyi 1963a) reported replacement of a thumb metacarpo-phalangeal (MP) joint with an MTP joint. Graham (Wray et al 1981) in 1954 described transfer of an MTP joint to thc thumb.

In the 1960s, research efforts were directed to the study of joint survival and viability in non-vascularised autografts. Entin et al (1962) demonstrated in dog studies that non-vascularised composite grafts did poorly, with hyaline articular cartilage ultimately being replaced by an inferior fibrocartilage. Erdelyi (1963b) reported his clinical experience with non-vascularised joint transplants of small joints of the foot to the fingers. He described the histological findings of a transplanted joint resected 9 months after transfer with apparent necrosis of cartilage, capsule, and bone. The cartilage, however, was noted to be substituted with a tissue 'adequate in a functional respect', although 'morphologically inferior'. Kettelcamp (1972) reported the results of experimental autogenous joint transplantation in monkeys, in which he demonstrated cartilage survival but inadequate bone repair.

The development of microvascular surgery made successful free tissue transfer a reality. Buncke et al (1967) reported the successful experimental replantation of extremities in rats with the preservation of articular cartilage architecture and function. He further demonstrated the survival of vascularised toe-to-hand transfers in monkeys. In that same article, Buncke et al reported the first successful clinical vascularised joint transfer, when he transferred an MP joint of a severely traumatised index finger to the PIP joint of the adjacent long finger in a 19-year-old patient.

Hurwitz (1979) successfully transferred free vascularised MP joints in the dog and demonstrated well-preserved articular cartilage up to four months after transfer, with the vascularised joints histologically 'indistinguishable from normal joints'. Tsai et al (1982a) reported the results of a primate study in which vascularised total joint transfers were performed in Macaca monkeys.

This data confirmed the advantages of vascularised transfer, as opposed to non-vascularised, with maintenance of hyaline cartilage and preservation of joint space up to seven months after transfer.

CLINICAL EXPERIENCE

Following Buncke's first successful transfer, few clinical cases have been reported. Foucher et al (1980) reported the first free vascularised joint transfer. Mathes et al (1980) reported a free microvascular transplant of a second MTP joint to the MP joint of the ring finger in a four-year-old. Follow-up at two and one-half years revealed continued epiphyseal growth.

Tsai et al (1982b) reported the first clinical series of vascularised joint transfer. They performed nine vascularised joint transfers in six patients for the reconstruction of traumatised joints. All joints were harvested from the foot, except for a single MP joint taken from a severely traumatised finger. The average follow-up was 24 months, and the mean range of active motion was 22°/55°. The authors concluded from this study that vascularised joint transfer provided a viable method for joint reconstruction in the young patient. Subsequent studies have demonstrated the usefulness of vascularised joint transfer in the reconstruction of traumatised finger joints, particularly in children and young adults (O'Brien et al 1984, Kuo et al 1984, Tsai & Bobb 1987, Foucher et al 1986, Yoshizu et al 1985).

ANATOMY

An understanding of the pertinent anatomy of the foot is essential for the successful harvest of a toe joint with its vascular pedicle. Our understanding of the pertinent anatomy has been greatly enhanced by Gilbert (1976) and May et al (1977) who have described in detail the anatomy of the first web space. The PIP joint of the second toe is the preferred joint for transfer in the majority of cases, using a pedicle based most often on the first dorsal metatarsal artery and venae comitantes (Fig. 12.1).

The dorsalis pedis artery descends from the anterior leg and passes beneath the extensor retinaculum between the tendons of the extensor hallicus longus (EHL) and the extensor digitorum

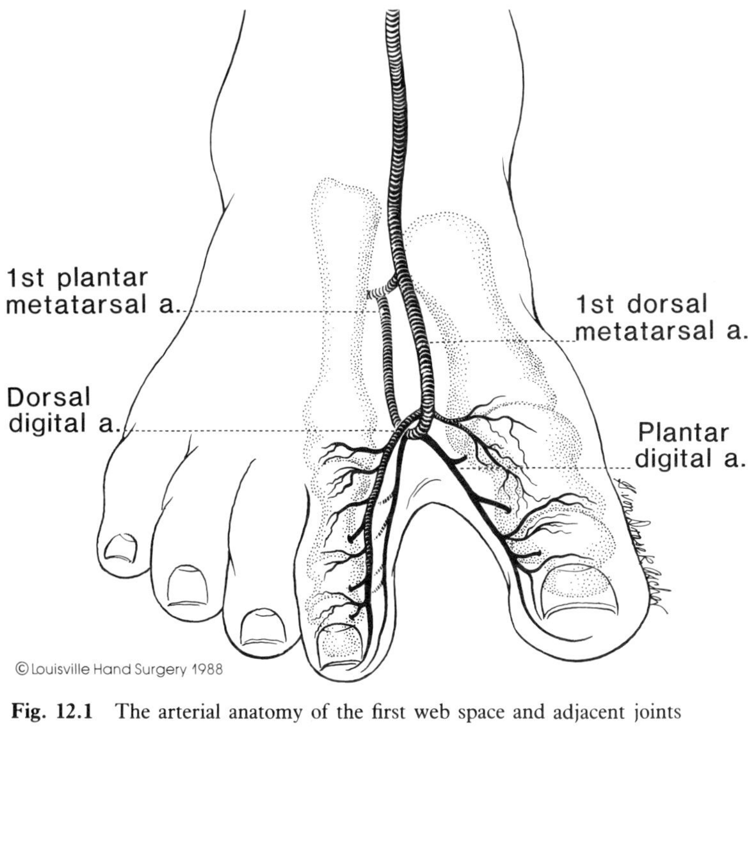

Fig. 12.1 The arterial anatomy of the first web space and adjacent joints

longus (EDL). At the level of the tarsometatarsal joint, it gives off a branch which dives plantarly to anastomose with the plantar arch. This in turn branches to form the first plantar metatarsal artery, which continues distally in the first web space. The dorsalis pedis artery itself continues distally in the first web space as the first dorsal metatarsal artery. This vessel courses between the EHL and the EDL, crossing under extensor hallucis brevis. At the level of the MTP joint, the first dorsal metatarsal artery gives off a communicating branch which again dives plantarly to anastomose with a branch from the first plantar metatarsal artery. The first dorsal metatarsal artery, after giving off the communicating branch, then divides to send branches to the fibular aspect of the great toe and tibial aspect of the second toe.

The first dorsal metatarsal artery provides the primary pedicle in the majority of cases and therefore requires close study of its course and anatomical relationships. May et al (1977) reported studies of 50 cadaveric specimens noting two basic patterns in the first dorsal metatarsal artery. In Type I (78%), the first dorsal metatarsal arose from the dorsalis pedis artery and coursed distally superficial to the first dorsal interosseous muscle. In Type II (22%), the first dorsal metatarsal artery arose deeply and coursed distally either within the substance of the interosseous muscle or deep to it. In both types, the vessel passed dorsal to the transverse metatarsal ligament before giving off branches to the great and second toes. In all specimens, the first dorsal metatarsal sent a branch plantarly (the distal communicating artery) that anastomosed with the first plantar metatarsal artery.

Gilbert (1976) performed latex studies of the vascular anatomy of 50 cadaveric specimens. He noted the lateral plantar artery of the great toe to be the dominant vessel supplying that toe in the majority of cases. The medial plantar collateral artery of the second toe, however, is often insignificant, with the medial dorsal digital artery being dominant.

Gilbert classified the anatomical variations of the first dorsal metatarsal as follows:

1. In Type Ia, the artery is superficial and separated from the skin by only the 'small posterior body of the interosseous muscle'. In Type Ib, the artery lies within the substance of the interosseous muscle, but is 'superficial enough to be easily dissected'. Of the specimens in his study, 66% were Type Ia or Ib.
2. In Type II, the artery lies deep to the first interosseous muscle and becomes superficial at the deep transverse metatarsal ligament, passing dorsally to it. Type II is further divided into Type IIa and b, depending on the presence or absence of a small superficial branch lying on the dorsum of the first interosseous muscle. Type II occurred in 22% of the cases.
3. In Type III, the dorsal metatarsal artery, although located superficially, is smaller and is a non-dominant vessel with minimal contribution to the first and second toes. This pattern was found by Gilbert in 10% of the specimens.

Thus, based on this study, Gilbert concludes that the first dorsal metatarsal artery is of adequate size and position to be harvested from a dorsal approach as a vascular pedicle in 88% of patients. In the remaining patients, dissection of the first plantar metatarsal artery may be necessary. According to Gilbert, the diameter of the first dorsal metatarsal artery ranges from 1 to 1.5 mm, and is easily anastomosed using microscopic technique.

May et al (1977) demonstrated the existence of a distal communicating artery connecting the first dorsal and first plantar metatarsal arteries in 100% of specimens. Either vessel is of adequate size to serve as the pedicle supplying the first web space.

JOINT SELECTION

Following the work of May et al, which demonstrated the use of the first web space of the foot as an appropriate source for a free neurovascular flap, Tsai et al (1982a) successfully performed vascularised joint transfers in an experimental primate model. Nine vascularised second-toe PIP joints were transferred to the hand of Macaca monkeys. Seven of these survived and were noted to have preservation of hyaline cartilage up to 10 months later. The study was designed to demonstrate the clinical applicability to man. The technique included harvest of a skin island from the dorsum of the second toe to serve as a 'patency monitor'. Although the authors noted that either the MTP or PIP joints could be transferred, the PIP joint was preferred because 'it can be transferred with its extensor mechanism, which is fitted to the joint well, and offers attachment of the central slip for extension of itself and lateral bands for extension of distal recipient site joints'. In addition, the PIP joint was preferred on the basis of donor site morbidity, with less disability noted at the PIP joint level.

O'Brien et al (1984) have previously noted that the metatarsal is comparatively longer than the corresponding metacarpal. The proximal phalanx of the finger, however, is longer than the corresponding toe proximal phalanx. Consequently, the distance from the base of the metacarpal to the articular surface of the proximal phalanx is approximately equal to that from the base of the corresponding metatarsal to proximal phalanx joint surface. The authors also emphasise that transfer of an MTP joint includes two epiphyseal growth centers, whereas a toe PIP joint contains a single growth center. Epiphyseal growth plates in the foot, however, may close earlier than those of the fingers. These points must be considered in donor joint selection where further growth is required.

Although the second toe is generally favoured for joint harvest, extensor lag has been reported frequently. Foucher et al (1986), for instance, note the common pre-existence of second toe claw deformity due to shoe wear in our population. He further states that the thicker volar plate of the toe provides an increased lever arm for the flexor tendons. This is compounded by an inadequate pulley system allowing for flexor tendon bowstringing and further increase in flexor mechanical advantage over the extensors.

Tsai and Bobb (1987), stimulated by common extensor lag in their early patients, evaluated the range of motion of the PIP joint in the second toe of 50 normal individuals. Their results (Table 12.1) suggest a significant difference according to the patient's age. Thus, the age of the patient and existing range of motion of the donor toe must be considered and may directly affect the final range of motion of the joint in the recipient finger.

Table 12.1 Average range of motion of the proximal interphalangeal joint of the second toe of 50 normal individuals (Tsai & Bobb 1987).

Age (years)	*Active motion*	*Passive motion*
0–10	20°/47°	−5°/72°
11–20	16°/48°	−3°/80°
21–30	0°/69°	−2°/76°
>40	14°/46°	0°/71°

PREOPERATIVE EVALUATION

Radiographic evaluation is an essential part of the preoperative assessment. Plain radiographs must be obtained of the donor foot as well as of the recipient hand to assure the presence of a non-arthritic donor joint. The relative lengths of the metatarsal, metacarpal and phalanges must be determined, to aid in preoperative planning of osteotomy sites.

The blood supply of the donor foot must be evaluated preoperatively. Physical examination for palpable pulsation of the dorsalis pedis artery is essential; it is, perhaps, the only necessary preoperative test. Although absence of a palpable dorsalis pedis pulse warrants concern, the pulse may be absent in 8% of normal feet (May et al 1977). May advises that the absence of a dorsalis pedis pulse does not exclude the use of the flap 'unless peripheral vascular disease is the cause and is confirmed by other means'.

The use of preoperative arteriography of the lower extremity is somewhat controversial. Although recommended by some authors, the trend is to evaluate lower extremity blood flow by physical examination and Doppler study, reserving the use of arteriography for difficult or unusual cases. Similarly, arteriographic evaluation of the upper extremity is seldom indicated, with adequate evaluation provided by physical examination, including the Allen test.

OPERATIVE TECHNIQUE

The transfer of a second-toe PIP joint to the PIP joint of a finger, the most commonly performed vascularised joint transfer, will be described. The procedure is performed under general anaesthesia, preferably with two surgical teams operating simultaneously. When a single team is available, the recipient site is prepared first.

The recipient site is approached via a dorsal incision under tourniquet control with excision of the arthritic joint, removing all sclerotic bone to healthy bleeding bone. The original technique included a transverse saw cut through the proximal phalanx. The technique has recently been modified, however, to preserve the recipient finger extensor mechanism. A step-cut osteotomy through the midshaft of the middle phalanx of the finger is used to preserve the dorsal cortex and thus maintain the extensor tendon attachments (Fig.12.2). The neurovascular bundles must be protected at all times.

An incision is made dorsally over the anatomical snuffbox to expose the dorsal branch of the radial artery and venae comitantes or branches of the cephalic vein. These vessels are isolated and prepared for subsequent anastomosis with the joint pedicle. An interposition vein graft may be required and can readily be harvested from the forearm or foot.

The foot is likewise approached dorsally for dissection of the vascularised joint. The design of the skin incision includes harvest of a skin island as a marker of vascular patency. The original technique described by Tsai et al (1982b) harvested an ellipse of skin over the dorsum of the PIP joint of the second toe. This technique has recently been revised. The new technique entails taking the skin island from the fibular aspect of the great toe (Fig. 12.3). It is expected that this change will reduce postoperative extensor tendon adhesions.

The incision begins over the dorsum of the foot, running longitudinally to expose the dorsalis pedis artery and saphenous vein. It continues distally over the first dorsal metatarsal artery, to the first webspace, and on to the dorsum of the second toe. A second limb of the incision extends over the fibular aspect of the great toe for harvest of the skin island.

The first dorsal metatarsal artery is dissected beginning at its origin off the dorsalis pedis and continuing distally, taking care to ligate its branches. If a longer pedicle is required, the dissection may include the distal aspect of the dorsalis pedis artery. The first dorsal metatarsal artery dissection continues distally into the web space and should include the distal communicating branch and a portion of the first plantar metatarsal artery. In the event the first dorsal metatarsal artery is inadequate, the first plantar metatarsal artery may be relied upon as the pedicle. The branch of the first dorsal metatarsal to the tibial aspect of the second toe is carefully dissected, protecting its branches to the PIP joint. It is ligated at the level of the DIP joint. The fibular digital artery and vein of the second toe are carefully preserved to provide vascularity to the remaining distal aspect of the toe. Its branches to the PIP joint, however, must be ligated to provide for joint harvest. Branches from the fibular digital artery of the great toe to the skin island must be carefully preserved and can be taken with surrounding subcutaneous tissue.

Upon completion of both pedicle exposure and initial dissection, attention is directed toward harvest of the joint. The bone length necessary for transplant is determined by measuring the bone defect remaining after resection of the arthritic

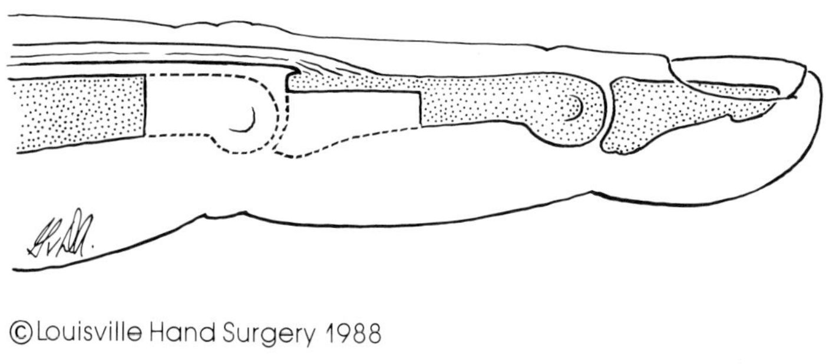

Fig. 12.2 Technique of resection of arthritic finger joint with shelf of bone to preserve attachment of extensor tendon. (Reproduced from Ellis P R, Tsai T M 1989 Management of the traumatized Joint of the finger from Clinics in Plastic Surgery 16.)

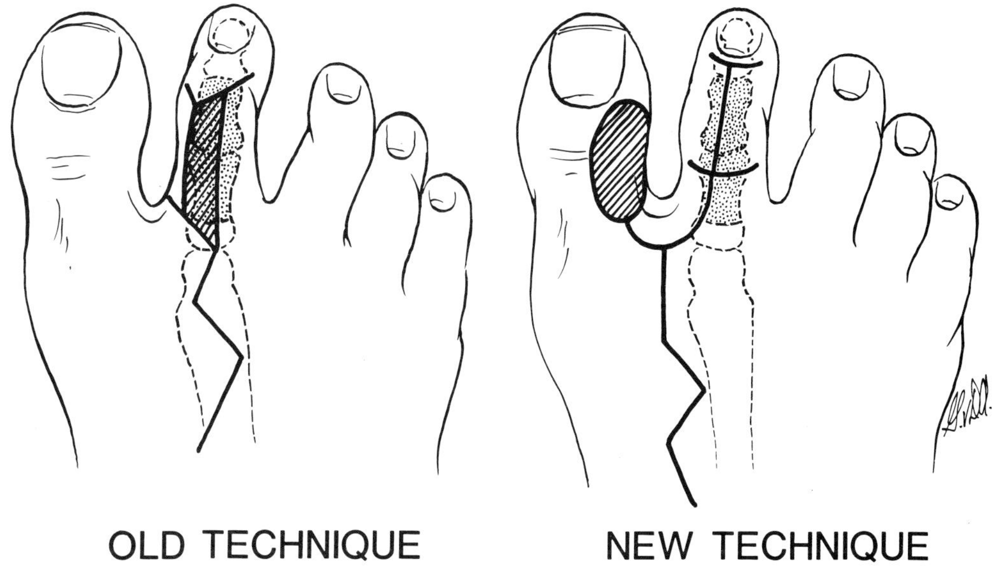

Fig. 12.3 The new technique entails harvest of the skin island from the fibular aspect of the great toe.

joint. The extensor mechanism of the toe may be transferred with the joint where necessary. When possible, however, the extensor tendon of the PIP joint of the finger is preserved and used preferentially. The DIP joint of the second toe is disarticulated. An osteotomy is made through the proximal phalanx of the toe at the level determined above. The graft is then elevated taking great care to protect the skin island and harvested joint pedicles. The tourniquet is released for approximately half an hour to assure adequate blood flow through the pedicle, to reduce ischaemia time prior to pedicle ligation, and to allow the arterial spasm to subside.

The joint is now ready for transfer. The pedicle is ligated and the composite graft is transferred to the recipient hand. Bone stabilisation is achieved initially using Kirschner wires supplemented with intraosseous or cerclage wires. The extensor tendons are repaired using the tendon of the finger or, as necessary, harvested toe extensor (Fig. 12.4).

The arterial pedicle of the joint is anastomosed most commonly to the dorsal branch of the radial artery in an end-to-side fashion. A reverse interposition vein graft is often required when pedicle length is inadequate. Vein anastomosis is accomplished using a branch of the cephalic vein in an end-to-end fashion. The skin is closed, taking care to avoid excessive tension. The skin island is incorporated in the closure and is monitored for capillary refill. Split-thickness skin grafts are used to avoid tension when necessary.

The donor toe may be treated as a resection arthroplasty, but is more commonly arthrodesed using an iliac graft or bone resected from the hand. A bone peg, harvested from the iliac crest and fashioned to fill the defect, restores toe length. Longitudinal Kirschner wire fixation provides adequate stabilisation.

CASE REPORT

A 22-year-old male presented for treatment approximately three weeks after sustaining a human bite over the right long MP joint (Fig. 12.5). Despite surgical debridement and intravenous antibiotic therapy, the joint was destroyed. The joint was subsequently resected, stabilised with an external fixator, and packed with antibiotic-impregnated polymethyl methacrylate beads. The infection responded to this treatment, and the

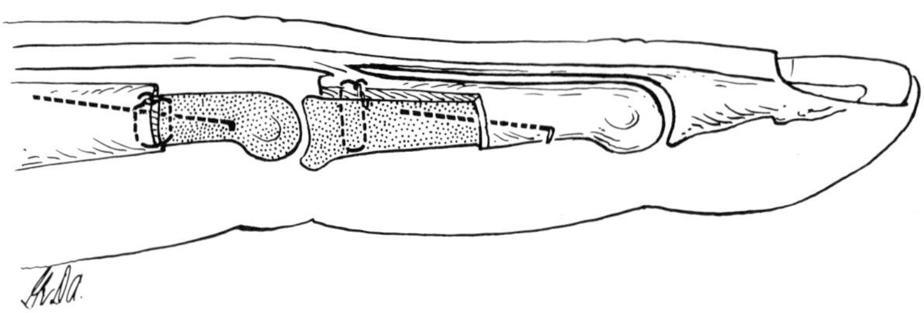

Fig. 12.4 Transferred joint with internal fixation. (Reproduced from Ellis & Tsai 1989.)

placement of a vascularised toe joint was selected as the technique for reconstruction.

A vascularised PIP joint was harvested from the second toe and successfully transferred to the MP joint. The patient's operative course was without complication. At 9 months after surgery, he had a range of motion of 15°/75°.

DISCUSSION

Reconstruction of the traumatised MP and PIP joints of the hand remains a significant problem. No single technique offers a solution in all cases. The technique of vascularised joint transfer, however, provides an acceptable alternative in properly selected cases.

Increasing clinical experience in the use of vascularised joint transfer has demonstrated acceptable results. O'Brien et al (1984) reported seven vascularised joint transfers to finger MP and PIP joints. Six of the seven transfers were considered successful. Growth centres transferred demonstrated continued growth. The average range of motion for the series was 33°. Reported complications included frequent extensor tendon adherence.

Kuo et al (1984) reported six cases of free vascularised second-toe MTP joints to finger and thumb MP joints. The authors used a technique, previously described by Erdelyi (1963a), in which the graft is rotated 180° on its longitudinal axis to increase palmar flexion of the transferred joint. The transferred joints of this series developed an average arc of approximately 30° active flexion. The only reported complication was a single malunion necessitating corrective osteotomy.

Foucher et al (1986) presented a series of ten vascularised toe joint transfers. Nine joints were transferred to the PIP joint, and one to the MP joint, with an average arc of active motion of 32.2° for the PIP joint and an arc of 65° for the single MP joint. Again, the most significant complication noted was an extension deficit averaging 37° for the nine recipient PIP joints.

Yoshizu et al (1985) reported on nine vascularised joint transfers in eight patients. Range of motion, reported for four of the patients, averaged 50°.

Since the original report of Tsai et al (1982b), these authors have performed an additional 47 vascularised joint transfers to the hand. The results of this large series will be reported elsewhere. The preliminary results, however, are consistent with previous studies, with an average range of motion of transferred joints of approximately 31°.

Singer et al (1988) recently reported the long-term follow-up of four vascularised joint transfers previously described by O'Brien et al (1984). Two MTP and two PIP toe joints were transferred. An encouraging finding of their study was a progressive improvement in range of motion 3–8 years after surgery. Follow-up at an average of 6.6 years revealed significant growth and improved range of motion for the two MTP transfers, which averaged 75° active motion. The two PIP transfers, however, had a significant extensor lag and a minimal contribution to continued growth, with extension lags of 40° and 90°, and an average of 35° active motion. This series clearly demonstrates the advantage of MTP transfer over PIP transfer where continued growth is needed. The double epiphysis present at the MTP level, and the more significant growth contribution of the metatarsal, account for this discrepancy.

Other isolated case reports have noted preserved

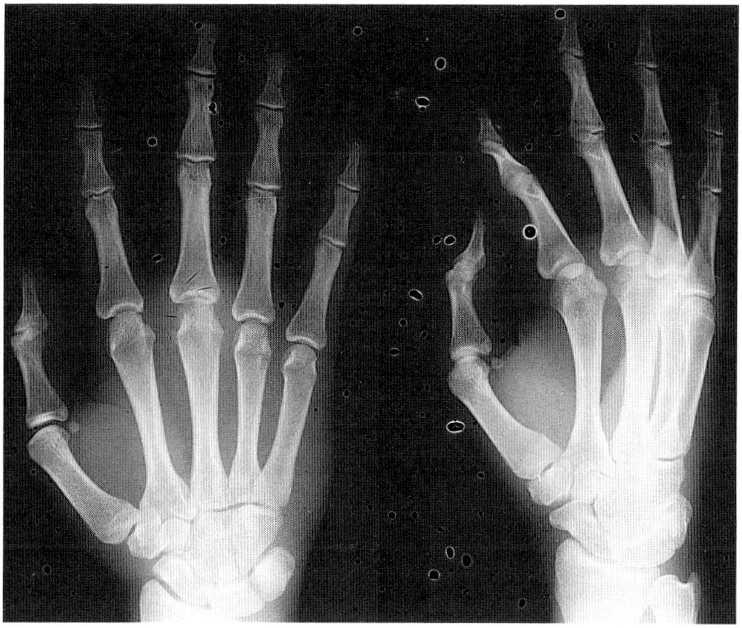

A

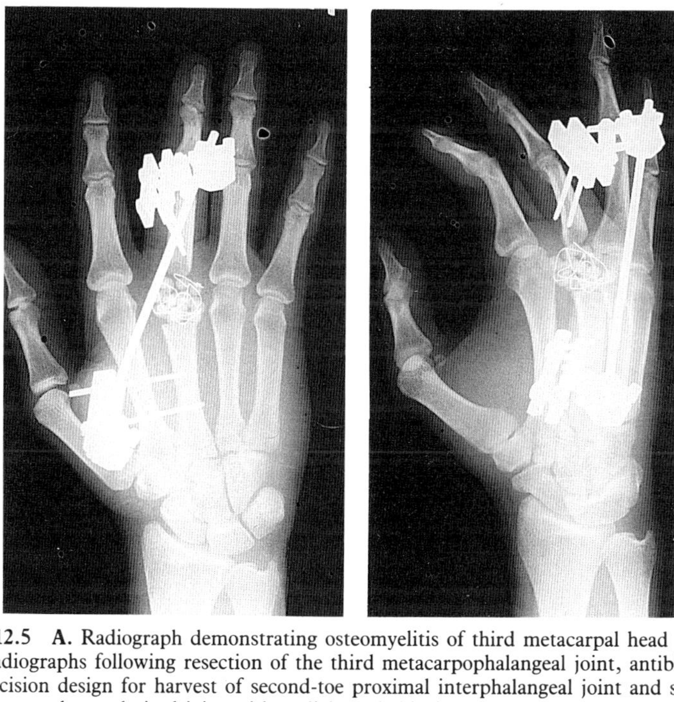

B

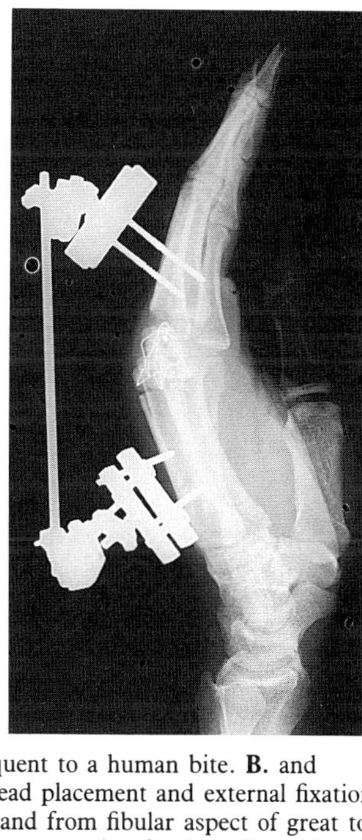

C

Fig. 12.5 **A.** Radiograph demonstrating osteomyelitis of third metacarpal head subsequent to a human bite. **B.** and **C.** Radiographs following resection of the third metacarpophalangeal joint, antibiotic bead placement and external fixation. **D.** Incision design for harvest of second-toe proximal interphalangeal joint and skin island from fibular aspect of great toe. **E.** Harvested vascularised joint with pedicle and skin island. **F.** and **G.** Radiographs demonstrating fixation of transferred joint. **H.** Radiograph of second toe with fixation of iliac crest graft. **I.** and **J.** Radiographs of joint 6 months after transfer. **K.** Radiographs of donor site 6 months after transfer demonstrating union of graft. **L., M., N.** and **O.** Final range of motion. (Reproduced from Ellis P R, Hanna D, Tsai T M 1991. Vascularized single toe joint transfer to the hand. Journal of Hand Surgery 16A.)

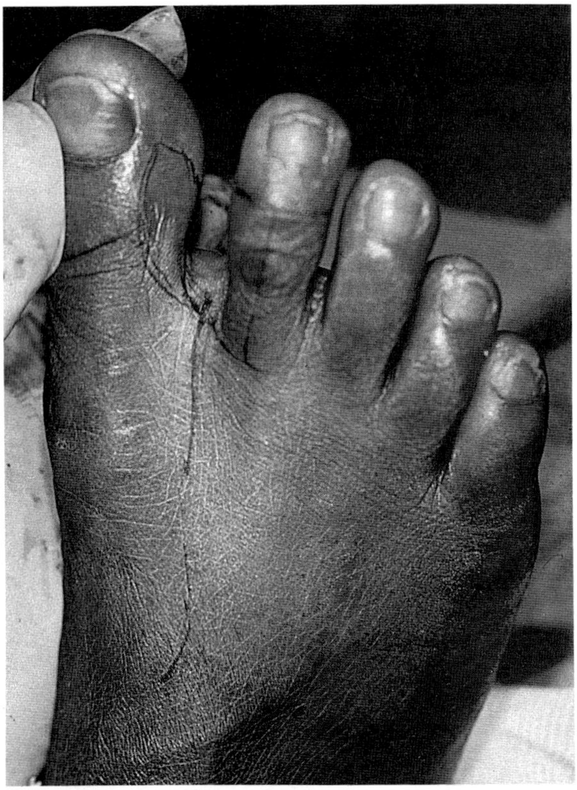

D

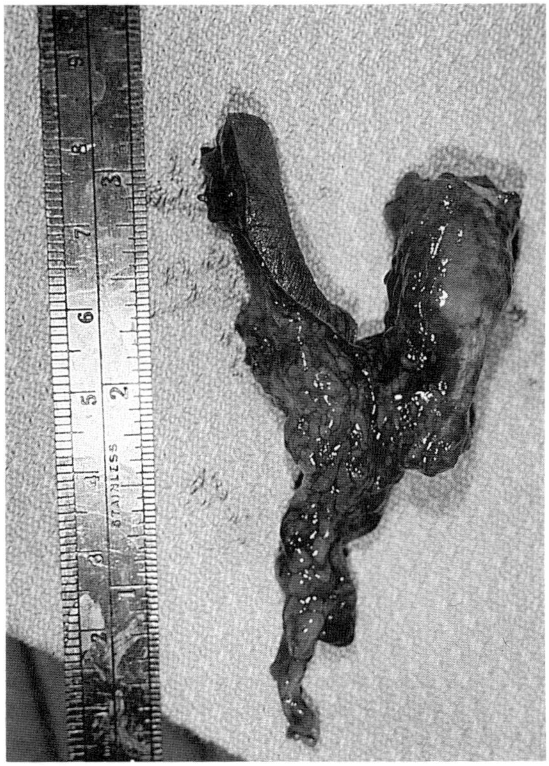

E

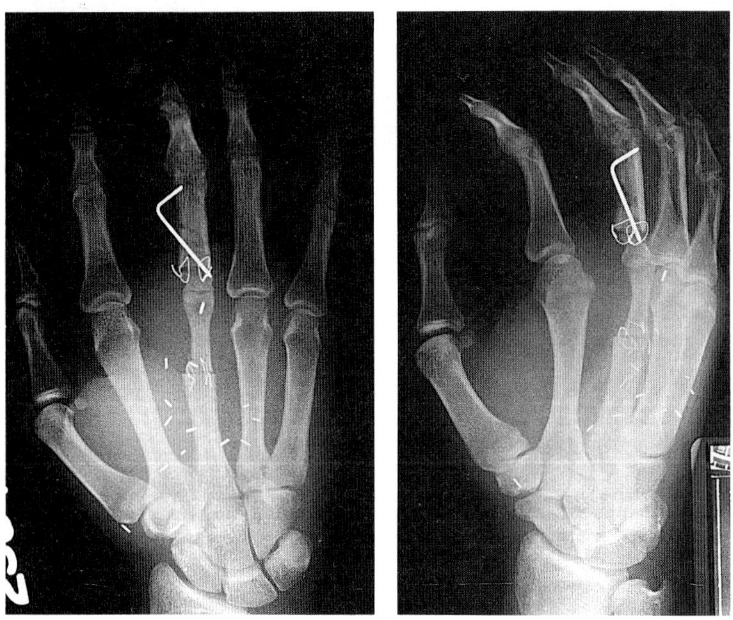

F

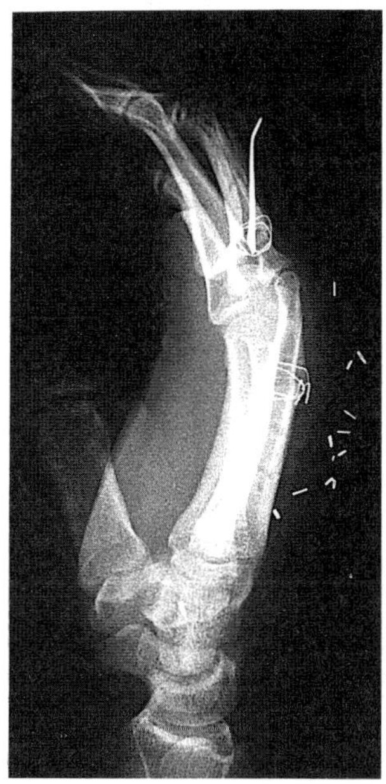

G

Fig. 12.5 (cont)

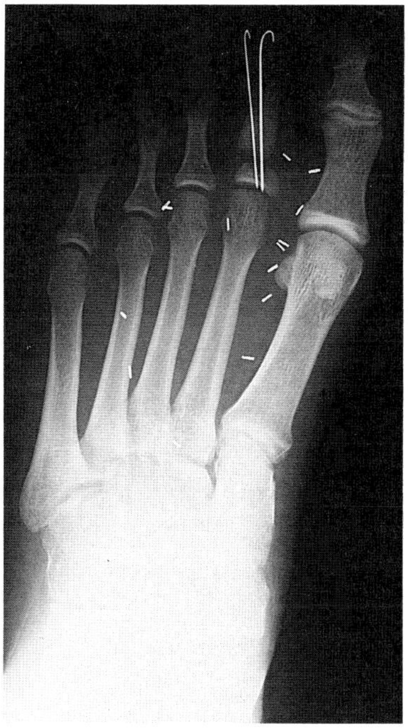

H

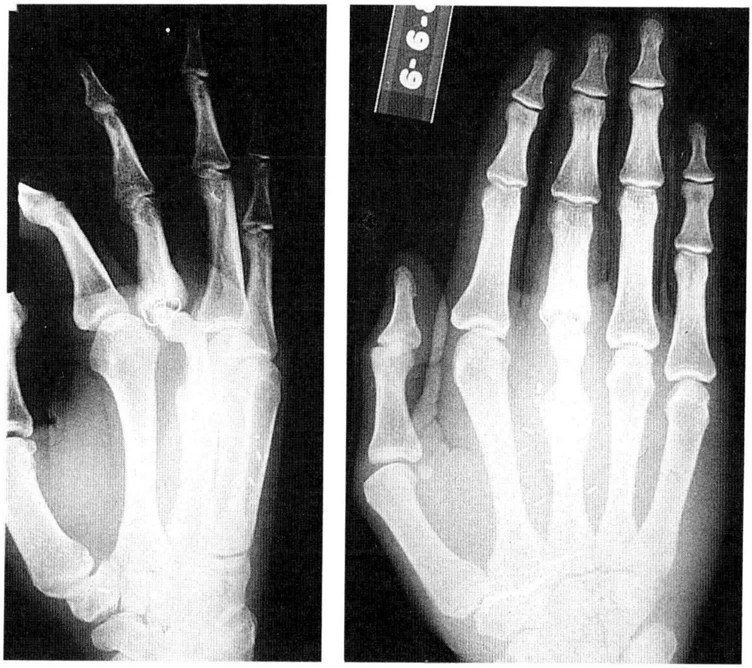

I

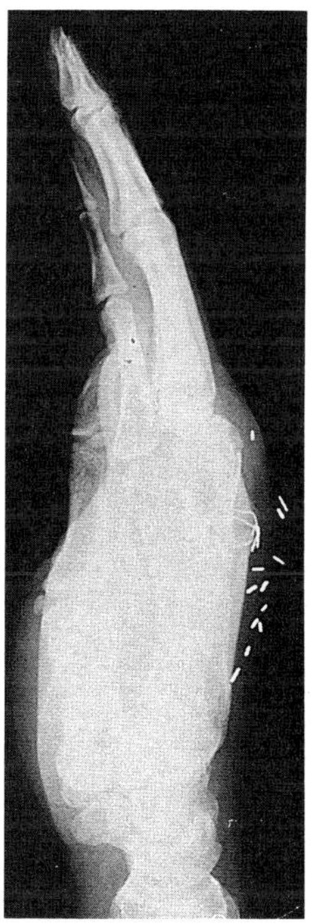

J

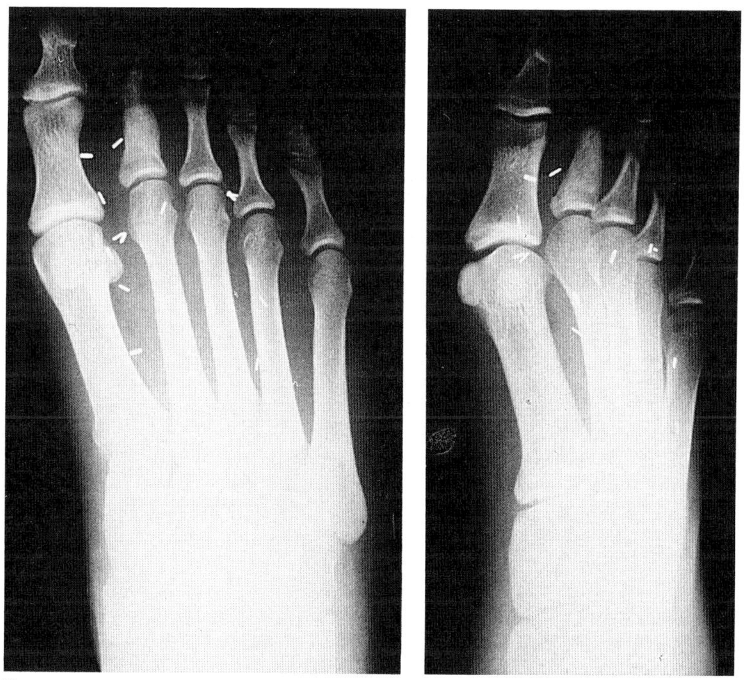

K

Fig. 12.5 (cont)

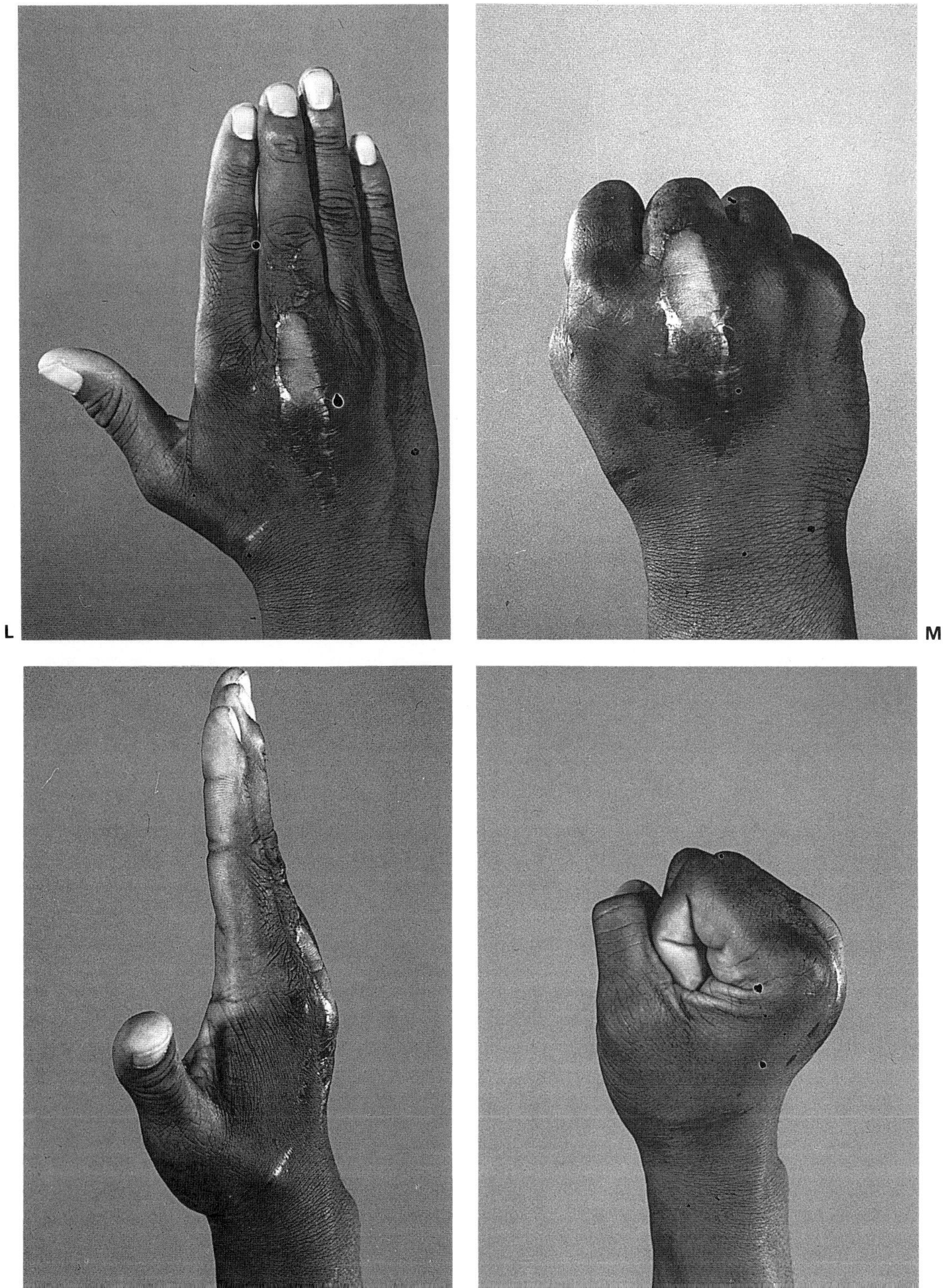

Fig. 12.5 (cont)

epiphyseal growth with both PIP and MTP joint transfer (Mathes et al 1980, Wray et al 1981, Tsai et al 1982b). MTP joint transfer, however, may be preferred where continued growth is necessary.

The most significant complication associated with vascularised joint transfer that recurs throughout the literature is persistent extensor lag (O'Brien et al 1984, Foucher et al 1980). This is perhaps a greater problem with PIP joint transfer than MTP transfer (Singer et al 1988). The factors contributing to this problem are diverse. The natural tendency for claw (flexion) deformity of the PIP joint of the toe is well established (Foucher et al 1986). Tsai et al (1985) have demonstrated the inherent limitations of range of motion of the second toe. As described by Foucher et al (1986), there are biomechanical mechanisms that contribute to flexion deformity. The transferred joint, therefore, has inherent limitations in movement. Reconstruction of the extensor mechanism of the finger is critical in obtaining good results. The recent changes in technique implemented by Tsai and designed to retain the extensor mechanism of the recipient finger, however, appear to result in improved extension in a preliminary series. Tenolysis may also improve overall range of motion, but should not be performed sooner than six months after initial transfer.

INDICATIONS AND ALTERNATIVES

Vascularised toe joint transfer has its strongest indication in the reconstruction of traumatised joints in young patients. This technique provides viable autogenous tissue to reconstruct small joints, replacing bone, cartilage, ligament, tendon and skin. Failed arthroplasties may also be reconstructed using this procedure. Unfortunately, results have been disappointing in reconstruction of congenital deformity or of joints in which flexor motor units are absent or compromised.

All joint-transfer series reviewed demonstrate the maintenance of articular cartilage and joint viability. This technique, therefore, provides a physiological alternative for joint reconstruction. Other reported procedures fail to demonstrate definite advantages over vascularised joint transfer. Post-traumatic silicone arthroplasty has resulted in limited range of motion and high complication rates (Iselin 1975, Riggs & Cooney 1983, Strickland 1974). Furthermore, silicone implants have not been recommended in young patients.

Resurfacing techniques also have limited application. Perichondrial arthroplasty as reported by Seradge et al (1984) provides only modest gains in range of motion. It is contraindicated in digits with significant bone defects or previous infection. Conversely, vascularised joint transfer provides additional bone stock in fingers with bone defects and increases vascularity.

As noted previously, transfer of vascularised joints with open physes can be used to reconstruct digits requiring further growth. This advantage is not offered by any other reconstructive technique.

Vascularised joint transfer has application for immediate reconstruction of severely traumatised joints. In cases of severe trauma to a digit, preserved MP or PIP joints of otherwise non-viable digits can be used as vascularised autografts to replace the damaged joints of the viable digits (Tsai et al 1982b). Under different circumstances, vascularised toe joints can be harvested as part of the emergency procedure to replace severely injured finger joints (Tsai et al 1985).

Various combinations of vascularised joint transfers have been reported with varying degrees of success. Although hemi-joint transfer has been reported (Tsai & Bobb 1987), experimental studies have shown inferior articular cartilage survival in vascularised hemi-joints as compared to that found in transferred whole joints (Hurwitz 1979). Double joint transfer has also been used successfully, including transfer of same-toe PIP with DIP joint (Tsai & Singer 1984) and double MTP joint transfer (Rose 1984). In the latter case, two MTP joints were fixed in series to replace two finger joints.

SUMMARY

At present, no technique has achieved universal success in the treatment of post-traumatic arthrosis of joints of the hand. Vascularised autogenous joint transfer provides a viable option in select cases where traditional techniques such as arthrodesis, silastic interposition arthroplasty or amputation are undesirable. Its use may be considered in the reconstruction of post-traumatic arthritis in young patients. The technique provides the potential for a painless, stable joint with a useful range of motion and the prospect for a long-term solution to a difficult problem.

ACKNOWLEDGEMENTS
The authors would like to give special thanks to Kell Julliard for his editorial assistance in preparing this manuscript, and to Grace von Drasek-Ascher, A. M. I., for her preparation of the artwork.

REFERENCES

Buncke H J, Daniller A I, Schulz W P, Chase R A 1967 The fate of autogenous whole joints transplanted by microvascular anastomoses. Journal of Plastic and Reconstructive Surgery 39: 333–341
Ellis P R, Tsai T M 1989 Management of the traumatized joint of the finger. Clinics in Plastic Surgery 16: 457–473
Ellis, P R, Hanna D, Tsai T M 1991 Vascularized single toe joint transfer to the hand. Journal of Hand Surgery 16A: 160–168
Entin M A, Alger J R, Baird R M 1962 Experimental and clinical transplantation of autogenous whole joints. Journal of Bone and Joint Surgery 44A: 1518–1536
Erdelyi R 1963a Reconstruction of ankylosed finger joints by means of transplantation of joints from the foot. Journal of Plastic and Reconstructive Surgery 31: 140–150
Erdelyi R 1963b Experimental autotransplantation of small joints. Journal of Plastic and Reconstructive Surgery 31: 129–139
Foucher G, Merle M, Maneaud M, Michon J 1980 Microsurgical free partial toe transfer in hand reconstruction: a report of 12 cases. Journal of Plastic and Reconstructive Surgery 65: 616–627
Foucher G, Hoang P, Citron N, Merle M, Dury M 1986 Joint reconstruction following trauma: comparison of microsurgical transfer and conventional methods: a report of 61 cases. Journal of Hand Surgery 11B: 388–393
Gilbert A 1976 Composite tissue transfer from the foot: anatomic basis and surgical technique. In: Daniller A I (ed) Symposium on Microsurgery. C V Mosby, St Louis, Ch 25, p 230
Hurwitz P J 1979 Experimental transplantation of small joints by microvascular anastomoses. Journal of Plastic and Reconstructive Surgery 64: 221–231
Iselin F 1975 Arthroplasty of the proximal interphalangeal joint after trauma. The Hand 7: 41–42
Kettelcamp D B 1972 Experimental autologous joint transplantation. Clinical Orthopaedics and Related Research 87: 138–145
Kuo E T, Ji Z L, Zhao Y C, Zhang M L 1984 Reconstruction of metacarpophalangeal joint by free vascularized autogenous metatarsophalangeal joint transplant. Journal of Reconstructive Microsurgery 1: 65–74
Mathes S J, Buchannan R, Weeks P M 1980 Microvascular joint transplantation with epiphyseal growth. Journal of Hand Surgery 5: 586–589
May J W, Chait L A, Cohen B E, O'Brien B M 1977 Free neurovascular flap from the first web of the foot in hand reconstruction. Journal of Hand Surgery 2: 387–393
O'Brien B M, Gould J S, Morrison W A, Russell R C, MacLeod A M, Pribaz J J 1984 Free vascularized small joint transfer to the hand. Journal of Hand Surgery 9A: 634–641
Riggs S A, Cooney W P 1983 Arthroplasty for the traumatized digital joint. Journal of Hand Surgery 8: 215
Rose E H 1984 Reconstruction of central metacarpal ray defects of the hand with a free vascularized double metatarsal and metatarsophalangeal joint transfer. Journal of Hand Surgery 9A: 28–31
Seradge H, Kutz J E, Kleinert H E, Lister G D, Wolff T W, Atasoy E 1984 Perichondrial resurfacing arthroplasty in the hand. Journal of Hand Surgery 9A: 880–886
Singer D I, O'Brien B M, McLeod A M, Morrison W A, Angel M F 1988 Long-term follow-up of free vascularized joint transfers to the hand in children. Journal of Hand Surgery 13A: 776–783
Strickland J 1974 Silicone replacement arthroplasty in post-traumatic disabilities of the proximal interphalangeal joint. Journal of Bone and Joint Surgery 56A: 1096
Tsai T M, Ogden L, Jaeger S H, Okubo K 1982a Experimental vascularized total joint autografts — a primate study. Journal of Hand Surgery 7: 140–146
Tsai T M, Jupita J B, Kutz J E, Kleinert H E 1982b Vascularized autogenous whole joint transfer in the hand — a clinical study. Journal of Hand Surgery 7: 335–341
Tsai T M, Singer R 1984 Elective free vascularized double transfer of toe joint from second toe to proximal interphalangeal joint of index finger: a case report. Journal of Hand Surgery 9A: 816–820
Tsai T M, Singer R, Elliott E, Klein H 1985 Immediate free vascularized joint transfer from second toe to index finger proximal interphalangeal joint: a case report. Journal of Hand Surgery 10B: 85–89
Tsai T M, Bobb D 1987 Vascularized whole, hemi-, and double-joint transfers in the hand. In: Urbaniak J (ed) Microsurgery for major limb reconstruction. C V Mosby Company, St Louis, Ch 37, p 282
Wray R C, Mathes S M, Young V L, Weeks P M 1981 Free vascularized whole-joint transplants with ununited epiphyses. Journal of Plastic and Reconstructive Surgery 67: 519–525
Yoshizu T, Watanabe M, Tajima T 1985 Experimental study and clinical application of free toe joint transplantation with vascular anastomosis. In: Tubiana R (ed) The Hand. W B Saunders Company, Philadelphia, Ch 70, p 685

M. Frey and H. Gruber

13 The vascularised nerve graft — consideration of indications on the basis of a review to the literature and of our own experimental investigations

The importance of an adequate blood supply to a nerve as a precondition for axonal regeneration has been shown by several authors (Smith 1966 a, b, Lundborg 1970, Lundborg & Rydevik 1973, Lundborg 1975). When a thicker nerve, such as the ulnar nerve, is used for grafting, fibrosis takes place if the nutrient vessels are not kept intact or anastomosed immediately. Spontaneous revascularisation from the recipient bed works well in thin nerve grafts, such as the sural nerve, but it is insufficient for thick nerve grafts. To overcome this problem, Strange used the ulnar nerve for 'nerve pedicle grafting' to a defect in the median nerve for the first time in 1946 (Strange 1947). Similar considerations led to the 'cross-arm nerve pedicle flap for reconstruction of major defects of the median nerve' reported by Edgerton in 1968. The use of these techniques is limited to rare cases, in which the use of the ulnar nerve as a graft for reconstruction of the median nerve is justified because it too is damaged distally, and irreparably so. The rapid development of microvascular surgery was required to apply the principle of immediate reconstruction of blood circulation also to more dispensable and usually thinner nerves.

The publication of the paper 'The free vascularized nerve graft — a further experimental and clinical application of microvascular techniques' by Taylor and Ham in 1976 initiated a discussion on improving the results of nerve grafting by immediate microsurgical re-establishment of the blood supply. This discussion is still going on, because even numerous experimental series and several clinical cases have not so far produced clear evidence for the superiority of vascularised nerve grafts (VNG) over conventional, non-vascularised nerve grafts (CNG). At first, Taylor and his co-workers transplanted the femoral neurovascular bundle to the contralateral side in pigs. Proximal anastomoses were performed to the femoral vessels. Later, distal anastomoses were performed in addition, to maintain high flow rates in the graft vessels. In this way, the danger of thrombosis at the microvascular anastomoses is reduced markedly. Besides the description of this important detail of microsurgical technique, the first clinical application of the use of the superficial part of the radial nerve as a free vascularised nerve graft was reported. A 24-cm-long nerve graft was used to bridge a 22 cm defect in the median nerve. The radial artery and its concomitant veins were used not only to re-establish the blood supply of the nerve graft immediately after transfer, but also to reconstruct a defect in the radial artery.

In his paper, Taylor summarises the advantages of the vascularised nerve graft in the following way:

1. A very long piece of the radial nerve may be grafted to a distant site.
2. A scarred recipient bed can be bridged with safety.
3. Survival of the nerve graft can be inferred early, by the presence of a peripheral pulse in its accompanying artery, and may be confirmed subsequently by angiography.
4. The accompanying vessels may be used to supplement the blood supply to the limb.
5. The increased vascularity may support additional cable grafts.
6. If the anastomoses should fail, then the nerve may still survive as an ordinary free graft.

The disadvantages are summarised as:

1. Some loss of sensation is inflicted at the donor site. (The patient had insignificant sensory impairment of her donor hand after two months, and there was no problem with neuroma tenderness at the donor elbow.) Seddon (1972) advises against using the superficial radial nerve as a donor nerve, but Sunderland (1968) concludes that the sensory loss is of no importance provided the nerve is taken from the other arm.

2. The superficial radial nerve has a relatively small diameter, as compared to the median. One or more supplementary cable nerve grafts may be desirable. (These were not available for use in this case.)

3. The operation is a long one, and a major blood vessel is sacrificed with the graft.

Summing up, Taylor estimated the advantages as greater than the disadvantages. In the following years, a lot of divergent reports on the efficiency and the superiority of vascularised nerve grafts over conventional nerve grafts were published. The increase of research work in this field reflects the attempt to improve the results of nerve reconstruction by nerve grafting, although the results with conventional grafts had already reached a relatively high level by a preceding improvement in microsurgical techniques, and a significant increase in knowledge of peripheral nerve regeneration.

Interestingly, a second tendency can be observed in papers published in the field of peripheral nerve regeneration where there is a gap. Are all the different kinds of conduits being investigated because we hope for improvement in the final functional results, or because we are seeking to replace nerve grafts by other conduits which do not involve the disadvantages and limitations of autologous nerve grafts? In recent papers, empty perineural tubes (Restrepo et al 1983), vein grafts (Chiu et al 1988, Rigoni et al 1983, Suematsu et al 1988), vascularised pseudosheaths (Mackinnon & Dellon 1988) or muscle (Glasby et al 1986, Smahel & Chen 1989) were used as conduits to bridge a nerve gap (Mackinnon 1989). Biodegradable nerve guides have also been used for this purpose (Seckel et al 1984, Merrell et al 1986). That nerve grafts should exactly match the diameter of the bridged nerve seems to be unnecessary, if we heed the experimental investigation of Jenq and Coggeshall (1987). In this study in the rat, an 8 mm gap in the sciatic nerve was bridged by the removed piece of sciatic nerve in one group and by a double sural nerve transplant in the other group. As a result of this study, we learn that the size of the transplant does not seem to determine the size of regenerated nerve. If these experimental results are relevant for clinical nerve grafting, a lot of basic principles of nerve surgery have to be called into question. If we try to understand the controversy surrounding the results of experimental studies and the difficulties in reproducing the results of enthusiastic reports of new operative techniques for nerve reconstruction, we have to consider several inherent problems:

1. In some experimental studies, wrong methods are used and as a consequence wrong conclusions are drawn.

2. The majority of experimental series are concentrated maximally upon the regenerative processes in the nerve graft, secondarily extended to the nerve proximal and distal to the graft. Only very few investigators pay enough attention to the function regained in the end-organ, but this is what we should be primarily interested in from a clinical standpoint.

3. The influence of the end-organ connected to the regenerating nerve is almost never included in studies. As an exception, Mackinnon and Dellon (1988) showed in a cross-face nerve grafting model in primates that regeneration across the nerve graft connected to the distal nerve was qualitatively superior to that which occurred across the nerve graft without any end-organ connection.

4. Unjustified correlations between morphological parameters, like number or diameter of regenerated nerve fibres in a nerve graft, and the final functional result, can be found frequently in publications on experimental work. In a recently published, extensive study of ipsilateral and cross-over nerve grafting in sheep (Frey et al 1990), it was shown that the functional recovery in the reinnervated muscle correlated only with the number of myelinated nerve fibres in the distal nerve segment behind the second suture line of the graft. At no stage of the study could a correlation be found between the morphology within

the graft and the function regained by the end-organ.

5. The complex process of nerve regeneration along a nerve graft makes the establishment of a standardised model extremely difficult. Even if experimental conditions can reduce the influencing factors to a minimum, one still ends up with a result that is a product of multiple factors, and that is difficult to analyse.

6. Reports of clinical applications of vascularised nerve grafts include, unfortunately, only a few cases.

7. The reported cases have completely different lesions, with different history and different ages of the patients. The time elapsed since onset of the palsy is never the same. As a result of these inhomogenous preconditions in a small group of patients, a definitive statement about the place for the vascularised nerve graft is impossible at this time.

8. A controlled prospective clinical study would be necessary to get any relevant and conclusive information about the value of the vascularised nerve graft.

Nevertheless, in the following, we will try to summarise the data presently available about the vascularised nerve graft, based on a survey of the specific literature. Then we will present some of our own experimental data on vascularisation of conventional nerve grafts in relation to functional recovery. The indications for the use of vascularised nerve grafts will be discussed, as we see them at the present time.

LITERATURE REPORTING THE SUPERIORITY OF VASCULARISED NERVE GRAFTS OVER CONVENTIONAL NERVE GRAFTS IN EXPERIMENTAL SERIES

Koshima and Harii (1985) compared vascularised and free (non-vascularised) nerve grafts transplanted into silicone tubes, using the sciatic nerve in rats as an experimental model. Morphometric studies of axonal regeneration in the 15-mm-long, silicon-covered segments were performed from the first to the 24th postoperative week. There was a significant increase in the number of large myelinated axons in the vascularised nerve graft group over those in the free nerve graft group at the distal ankle region. Furthermore, the diameters of myelinated axons in the vascularised nerve graft were larger than those in the free graft at all specimen sites during all postoperative weeks. The authors suggest that the preservation of the vascular system in vascularised nerve grafts would decrease the likelihood of fibrosis and result in better regeneration of axons. Using the identical model, the same authors (Koshima & Harii 1985) again investigated the differences between axonal regeneration in vascularised and conventional nerve grafts (n=37), but this time the sciatic nerve segments were grafted into an acute burn wound, thus reducing the vascular condition of the recipient bed. From the first to 24th postoperative week, the vascularised nerve grafts showed, once again, earlier axonal regeneration and a higher density of large regenerated axons. These findings correlated with a faster nerve conduction velocity and a higher action potential in the vascularised group.

Similar results were found by Restrepo et al (1985) in cross-sectioned sciatic nerves of rabbits after vascularised and conventional nerve grafting. In this comparison, the regenerated fibres in the vascularised grafts were surrounded by a thicker myelin sheath. This fact was interpreted as a more favourable regeneration when vascularised nerve grafts had been used.

Also, Kärcher (1985) stated the advantages of the preserved blood supply in nerve grafts. He used a segment of the femoral nerve to bridge a defect in the sciatic nerve of eight rats. The grafted segment was pedicled on the femoral artery and vein, which were shunted distally. The superiority of vascularised nerve grafts is supported by this author.

Blood flow to both conventional and vascularised canine saphenous nerve grafts was quantified by Lind and Wood (1986), using radionuclide-labelled microspheres. At 2, 24 and 72 hours postoperatively, vascularised nerve grafts demonstrated adequate blood flow equal to or exceeding normal nerve controls. In contrast, conventional nerve grafts exhibited no significant fascicular revascularisation in the first 24 hours, and only one of three dogs demonstrated adequate blood flow by three days postoperatively.

Similar results for the early postoperative blood flow in vascularised and non-vascularised nerve grafts were reported by Lux et al (1988). The saphenous nerve of dogs served as a model. The intravascular presence of India ink was not observed until the third day postoperatively in the non-vascularised grafts, while it was demonstrated in vascularised grafts on the first postoperative day. Quantitative microsphere studies showed that control blood flow in undisturbed nerves ranged from 0.06 to 0.16 ml/min per g dry weight. On postoperative day 1, flow was not detectable in any of the non-vascularised grafts, while flow in the vascularised grafts had reached a mean of 1.88 ml/min per g dry weight. By day 6, blood flow rate had increased to 7.63 and 4.72 ml/min per g dry weight for non-vascularised and vascularised grafts respectively. Although this study documented higher blood flow in non-vascularised nerve grafts than in vascularised grafts a few days after grafting, the authors conclude that it may be of advantage to avoid the 'up to 3 days of warm ischaemia', even in a well-vascularised bed.

The clinically most interesting parameter, the recovery of muscle function, has been included in only one experimental comparison of the two nerve grafting techniques so far. Shibata et al (1988) used the median nerve as a vascularised nerve graft in a group of 20 rabbits, and as a non-vascularised, conventional graft in another group of 20 rabbits. The contralateral side served as a control. Postoperative evaluation was performed at 10 and 24 weeks. Nerve conduction velocity, compound action potential area, axon diameter and muscle weight did not demonstrate statistically significant differences. Axon counts and muscle strength did show a superior value for vascularised nerve grafts at 24 weeks. One has to mention that the statistically significant difference in number of axons was not observed for all biopsy sites. Recently, we have been able to show that a correlation between axon number and functional recovery in the muscle can be found only in the biopsies distal to the nerve graft, and not in biopsies proximal or within the nerve graft (Frey et al 1990). Therefore, the varying results for the two nerve biopsies distal to the graft in the study of the Louisville group cannot decide the superiority of one of the two grafting techniques. Maximal contraction force was about 20% higher in the group with vascularised, than in the group with non-vascularised, nerve grafts at 24 weeks. This is not very much, when we consider that, for the non-vascularised nerve grafting procedure, a model was used which we know already to be inferior as judged by clinical application. So we are still missing a functional investigation of the question of whether immediate repair of vascular supply is advantageous in conventional grafts like the sural nerve graft. This question is open for the normal recipient bed as well as for the scarred region, which might mean problems for spontaneous vascularisation. Today, probably nobody would use a graft of the diameter of the ulnar nerve without microvascular anastomoses in the clinical situation. Schupeck et al (1989) investigated nerve regeneration in vascularised and conventional grafts of the sciatic nerve of the rat, using parameters like nerve action potential amplitude, the level of norepinephrine, prostacycline, malondialdehyde, and the blood–nerve barrier. This study showed that nerve blood flow was much greater in vascularised grafts, but the increase was confined to non-nutritive flow, deriving from arteriovenous shunt flow. The vascularised nerve grafts had larger nerve action potentials than conventional grafts at 1 month, but there was no longer a difference at 6 months, suggesting that there may be earlier regeneration in vascularised grafts without any ultimate advantage. There were no statistically different findings for the other parameters in the two groups, except for the 6-keto prostaglandin F1a. Its better restoration suggests that vascularised grafts may be more effective in restoring the vasoreactivity of peripheral nerve following grafting.

LITERATURE REPORTING NO SUPERIORITY OF VASCULARISED NERVE GRAFTS OVER CONVENTIONAL NERVE GRAFTS IN EXPERIMENTAL SERIES

In an extensive experimental study in the sciatic

nerve of the rat (n=57), McCullough et al (1984) called into question the advantages of the vascularised nerve graft. Three different groups of nerve grafts were investigated: vascular pedicled, devascularised, and devascularised and wrapped in a polythene sleeve. Micro-angiography, histological and electroneurographic assessment showed no differences between all groups. Vascularisation was significantly delayed in the devascularised nerve graft wrapped in the polythene sleeve, but with time vascularisation shows no differences. As a consequence, increased sprouting of axons can be observed in the avascular zone. Surprisingly, in this study there was no delay in the growth of the regenerating axons of the devascularised conventional nerve graft.

In 1985, Daly and Wood showed, in a series of nine dogs, that the blood flow in conventional saphenous nerve grafts was significantly higher than in vascularised grafts six months postoperatively. Using ^{85}Sr-marked microspheres, the endoneural blood flow in conventional grafts was shown to be six times that of the vascularised.

In 1984, Settergren and Wood pointed out that the blood flow is significantly higher in non-vascularised nerve grafts than in vascularised grafts. They performed their experimental series in rabbits.

Interesting results on the alterations with time in vascularised and conventional nerve grafts were published by Pho et al (1985). The 2-cm-long segment of the femoral nerve of the rat showed no differences between vascular pedicled and devascularised grafts. There was also no difference in the time course of vascularisation (2, 4, 6 and 12 weeks), the collapse of the reticulin framework, the axonal regeneration and the remyelination.

Morphometric studies of the sciatic nerve of the rat by Seckel et al (1986) showed no statistical difference for the number and the size of axons between the vascularised and the devascularised nerve grafts. In contrast to other reports, the myelin sheaths were thicker in the devascularised group. Even in the devascularised nerve graft, there were no structural differences between the centre and the periphery of the nerve cross-section. The intraneural scar formation was the same in both groups. As a conclusion, the clinical application of vascularised nerve grafts was recommended only in defects demanding a long (10–20 cm) or thick nerve graft, or in the case of an avascular recipient area.

RELATIONS BETWEEN VASCULARISATION, MORPHOLOGY OF NERVE FIBRES AND FUNCTIONAL RESULTS AFTER NERVE GRAFTING — AN EXPERIMENTAL STUDY IN SHEEP

Considering the divergent opinions about the influence of the vascularisation of a nerve graft on the final functional recovery, the basic question arises of whether the spontaneous vascularisation of conventional nerve grafts is insufficient or too late, and whether the vascularisation really is of crucial importance for successful neurotisation.

Radek (1986) investigated the blood supply of transected rabbit peripheral nerve after end-to-end suture or autogenous grafting. In a first group of 12 animals, an end-to-end suture of the tibial nerve was performed. In a second group of 15 rabbits, a 1.5 cm length was excised from the tibial, and 2 cm from the peroneal, division of the sciatic nerve at mid-thigh level, and the latter afterwards used to bridge the nerve defect in the tibial nerve. The results of the quantitative evaluation of the density of the vascular network showed that the average density for the control (non-operated nerves) was 31.97 ($\pm$2.15)/mm^2. After direct nerve suture it was 22.79 ($\pm$9.61)/mm^2, and after nerve grafting significantly higher, with 60.79 ($\pm$4.25) mm^2. These results indicate a great potential for revascularisation in fresh and thin autogenous grafts.

A further experimental study on revascularisation of conventional nerve grafts was performed by Penkert et al (1988). The revascularisation process after different postoperative intervals was demonstrated in the sciatic nerve of rabbits by the use of micro-angiography with roentgen-positive, water-soluble contrast medium. The third postoperative day was the earliest time for revascularisation of the autologous graft from the surrounding tissues. On the fourth postoperative day, a hyperaemia with extension to all parts of the intraneural vessel system existed, and this persisted to the fifth and sixth day. In one experimental group, revascularisation was allowed to occur only in a longitudinal direction. Revascularisation under these conditions proved to be poor, slow and obviously dependent on the length of the graft. The authors conclude that revascularisation from surrounding tissues occurs by the third postoperative day. Therefore, survival and subsequent function of free autologous nerve grafts may depend on the diameter of the grafts and the quality of the recipient site, but not on the length of the grafts.

Because there is still no answer to the question of whether a correlation exists between spontaneous vascularisation and nerve regeneration as well as functional recovery, we studied the role of vascularisation (Frey et al 1988) within an extensive experimental series, which was originally dedicated to the problem of elongation of a motor nerve beyond its natural length by nerve grafting (Frey et al 1990).

Material and methods

In 24 adult sheep the vastus nerve (motor branch of the femoral nerve) was elongated by nerve grafting as far as possible. The saphenous nerve was used as nerve graft with a length of 28 (±1.8)/cm on average. In one group, nerve grafting was performed as an ipsilateral procedure, in a second group as cross-over nerve grafting to the contralateral hind limb. The microsurgical nerve suture between the distal end of the nerve graft and the freshly cut rectus nerve supplying the rectus femoris muscle was performed after different intervals: 0, 3, 6 and 9 months. In the ipsilateral group, the contralateral side was used as a control by a direct nerve suture between the vastus nerve and the rectus nerve without interpositioning a nerve graft.

The final experiments consisted of neurographic studies, muscle force measurements and morphometric analyses of multiple nerve and muscle biopsies, at least 6 months after the last operation.

Stimulated by the open questions related to the vascularised nerve graft, we were interested in the correlations of the vascularisation of the conventional free nerve graft with the morphology of the regenerating nerve fibres and the functional recovery. Therefore, the total vascular area (area of all vascular lumina) was assessed by computer-supported planimetry on the nerve cross-sections of the ipsilateral group, and correlated to the total number and the diameter of axons, the total areas of nerve fascicles (areas within the perineurium) and to the maximal tetanic tension regained by the rectus femoris muscle re-innervated by the vastus nerve over the long saphenous nerve graft. Nerve biopsies were taken from the vastus nerve at the time of nerve grafting, and from the proximal and distal part of the nerve graft at the time of final assessment. Details of the histological and planimetric techniques are described elsewhere (Frey et al 1990).

Results

As one can see in Table 13.1, the number of axons in the proximal nerve graft is always higher than in the supplying vastus nerve at the time of the final experiment. Often there is even an increase in the number of axons found along the nerve graft from proximal to distal. Parallel to this increase in the number of axons, there is a decrease in the diameter of the axons (Figs 13.1–13.4). There is no correlation between the number of axons and the regained muscle force (Fig. 13.5). There is also no dependence of the maximal tetanic tension upon the diameter of the regenerated axons (Fig. 13.6). The vascular area related to the area of nerve fascicles is significantly higher in the nerve grafts than in the normal nerve (Table 13.1, Figs 13.8 and 13.9). Again, no correlation can be observed between the relative vascular area and the number of axons (Fig. 13.7) or the functional recovery (Table 13.1).

Discussion

After direct nerve suture, an increase in the number of nerve fibres and in the vascular area is found behind the nerve suture line. This phenomenon takes place to an even greater extent when a very long nerve graft is interposed. In the nerve graft, there are more nerve fibres and more vessels than in the normal nerve used as a supplying donor nerve. At least in this experimental series, the degree of vascularisation cannot be limiting the functional result of re-innervation.

Table 13.1 Quantitative analysis of cross-sections of nerve biopsies of ipsilateral nerve grafts and of the contralateral control side (= direct nerve suture) in 6 sheep. Months = interval between proximal nerve suture of the nerve graft to the donor nerve (N. vastus) and the distal nerve suture of the nerve graft to the recipient nerve (N. rectus femoris). N. vastus = motor branch of the femoral nerve to the vastus muscle, used as source of re-innervation. Prox. graft = proximal end of the nerve graft. Dist. graft = distal end of the nerve graft. N. vastus/C = motor nerve used as a source of re-innervation for the direct nerve suture on the control side. N. rectus/C = distal nerve used for direct nerve suture on the control side. Axons = total number of myelinated axons. Fascicle area = total amount of area surrounded by perineurium in the nerve cross-section (μm^2). Vascular area = total amount of area surrounded by perineurium in the nerve cross-section (μm^2). % = relation of the vascular area to the fascicle area (total fascicle area = 100%). Max. tetanic tension = maximal tetanic tension developed by the rectus femoris muscle under indirect, supramaximal electric stimulation (Newton).

Sheep Months	S17 0	S19 3	S20 3	S13 6	S14 6	S18 9
N. vastus						
Axons	1035	1587	1601	2100	2467	2174
Fascicle area	535005	574207	916816	810954	786123	750347
Vascular area	44259	40960	52665	32338	29295	55786
%	8.28	7.14	5.75	3.99	3.73	7.44
Prox. graft						
Axons	1487	2976	3146	3104	2857	3429
Fascicle area	237281	537548	1516780	866478	777504	749698
Vascular area	56775	244017	73198	41218	56632	155751
%	23.9	45.4	4.8	4.7	7.29	20.7
Dist. graft						
Axons	1426	1510	5967	1327	11269	4624
Fascicle area	211738	350627	1191033	210317	1712832	452404
Vascular area	9991	219359	185634	49685	460658	34380
%	4.72	62.57	15.59	23.63	26.9	7.6
N. vastus/C						
Axons		2033				
Fascicle area		611533				
Vascular area		58881				
%		9.63				
N. rectus/C						
Axons		3181		5942		
Fascicle area		577145		1587470		
Vascular area		104377		86382		
%		18.09		5.45		
Max. tetanic tension						
left	62.5	103	172	27	80	143
right/C	125	182.5	155	190	124	

The same is true for the total number of axons. Therefore mainly qualitative differences in the regenerating axons must be responsible for the functional result. The quality of a regenerating axon is not dependent upon the diameter of the axon. How far this kind of quality of regeneration of axons can be influenced by the immediate microsurgical reconstruction of the blood supply of the nerve graft, has not been answered by any experimental or clinical study so far.

CLINICAL APPLICATION OF VASCULARISED NERVE GRAFTS

In 1978, Taylor added two further clinical cases of nerve grafting with simultaneous microvascular reconstruction to his first initial case. One patient had sustained severe high voltage electrical burns to all limbs. The 20-cm-long defects in the median and ulnar nerve of the left forearm were repaired by transferring 26 cm unbranched lengths of the

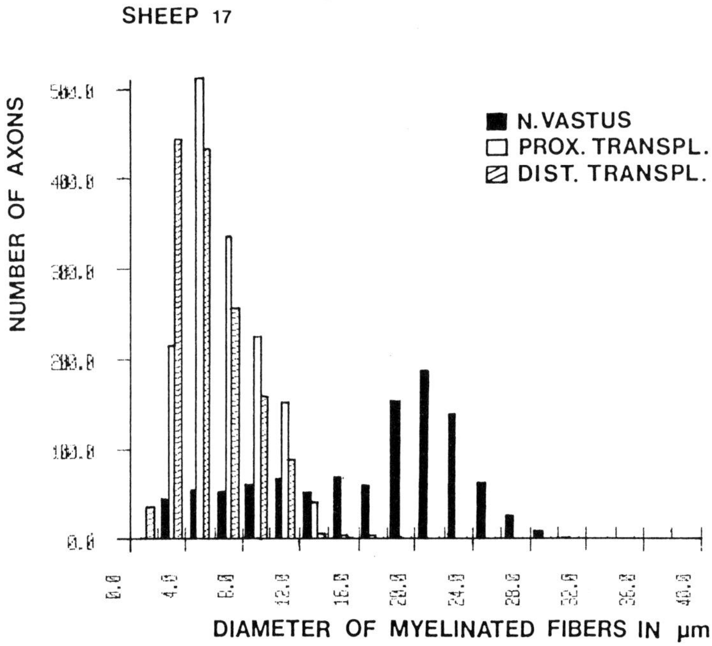

Fig. 13.1 Distribution of the diameters of myelinated nerve fibres in the vastus nerve compared to the proximal and distal ends of the nerve graft in a sheep 6 months after proximal and distal nerve suture at the same time (interval = 0 months). Note the marked reduction in fibre size and increased number of axons in the transplant.

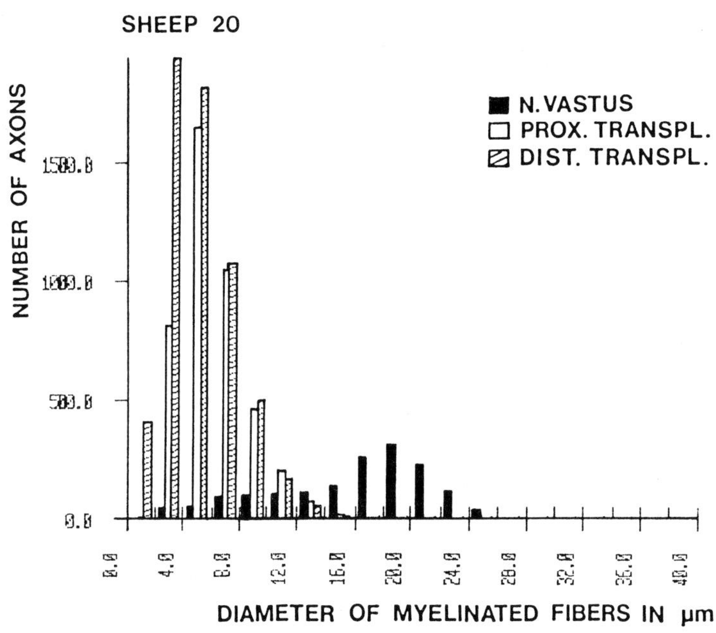

Fig. 13.2 Similar histogram as in Fig. 13.1, but the time interval between the proximal and the distal nerve suture was three months.

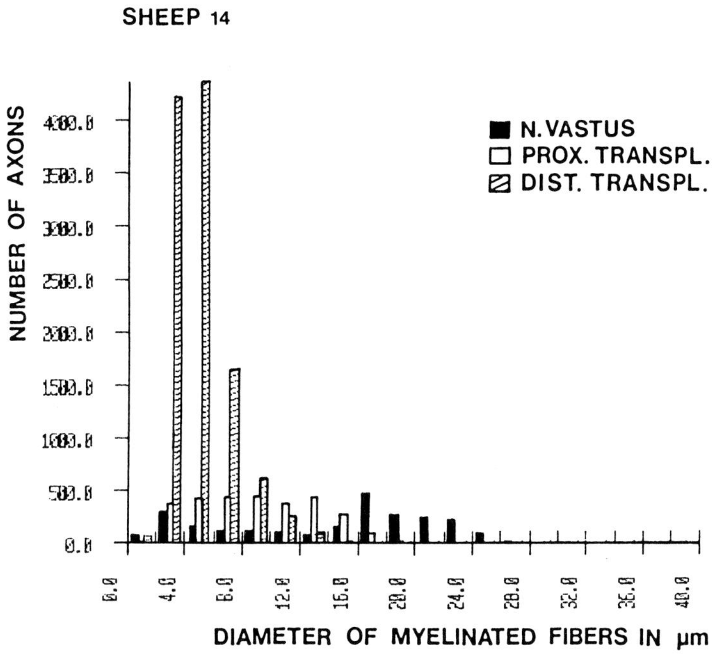

Fig. 13.3 Similar histogram as in Fig. 13.1, but the time interval between the proximal and the distal nerve suture was six months.

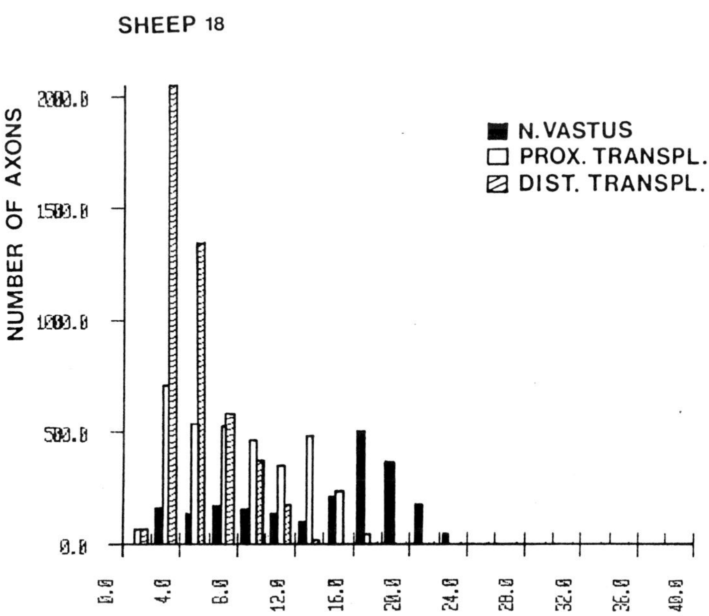

Fig. 13.4 Similar histogram as in Fig. 13.1, but the time interval between the proximal and the distal nerve suture was nine months.

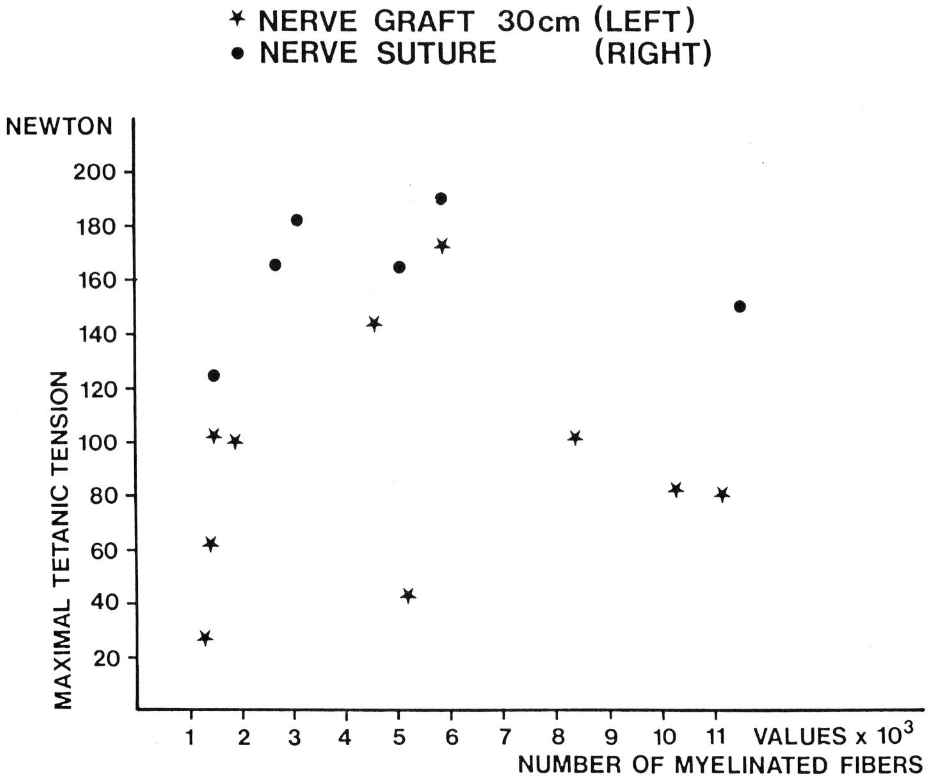

Fig. 13.5 Correlation between the total number of myelinated nerve fibres in the distal end of the graft or distal to the direct nerve suture, and the maximal tetanic tension of rectus femoris muscle.

median and ulnar nerves, vascularised by the brachial vessels, from the amputation stump of the right arm. The other patient had suffered a Volkmann's ischaemia of the right forearm as a complication of a tight plaster. Massive necrosis of all flexor muscles in the forearm resulted, together with a 20 cm segment of the median nerve just beyond its anterior interosseous division. The radial nerve was compressed in the spiral groove, and 11 months later only partial recovery of the forearm extensors was evident; this seriously restricted the possibilities of tendon transfer. The ulnar nerve had been damaged at the elbow, and was subsequently repaired after transposition. This extensive destruction of the median nerve and forearm flexors was reconstructed by a combination of extensor tendon transfers and a microvascular free transplant of the superficial radial nerve and the brachioradialis muscle, taken from the opposite arm with their radial vessel supply. In this patient, two sural nerve cables were added to the radial nerve graft to match the median nerve stumps. In both cases, nerve regeneration could be attested by Sir Sydney Sunderland beyond the distal nerve graft repair, with protective sensation in both cases, and strong contraction of the grafted muscle in the second case, 9 and 10 months postoperatively. The author sees the rapid rate of re-innervation as the greatest advantage of the procedure, but restricts the indication to those cases where conventional techniques carry high risk of graft necrosis, situations in which the nerve gap is large, the recipient bed is scarred, or the free transfer of a thick nerve is desired.

Later, Townsend and Taylor (1984) presented their experience with the composite arterialised neuro-venous systems. This composite graft offers the possibility of long distance vascular reconstruction at the same time as the vascularised nerve

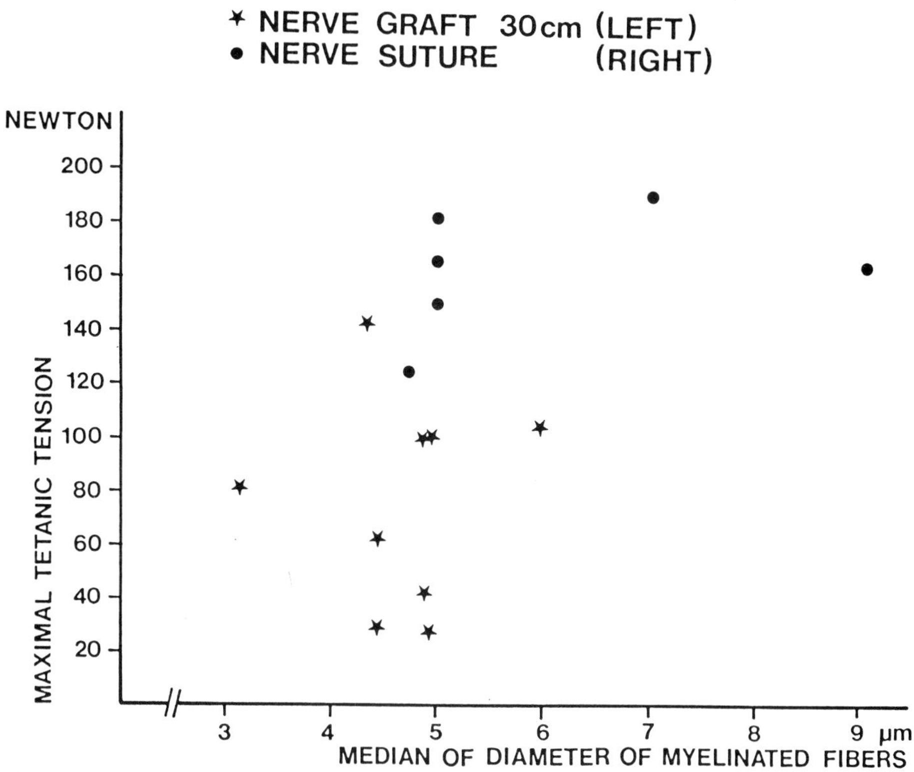

Fig. 13.6 Correlation between the median of the diameters of the nerve fibres in the distal end of the nerve graft or distal to the direct nerve suture, and the maximal tetanic tension.

graft is performed. At first, the results of a series of 15 dogs were reported, in which the saphenous nerve was vascularised by a proximal anastomosis of the saphenous vein to the artery. Regeneration was 2 mm per day in the vascularised nerve grafts, and 1.5 mm in the non-vascularised grafts. Electron microscopy showed that the phagocytosis was completed after nine weeks in the vascularised grafts. At that time, old myelin was still found in the non-vascularised grafts. These positive results were transferred to human conditions. In cadaver dissections, the sural nerve together with the saphenous vein was found to be suitable for reconstruction of nerve and artery at the same time, over a longer distance. Clinically, 6 cases of bridging nerve defects in the median nerve, the ulnar nerve and the facial nerve are reported. Besides the advantage of vascular reconstruction, the authors discuss an acceleration of nerve regeneration caused by a faster destruction of the myelin and by faster remyelinisation.

This concept of the arterialised venous free sural nerve graft was also used by Gu Yu-dong et al from August 1980. In the publication of 1985, it is proposed that the vein be used as a bypass, providing the possibility of interposition for reconstruction of the artery. In a comparison of a group of 12 patients with vascularised nerve grafts, the vascularised group were shown to be superior. In an experimental study in 76 rabbits, 2 cm of the median nerve together with the brachial artery and vein served as a model. The arterialised venous nerve graft showed similar results as the grafts with restored arterial and venous supply. Both forms of vascularised grafts had better results than the non-vascularised, and thin grafts fared better than thick in the latter group.

In an extensive cadaver dissection study, the blood supply of 13 different potential donor nerve grafts were examined by Breidenbach and Terzis (1986). Six of the 13 nerves were then further investigated with injection studies, revealing that

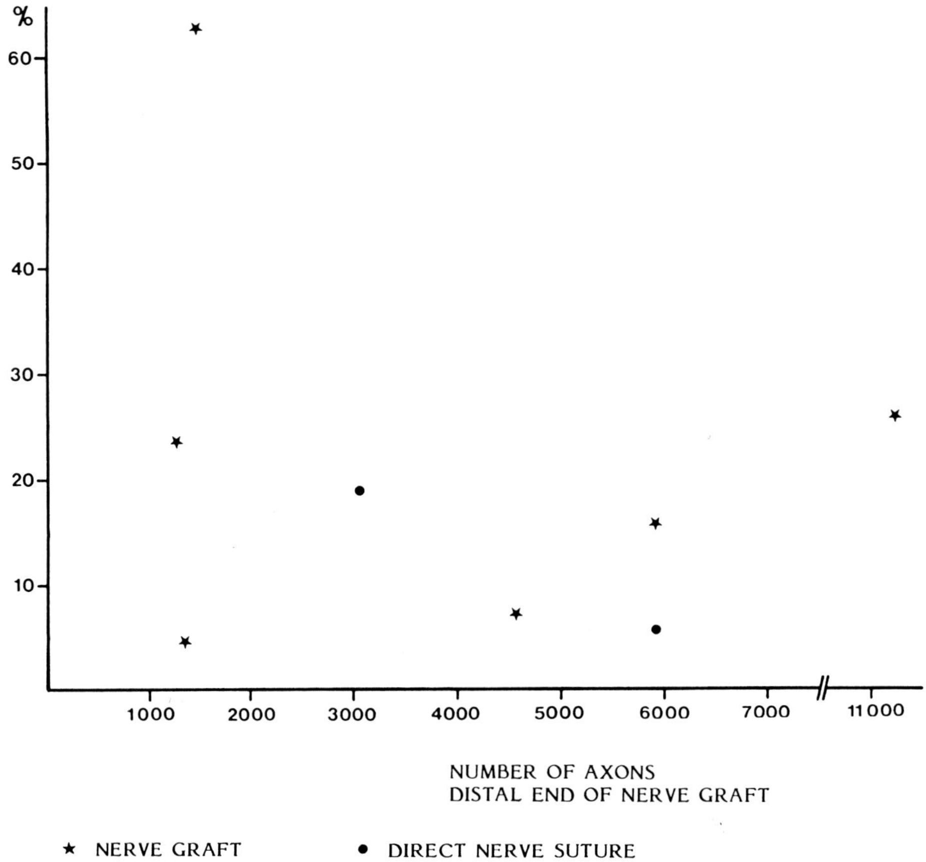

Fig. 13.7 Correlation between the number of axons, and the relative vascular area in the distal end of the nerve graft or distal to the direct nerve suture.

long lengths of the nerves may survive on the intrinsic supply alone. The saphenous nerve is believed to be best suited as a donor vascularised nerve graft. Finally, a method is proposed for forming cable grafts from segments of vascularised nerve grafts that are supplied solely by the intrinsic blood supply.

In 1984, these authors (Breidenbach & Terzis 1984) described the anatomy of six favourable nerves, which are suitable for grafting with microvascular reconstruction of their vascular supply. They saw the proximal nerve lesion, the long defect and the poorly vascularised recipient bed as indications for vascularised nerve grafting.

A modification of the vascularised sural nerve graft was used by Doi et al (1984) in four clinical cases. Pedicled on a skin branch of the peroneal artery or on a perforating muscle branch of the posterior tibial artery, the sural nerve can be used as a double or threefold transplant. A skin island can be included to cover a soft tissue defect. By the use of this vascularised nerve graft, a quicker advancement of the Tinel's sign was observed.

The anatomy and the surgical approach was described for the vascularised sural nerve graft by Fachinelli et al in 1981. He proposed the division of the sural nerve to use it still vascularised in all strands as a folded graft for the first time. The vascularised sural nerve graft was also applied by Gilbert; he reported his experiences in 1984.

In 1983, Comtet reported nine cases, seven of which had a postoperative period of more than one year. The ulnar nerve and the medial cutaneous nerve of the arm served as donor nerves. One

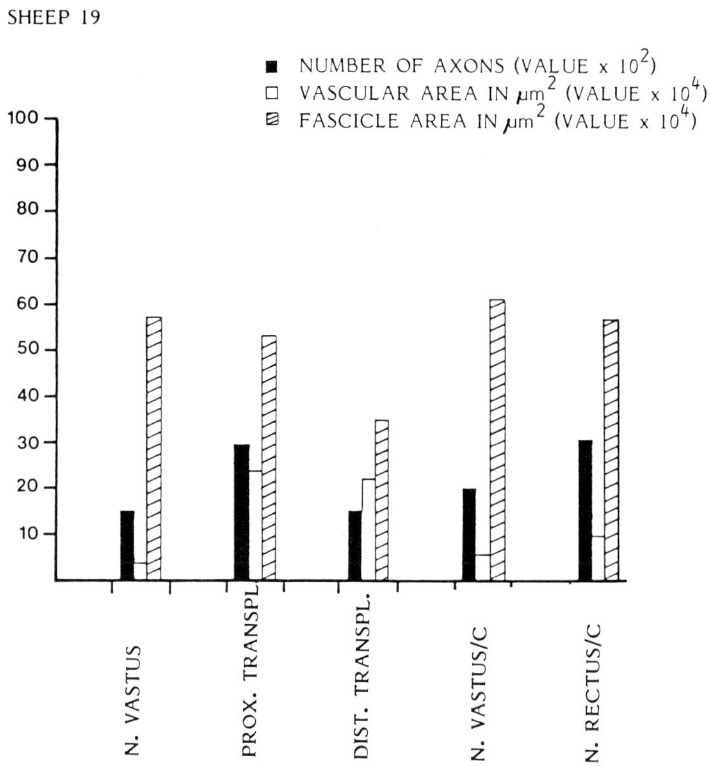

Fig. 13.8 Comparison between number of axons, vascular area and fascicle area in the normal donor nerve (N. vastus, N. vastus/C), in the recipient nerve distal to the direct nerve suture (N. rectus/C), in the proximal and in the distal end of the nerve graft. Sheep No. 19 is shown as an example nine months after the proximal suture of the graft to the vastus nerve, and six months after the distal suture of the graft to the rectus nerve.

venous thrombosis, three partial innervations and three failed innervations were described as complications.

Rose and Kowalsky (1985) tried to reconstruct sensibility in fingers by vascularised nerve grafts from the dorsum of the foot after conventional nerve grafts had failed. The deep peroneal nerve pedicled on the dorsalis pedis artery was used for microvascular transfer, with a length of 6.6 cm on average. The five clinical cases showed a moving two-point discrimination of 7.2 mm, and a static one of 9.5 mm at the assessment 4–5 months postoperatively on average. Important donor morbidity was reported in two of the five patients. One developed a neuroma and another a superficial skin loss.

The arterial blood supply of the different anatomical segments of the ulnar nerve was described by Kunzel et al (1986) in respect of the use of the ulnar nerve as a vascularised nerve graft.

The superiority of vascularised ulnar nerve grafts over conventional sural nerve grafts or avascular ulnar nerve grafts for brachial plexus reconstruction was postulated by Bonney et al (1984), who reported 30 vascularised ulnar nerve grafts out of 100 repairs of brachial plexus injuries. Unfortunately, besides the personal impression of the authors, no objective comparison of the different groups of patients was included in this paper. Four years later, the same group (Birch et al 1988) published the results in this group of patients, enlarged to 63 patients. Forty two patients were reviewed at a minimum of 30 months after operation. The ulnar nerve based on the ulnar vessels in the arm was used in 33 patients, while the nerve based on collateral vessels in the arm was used in nine. The free vascularised ulnar nerve graft was used in one-quarter of this series of repairs of supraclavicular lesions. Although the authors describe their results with the vascularised graft as no better than those from Narakas and Sedel, the following statement can be found in the discussion of this paper: 'The vascularised nerve graft has proved to be better than avascular ulnar trunk and marginally better than cutaneous nerve grafts in unfavourable lesions'.

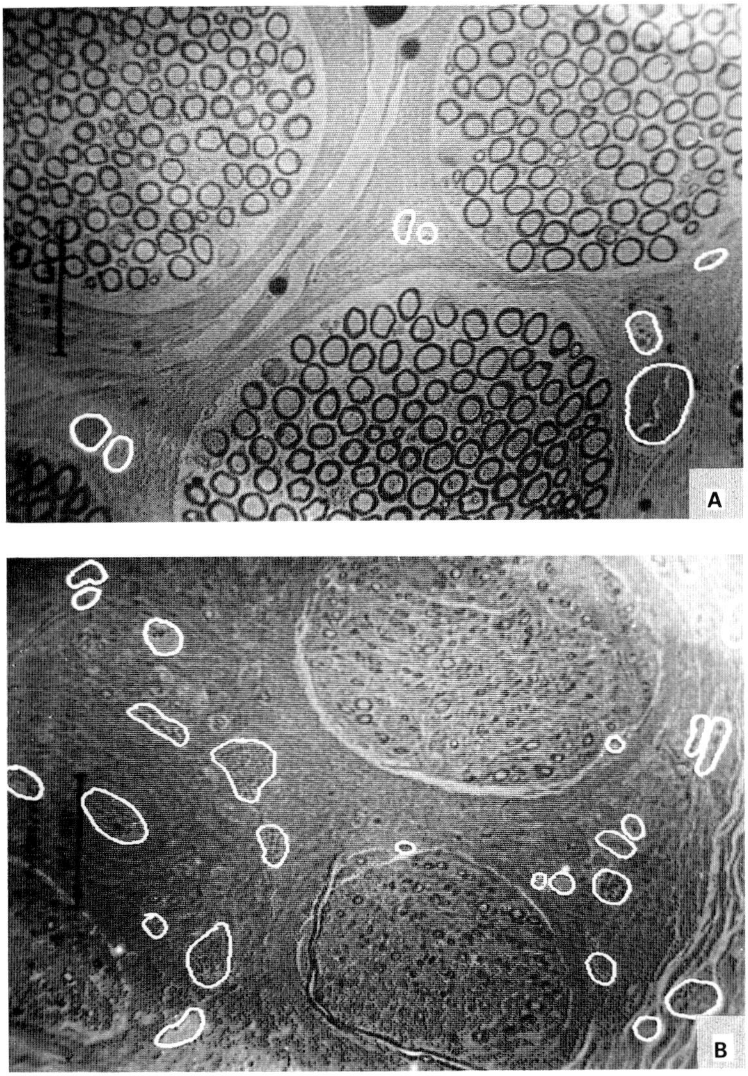

Fig. 13.9 Microscopic picture from the monitor screen. Sample of a normal N. vastus (**A**) and the distal end of a nerve graft nine months after proximal suture of the saphenous nerve graft to the vastus nerve and six months after the distal suture of the graft to the rectus femoris nerve (**B**). During planimetric assessment the vessels are marked by white lines. Calibration bars = 100 μm.

Again, the authors believe in this superiority, but could not prove it. Until now, a real clinical comparison of vascular pedicled ulnar nerve grafts and free non-vascularised sural nerve grafts in patients with brachial plexus lesions was performed only by Millesi (1988). In eight cases, the author compared the neurotisation of the biceps via vascularised nerve grafts, and the neurotisation of the triceps via free nerve grafts. In four cases, the regeneration was equal, in two cases the result was more favourable with the vascularised nerve grafts, and in two cases the free nerve grafts had better results. These results do not show any superiority of the vascularised nerve grafts, but one has to consider that the number of cases is rather low and that the presuppositions for neurotisation of the biceps muscle and the triceps muscle are somewhat different. Other differences between the individuals and in the extent of the plexus lesion may influence the functional result.

In 1988, Mackinnon et al reported a single clinical case of a histological and functional comparison of regeneration across a vascularised and a conventional nerve graft. The superficial branch of the radial nerve (vascularised nerve graft) and a conventional sural nerve graft were used as the interposition grafts between the two branches of the medial cutaneous nerve of forearm and the median nerve. This nerve grafting procedure was carried out in two stages. Biopsies were taken from the distal portions of the vascularised radial sensory nerve and the conventional sural nerve at the time of the distal nerve repair, which was performed seven months after the proximal neurorrhaphy. Histological evaluation demonstrated superior regeneration across the vascularised nerve graft. Subjectively, the patient described better sensory recovery in the territories innervated by the vascularised nerve graft. Sensory testing in the two territories demonstrated better sensibility in the territory innervated by the vascularised nerve graft. The conclusions drawn in this paper rely on three weak points: 1) the comparison is carried out only in one single clinical case; 2) there is no correlation between the number of regenerated nerve fibres in the distal end of nerve grafts and the final result of recovery, as we could show in an above mentioned experimental series (Frey et al 1990); and 3) at the level of the distal forearm the fascicle groups cannot be identified to supply certain territories distally in the fingers. Therefore, it is not possible to ascribe successful sensory recovery in certain territories to one or other nerve grafts. In a review article, Breidenbach (1988) gives a good conclusion with the still limited knowledge about the role of microvascular reconstruction in nerve grafting: 'We see that there is some evidence that VNGs may be superior to CNGs in peripheral nerve reconstruction (excluding reconstruction of digital nerves) in moderately to severely scarred recipient beds. This conclusion, however, is based on studies without controls and often with inadequate numbers of patients and follow-up. With digital nerve reconstruction, however, there appears to be good evidence that vascularised nerve grafting may be beneficial. It will be interesting to see, if other investigators can substantiate the results of Rose and Kowalsky, and Rose et al.'

DISCUSSION OF THE THEORETICAL ADVANTAGES AND DISADVANTAGES OF THE VASCULARISED NERVE GRAFT

By summarising the divergent opinions of different authors in the literature concerning vascularised nerve grafting, the advantages and disadvantages can be listed. The advantages are:

1. Faster vascularisation
2. Independence from the recipient area
3. Thicker nerves can be used as grafts
4. Combination with conventional nerve grafts also improves the conditions of vascularisation for the non-vascularised free grafts
5. Earlier degeneration and phagocytosis
6. Preservation of the arrangement of the Schwann cells
7. Faster regeneration of axons
8. Earlier arrival of the regenerating nerve fibres at the distal nerve suture line
9. Improved myelinisation
10. Less connective tissue
11. Better re-innervation
12. Faster nerve conduction velocity
13. Faster and better recovery of motor or sensory function.

The disadvantages are as follows:

1. Longer operation
2. Difficult dissection for taking the nerve graft
3. Microvascular surgery necessary
4. Selection of the nerve graft is dependent on the anatomy of its vascular supply
5. Risk of thrombosis at the microvascular anastomoses
6. In the case of microvascular failure worse than conventional grafts
7. Number, diameter and length of vascularised nerve grafts limited
8. Improvement of re-innervation has not been sufficiently shown so far.

These advantages and disadvantages are rarely proved by the published data in a scientific way. Usually, they reflect the opinion of the authors, and are merely a kind of hypothesis. This fact is underlined by our experimental work, which showed the functional result of a nerve grafting procedure independent from the number and morphology of the regenerated nerve fibres in the graft. But a change in these parameters is often used as an argument for the superiority of vascularised nerve grafts. The vascular density or the blood flow has to be seen in a similar light. As long as research cannot give a definite answer to the question of superiority of vascularised nerve grafts under normal conditions as well as under the condition of reduced vascularity in the recipient bed, we want to limit the clinical application to the following indications:

1. The insufficiently vascularised recipient bed. One should consider also in this situation that the vascularised nerve graft could be damaged by the constrictive scar formation. The improvement of the local vascularity by a transfer of enough well-vascularised soft tissue into the problem region might be of more advantage than the microsurgical repair of the vascular supply of the nerve graft.

2. The use of a thick nerve as a graft. There is no doubt about the necessity to maintain or to reconstruct immediately the blood supply of the ulnar nerve, when it is used as a graft in the reconstruction of brachial plexus lesions. We still cannot be sure that the use of a thick vascularised nerve graft is as good as, or even better than, the use of thin conventional nerve grafts for the same purpose.

3. Conventional nerve grafting has been tried already without success.

4. There is the demand for vascular reconstruction at the same time. In these cases, vascularisation has to be improved also for the end organ, which is to be re-innervated later on by the nerve graft. Often, too little attention is paid to the aspect of reduced vascularisation of the end organ, when we try to improve re-innervation. The arterialised venous-nervous graft shows convincing qualities. No bigger artery has to be sacrificed. The nerve component of such a venous nerve complex is usually not thinker than a conventional graft. Even when the reconstructed blood supply is stopped by thrombosis, the thin nerve has almost the same chances as it would if used as a conventional graft.

Future research will show whether or not further indications for vascularised nerve grafting should be added.

ACKNOWLEDGEMENTS

Our own experimental study presented in this chapter was supported by the Jubilaumsfond der Osterreichischen Nazionalbank Project No. 2274, and the Medizinisch-wissenschaftlischen Fond des Burgermeisters der Bundeshauptstadt Wien, for which we are most grateful.

REFERENCES

Birch R, Dunkerton M, Bonney G et al 1988 Experience with the free vascularized ulnar nerve graft in repair of supraclavicular lesions of the brachial plexus. Clinical Orthopaedics and Related Research 237: 96–104

Bonney G, Birch R, Jamieson A M et al 1984 Experience with vascularized nerve grafts. Clinics in Plastic Surgery 11: 137–142

Breidenbach W C, Terzis J K 1986 The blood supply of vascularized nerve grafts. Journal of Reconstructive Microsurgery 3(1): 43–55

Breidenbach W C 1988 Vascularized nerve grafts — a practical approach. Orthopedic Clinics of North America 19: 81–89

Chiu D T W, Lovelace R E, Yu L T et al 1988 Comparative electrophysiologic evaluation of nerve grafts and autogenous vein grafts as nerve conduits: an experimental study. Journal of Reconstructive Microsurgery 4(4): 303–309

Comtet J J 1983 Les greffes nerveuses vascularisées. Acta Chirurgica Belgica 83: 293–297

Daly P J, Wood M B 1985 Endoneural and epineural blood flow evaluation with free vascularized and conventional nerve grafts in the canine. Journal of Reconstructive Microsurgery 2: 45–49

Doi K N, Kuwata N, Kawakami F et al 1984 The free vascularized sural nerve graft. Microsurgery 5: 175–184

Edgerton M T 1968 Cross-arm nerve pedicle flap for reconstruction of major defects of the median nerve. Surgery 64: 248–263

Fachinelli A, Masquelet A, Restrepo J et al 1981 The vascularized sural nerve — anatomy and surgical approach. International Journal of Microsurgery 3: 57–62

Frey M, Girsch W, Gruber I et al 1988 Vaskularisiertes Nerventransplantat — theoretische Vorteile und Nachteile. Handchirurgie 20: 79–82

Frey M, Gruber H, Happak W 1990 Ipsilateral and cross-over elongation of the motor nerve by nerve grafting: An experimental study in sheep. Plastic and Reconstructive Surgery 85(1): 77–89

Gilbert A 1984 Vascularized sural nerve graft. Clinics in Plastic Surgery 11: 73–77

Glasby M A, Gschmeissner S E, Hitchock R J I et al 1986 A comparison of nerve regeneration through nerve and muscle grafts in rat sciatic nerve. Neurology and Orthopaedics 2: 21

Glasby M A, Gschmeissner S E, Huang C L H et al 1986 Degenerated muscle grafts used for peripheral nerve repair in primates. Journal of Hand Surgery 11B: 347

Gu Yu-dong, Min-ming Wu, Yi-liu Heng et al 1985 Annals of Plastic Surgery 15: 332–339

Jenq Chung-Bii, Coggeshall R E 1987 Sciatic nerve regeneration after autologous sural nerve transplantation in the rat. Brain Research 406: 52–61

Kärcher H 1985 Das gefässgestielte Nerventransplantat, eine

neue experimentelle Technik an der Ratte. Deutsche Zeitschrift für Mund-, Kiefer- und Gesichtschirurgie 9: 380–382
Koshima I, Harii K 1985 Experimental study of vascularized nerve grafts: morphometric study of axonal regeneration of nerves transplanted into silicone tubes. Annals of Plastic Surgery 14: 235–243
Koshima I, Harii K 1985 Experimental study of vascularized nerve grafts: multifactorial analyses of axonal regeneration of nerves transplanted into an acute burn wound. Journal of Hand Surgery 10A: 64–72
Künzel K H, Fischer C, Anderl H 1986 The ulnar nerve as vascularized nerve transplant. Part 1: Anatomy: arterial vascular supply. Journal of Reconstructive Microsurgery 2: 175–179
Lind R, Wood M B 1986 Comparison of the pattern of early revascularization of conventional versus vascularized nerve grafts in the canine. Journal of Reconstructive Microsurgery 2/4: 229–232
Lundborg G 1970 Ischemic nerve injury. Scandinavian Journal of Plastic and Reconstructive Surgery Supplementum 6: 1–113
Lundborg G, Rydevik B 1973 Effects of stretching the tibial nerve of the rabbit. Journal of Bone and Joint Surgery 55B: 390–400
Lundborg G 1975 Structure and function of the intraneural microvessels as related to trauma, edema formation, and nerve function. Journal of Bone and Joint Surgery 57A: 938–948
Lux P, Breidenbach W, Firrell J 1988 Determination of temporal changes in blood flow in vascularized and nonvascularized nerve grafts in the dog. Plastic and Reconstructive Surgery 82(1): 133–142
McCullough C J, Gagey O, Higginson D W et al 1984 Axon regeneration and vascularization of nerve grafts — an experimental study. Journal of Hand Surgery 9B: 323–327
Mackinnon S E, Dellon A L, Hunter D A 1988 Histological assessment of the effects of the distal nerve in determining regeneration across a nerve graft. Microsurgery 9: 46–51
Mackinnon S E, Dellon A L 1988 A comparison of nerve regeneration across a sural nerve graft and a vascularized pseudosheath. Journal of Hand Surgery 13A: 935–942
Mackinnon S E, Kelly L, Hunter D 1988 Comparison of regeneration across a vascularized versus conventional nerve graft: case report. Microsurgery 9: 226–233
Mackinnon S E 1989 Surgical management of the peripheral nerve gap. Clinics in Plastic Surgery 16: 587–603
Merrell J C, Russell R C, Zook E G 1986 Polyglycolic acid tubing as a conduit for nerve regeneration. Annals of Plastic Surgery 17: 49–58
Millesi H 1988 Brachial plexus injuries — nerve grafting. Clinical Orthopaedics and Related Research 237: 36–42
Penkert G, Bini W, Samii M 1988 Revascularization of nerve grafts: an experimental study. Journal of Reconstructive Microsurgery 4(4): 319–325
Pho R W H, Lee Y S et al 1985 Histological studies of vascularized nerve graft and conventional nerve graft. Journal of Hand Surgery 10B: 45–48
Radek A J 1986 Blood supply of transected rabbit peripheral nerve after end-to-end suture or autogenous grafting. Scandinavian Journal of Plastic and Reconstructive Surgery 20: 273–277
Restrepo Y, Merle M, Michon J et al 1983 Fascicular nerve graft using an empty perineurial tube: an experimental study in the rabbit. Microsurgery 4: 105–112
Restrepo Y, Merle M, Michon J et al 1985 Free vascularized nerve grafts: an experimental study in the rabbit. Microsurgery 6: 78–84
Rigoni G, Smahel J, Chiu D T W et al 1983 Veneninterponat als Leitbahn für die Regeneration peripherer Nerven. Handchirurgie 15: 227–231
Rose E H, Kowalsky T A 1985 Restoration of sensibility to anaesthetic scarred digits with free vascularized nerve grafts from the dorsum of the foot. Journal of Hand Surgery 10A: 514–521
Schupeck M, Ward K K, Schmelzer J D et al 1989 Comparison of nerve regeneration in vascularized and conventional grafts: nerve electrophysiology, norepinephrine, prostacyclin, malondialdehyde, and the blood-nerve barrier. Brain Research 495: 225–230
Seckel B R, Chiu T H, Nyilas E et al 1984 Nerve regeneration through synthetic biogradable nerve guides: regulation by the target organ. Plastic and Reconstructive Surgery 74: 173–181
Seckel B R, Ryan S E, Simons J E et al 1986 Vascularized versus nonvascularized nerve grafts: an experimental structural comparison. Plastic and Reconstructive Surgery 78: 211–220
Seddon H J 1972 Surgical disorders of the peripheral nerves. Churchill Livingstone, Edinburgh,
Settergren C R, Wood M B 1984 Comparison of blood flow in the free vascularized versus nonvascularized nerve grafts. Journal of Reconstructive Microsurgery 1: 95–101
Shibata M, Tsai T M, Firrell J et al 1988 Experimental comparison of vascularized and nonvascularized nerve grafting. Journal of Hand Surgery 13A: 358–365
Smahel J, Chen L E 1989 Muskelgewebe als Leitbahn für die Regeneration peripherer Nerven. 27. Jahrestagung der Österreichischen Gesellschalt für Plastische Chirurgie, Graz
Smith J W 1966a Factors influencing nerve repair I. Blood supply of peripheral nerves. Archives of Surgery 93: 335–341
Smith J W 1966b Factors influencing nerve repair II. Collateral circulation of peripheral nerves. Archives of Surgery 93: 433–436
Strange F G StC 1947 An operation for nerve pedicle grafting — preliminary communication. British Journal of Surgery 423–425
Suematsu N, Atsuta Y, Hirayama T 1988 Vein graft for repair of peripheral nerve gap. Journal of Reconstructive Microsurgery 4: 313–318
Sunderland S 1968 Nerves and nerve injuries, E & S Livingstone Ltd, Edinburgh, p 705–706
Taylor G I, Ham F J 1976 The free vascularized nerve graft. A further experimental and clinical application of microvascular techniques. Plastic and Reconstructive Surgery 57: 413–425
Taylor G I 1978 Nerve grafting with simultaneous microvascular reconstruction. Clinical Orthopaedics and Related Research 133: 56–70
Townsend P L G, Taylor G I 1984 Vascularized nerve grafts using composite arterialized neuro-venous systems. British Journal of Plastic Surgery 37: 1–17

M. E. Jabaley

14 Peripheral nerve repair by direct suture and graft

When the application of microsurgery techniques to reconstructive problems of the extremities became an everyday reality in clinical practice, a substantial improvement in results was anticipated. This is exactly what occurred in small vessel surgery, and operations such as replantation and free tissue transfer became a reality. The availability of high quality optics, precision instruments, and miniaturised suture material have also permitted surgeons to visualise and join nerve ends more accurately than ever before. Despite these advances, however, the results of nerve suture are still sometimes disappointing, and the feeling is that any improvement in results that has occurred has resulted more from general improvements in technique and patient care than from alteration of the underlying processes; fundamental problems of nerve repair remain to be solved. Clearly, there are factors which come into play besides technical nerve union.

One can fairly say now, in the last decade of the 20th century, that technical improvements in nerve suture have taken us as far as they can and that future advances will only come from a better understanding of the basic biological processes and their manipulation. In this regard, *peripheral nerve surgery remains the last major frontier in extremity reconstruction* (Jabaley 1981).

Although exciting ideas are being pursued in the laboratory, surgeons working in the present day must still rely on available techniques to treat patients with transected nerves. For this reason, the main thrust of this chapter will be a description of current methods and the results obtainable by their use, but the reader should keep in mind that the final chapter on nerve repair remains to be written — we cannot be complacent with results as we now see them.

The current situation with nerve injury and repair is one whereby muscle and soft tissue atrophy occur rapidly, while regeneration proceeds at an agonisingly slow pace. Our very best technical efforts are good and may result in strong muscle recovery and sensory return. On the other hand, patients with proximal injuries or complex wounds, patients with underlying diseases or advancing age may never reach clinically acceptable results. Although we know many of the factors which influence outcome, others are poorly understood, and it is impossible to project outcome with certainty when first evaluating an injury (see Fig. 14.6).

The intent here is to describe in some detail the terminology and its application in a description of the anatomy of peripheral nerves. Nerve healing and function will be outlined, as well as those factors which affect them, and these principles will be applied to specific clinical problems at distinct levels. They will be illustrated by a few clinical cases, selected to show the quality of results which are possible and to illuminate some of the problems.

NOMENCLATURE AND ANATOMY

The nomenclature employed in this text has been recommended by the International Society of Reconstructive Microsurgery (Millesi & Terzis 1983). Its use is commended to the reader as part of the effort to develop a common language for nerve surgery and thereby avoid confusion.

A *peripheral nerve* (Fig. 14.1) is comprised of two main components: those elements which conduct impulses and are neuroectodermal in origin, and those portions which are non-conducting and are mesodermal in origin. Conduction occurs along afferent or efferent *axons* which originate in the cell bodies of the anterior horn or the dorsal root ganglia. The axon, together with the axolemma, the Schwann cell, its sheath and myelin constitutes the *nerve fibre*. Conduction along nerve fibres can be measured electrically as the action potential. When axons are *myelinated*, the surrounding Schwann cell envelops them with one or more layers of myelin, thereby forming a sheath. If *unmyelinated*, the axon is enveloped in the Schwann cell cytoplasm only. It is not uncommon for several unmyelinated axons to lie within a single Schwann cell. Within each axon is its axoplasm. Through this axoplasm, nutrients and the products of cell metabolism are carried both proximally and distally by the process of axon transport. Axon transport may be either 'slow' or 'fast'. When transected, the distal portion of a fibre undergoes Wallerian degeneration and dies, leaving empty tubules which may eventually be entered by regenerating axons.

Axons, both myelinated and unmyelinated, are surrounded by *endoneurium*. This material forms the chemical milieu in which the axons function and it is characterised by a slight positive pressure. A group of axons and their endoneurium are wrapped in *perineurium*, a structure of variable thickness consisting of several individual laminae, each arranged in a longitudinal, diagonal or transverse fashion. Perineurium is orderly, dense, tough and visible to the naked eye. It serves a barrier function, and the pressure within it is slightly higher than that on the outside. A group of axons, their endoneurium, and encircling perineurium are collectively called a *fascicle* (or funiculus). Two or

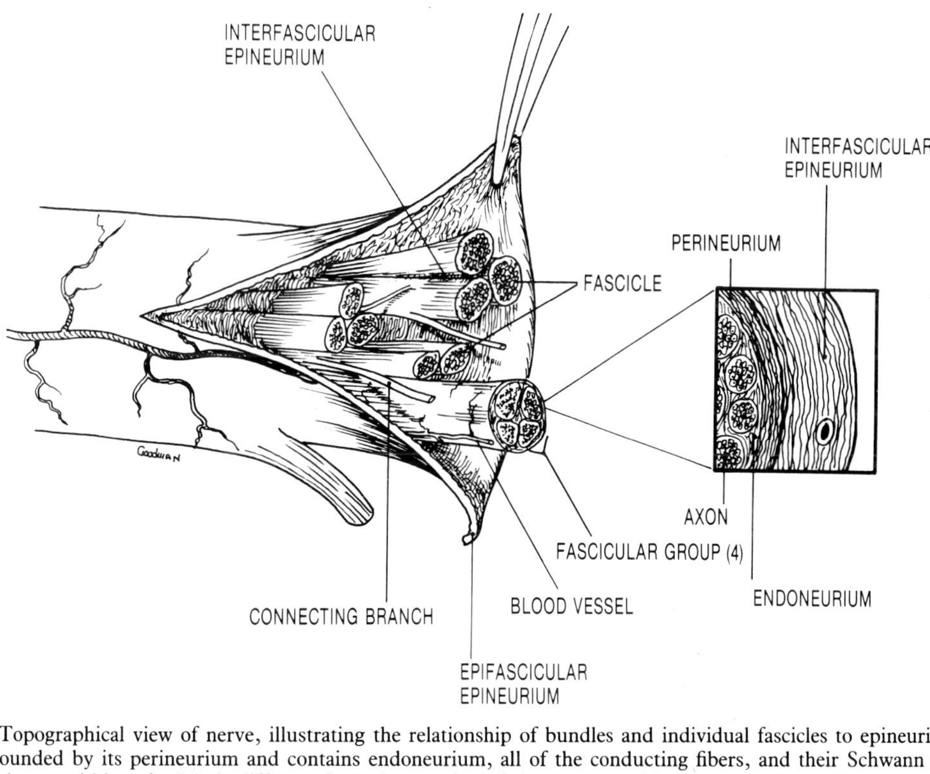

Fig. 14.1 Topographical view of nerve, illustrating the relationship of bundles and individual fascicles to epineurium. Each fascicle is bounded by its perineurium and contains endoneurium, all of the conducting fibers, and their Schwann cells. The chemical make-up within a fascicle is different from that portion of the nerve outside the perineurium. Outside the fascicles lies the *interfascicular* and *epifascicular* epineurium. Epineurium contains the major vessels and lymphatics, provides structural support, and is the gliding material of nerves. Within limits, epineurium can be incised or excised (provided the perineurium is not damaged). Epineurium is the plane of surgical dissection and suture of peripheral nerves.

more fascicles may form a *bundle* or *group of fascicles*. When transected, the contents of a fascicle bulge beyond the cut end (Fig. 14.2), evidence of the positive pressure contained within. The perineurium is semipermeable, and the chemical environment within it is different from that on the outside. In part, its role is to provide an environment within which conduction can occur. It is likely that axons adjacent to damaged or torn perineurium either function poorly or do not function at all. Fascicles may branch to join with adjacent fascicles. Axons may follow them, of course, so that the contents of a fascicle at any specific level as well as the fascicular configuration in cross-section, may be quite different from that at other levels. The surgical significance of such an arrangement is evident when the fascicles are selected for a *group fascicular repair*.

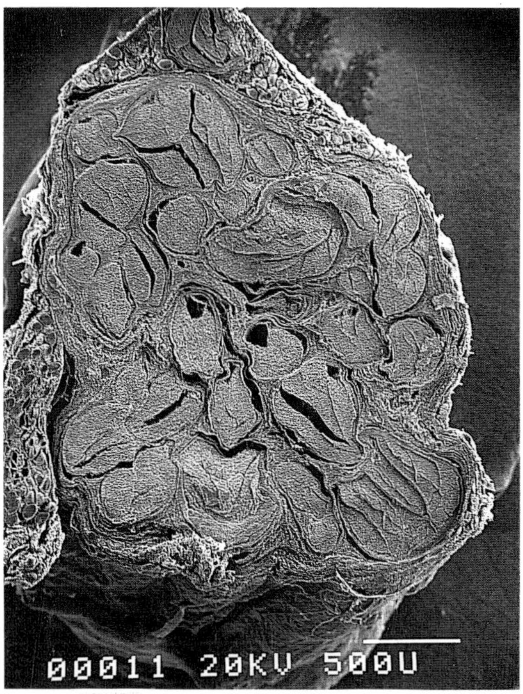

Fig. 14.2 Scanning electron micrograph of human median nerve, 30×. Several individual fascicles and bundles are clearly visible, lying within the epifascicular and interfascicular epineurium. The clefts are artefacts. The resemblance to Figure 14.1 is obvious. (Scanning electron micrograph reprinted with kind permission of Robert C Russell, M.D., Southern Illinois University, and the W B Saunders Co., Philadelphia).

Fascicles lie within and are surrounded by the *epineurium* (Fig. 14.2). Epineurium may be epifascicular (external) or interfascicular (internal), depending on its location. In either case, it is loosely organised, easily separated, and slides back and forth over the underlying fascicles in prepucal fashion. It consists mostly of collagen, contains large blood and lymphatic vessels, and serves both a supportive and a nutritional role. The blood vessels of the epineurium are mostly longitudinal in arrangement, and the circulation from them to the fascicles is segmental.

From a surgical standpoint, *the epineurium can be incised, excised, or dissected away from the fascicles*. Although this creates a measure of obligatory scarring, it appears not to hamper the function of the underlying fascicles so long as their perineurium is intact. Epineurium has been incriminated as the primary source of fibroblasts in neuroma formation, and its removal in nerve grafting operations has been advised for this reason (Millesi et al 1972). The recognition of the epineurium and its role is surgically important because it allows surgeons to perform epineurotomies to decompress intact nerves as part of a neurolysis, or to expose the underlying fascicles for purposes of identification and eventual union, either by direct suture or by graft (Fig. 14.3).

When a peripheral nerve is transected, a chain of rather complicated events ensues. Not all will be described, but certain aspects will be emphasised because of their surgical importance.

Under normal circumstances, a peripheral nerve is under slight longitudinal tension and the ends naturally retract a short distance when it is transected (Sunderland 1978). This natural shortening can be overcome easily by surgical mobilisation, joint flexion or both. If allowed to remain apart, shortening of the ends becomes associated with fibrosis and is more difficult to overcome. In discussing nerve gaps, one must distinguish between those resulting from loss of nerve substance and those occurring after retraction (as explained in the section on nerve grafting) (Millesi 1986).

Nerve transection initiates the process of Wallerian degeneration. In the distal portion of the nerve, the axon and axoplasm undergo phagocytosis by Schwann cells. This is characterised first by breakdown and clumping of myelin and

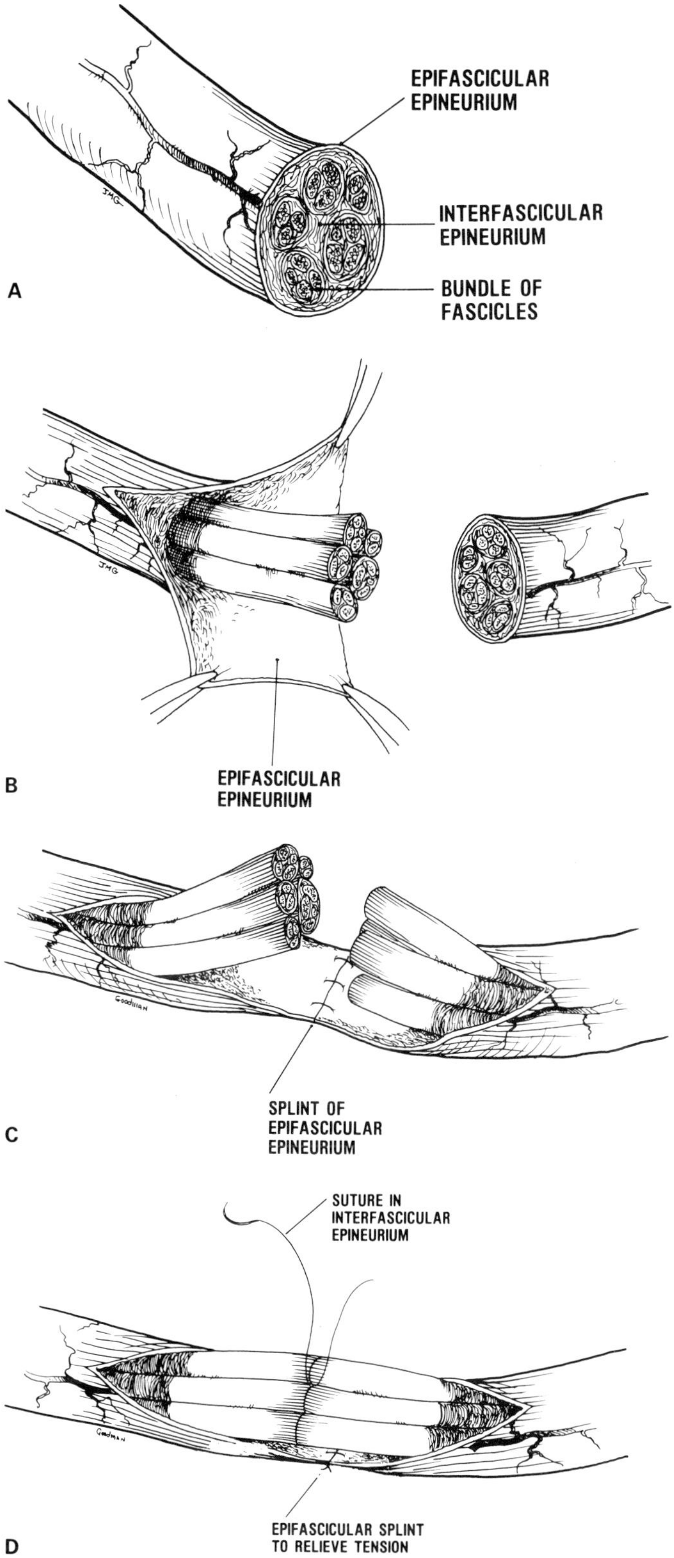

Fig. 14.3 A technique of nerve repair using an epineurial splint. Transected nerve ends naturally retract because of their elasticity. The small calibre suture material used in microsurgical repair is sometimes inadequate to overcome this retraction, even when no loss of nerve tissue has occurred. A strip of epineurium can be used as an autogenous tension-relieving device, allowing tension-free alignment of fascicles. Drawings were taken from actual repair of a transected ulnar nerve in the upper arm. Surgery was approximately 18 hours after injury. **A.** The nerve end is held by its external epineurium. The fascicle ends are bulging. Sometimes these must be trimmed. **B.** The epifascicular epineurium has been incised longitudinally and stripped back from the underlying fascicles (forceps are holding interfascicular epineurium). No epineurium has been removed. **C.** The splint has been constructed by suturing the epifascicular epineurium on the *deep surface only* with 8–0 nylon. Three or four sutures are usually sufficient. **D.** Tension has now been relieved by the splint, and the bundles are allowed to fall together. A few sutures of 10–0 or 11–0 nylon are placed in the interfascicular epineurium for alignment, not for strength. *Importantly*, the epifascicular epineurium has been sutured on the deep surface only and has not been closed around the periphery of the nerve. (Reprinted from: Jabaley M E Peripheral nerve repair. In: McCarthy J G & May J W Jr (eds) Reconstructive plastic surgery. W B Saunders & Co, Philadelphia (In press)).

axoplasm, then by phagocytosis and absorption by the Schwann cells. Importantly, endoneurial tubes persist as they are cleared by the Schwann cells, as do the perineurium and epineurium. There occurs a progressive contracture with time, and all who operate on nerves are familiar with the decreasing diameter of the distal portion which occurs after the first several weeks. This process is progressive for the first few months and is accompanied by an increased amount of collagen.

In the proximal nerve stump, there occurs a variable period of metabolic shock. Thereafter, the cell body (if it survives) goes into a hypermetabolic state very soon after regeneration begins. It is characterised at the site of transection by elongation and sprouting of regenerating axons so that their number may increase several-fold. If nerve union has not been accomplished, regenerating axons grow into a mass of collagen and fibroblasts to form the well-known neuroma. If union has been accomplished, axon sprouts enter the distal stump and grow along whatever substrate they encounter. They may grow along blood vessels, collagen fibers or any other solid substrate which is available, but their preference is clearly for the Schwann cell and its apparatus.

Considerable research effort is underway to determine whether, and to what extent, neuronotrophic factors in the distal stump play a role in attracting axons. Those axon sprouts which enter an endoneurial tube can follow it to its eventual destination and, ultimately, may function again. Those which do not, probably atrophy and either do not function or function in an abnormal way.

Nerve healing is a completely unique phenomenon. Unlike blood vessels, tendons and other such structures, nerve ends must first 'heal' by forming a bond of scar which must then serve as a bridge for regenerating axons. The local events at the site of nerve union are like those of mesodermal structure in other areas: epineurial fibroblasts appear, and begin to form a collagen scar between the nerve ends. This collagen milieu can be of variable thickness, depending on several factors, chief among them being tension. Regenerating axons must eventually find their way through this collagen mass to the distal stump. Their ability to do this is directly related to the thickness of the collagen scar; tension thus becomes critical.

A tension-free repair is analogous to a *primary union* between skin wound edges. It should heal with a thin scar. Such a scar offers minimal resistance to axonal regeneration. If tension is increased or if a gap exists, the width of the scar may become considerably greater and the collagen more dense; axon penetration will be correspondingly poorer. For these reasons, *a primary goal of nerve repair is a tension-free union*, so that the intervening scar will be as narrow as possible.

Although tension is possibly the most important factor in determining the width of the scar, other important considerations should be borne in mind: non-viable nerve ends are easily converted to scar; desiccation, trauma, and abusive handling of the nerve stumps will also damage them and further increase scarring; debris and foreign material from the injury is particularly noxious and stimulates excessive fibroplasia; finally, sutures and their insertion result in local damage and are a factor as well. For all these reasons, handling of the nerve ends is especially critical and should be done in such a way as to promote direct healing with a minimum of scar. (These factors should be kept in mind while reading the section on other methods of nerve union.)

In the clinical setting, surgeons have few tools for judging the quality, speed and completeness of regeneration following nerve repair (Dellon 1981). For this reason, it is important to perform a careful sensory and motor evaluation of all patients in the first several postoperative days. The findings may be quite different from the preoperative state, in that minimally damaged nerves which were non-functional may have recovered by this time.

This important baseline examination serves as the reference point for future tests to determine what structures are truly re-innervated. Should a question remain about possible crossover or dual innervation by other uninjured nerves, this is also the ideal time to perform selective blocks to further clarify matters. Thereafter, the surgeon's best tool to measure the speed of regeneration is *Tinel's sign*, the phenomenon by which paraesthesias are produced by lightly tapping over the ends of regenerating axons (Spinner 1978). Baseline photographs to document intrinsic muscle function can also be quite helpful.

THE IDEAL NERVE REPAIR

A diverse array of experimental and clinical observations are ample proof of the ability of the peripheral nervous system to regenerate and even reproduce itself under proper conditions: in lower species, such as the salamander and frog, for example, it is possible to completely regenerate an amputated part. This plasticity has been widely observed and studied in other species as well, and underscores the inherent potential of the nervous system to reproduce itself.

The quality of results in the best cases that surgeons have observed in humans has been practically perfect also (Fig. 14.4). For example, those cases with axonotmesis (Sunderland grade 3 lesions or lower) and recovery following stretch or compression injury are familiar to all. Many cases with the so-called 'Saturday night palsy' have been followed and observed to full recovery, for example. Furthermore, after transection and repair many patients have clearly recovered function in both extrinsic and intrinsic muscles, and sensation in the fingertips has been indistinguishable from normal. This is particularly true in younger patients. No paraesthesias are evident on tapping at the suture site or anywhere along the nerve. Such excellent results demonstrate the quality of

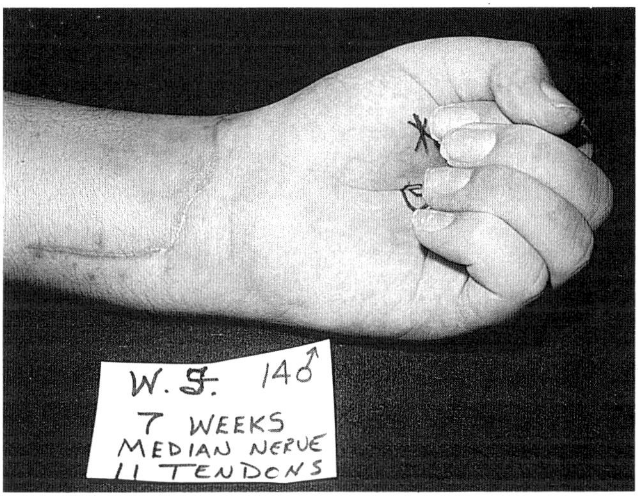

A

Fig. 14.4 This 14-year-old boy transected the radial artery, median nerve, and all tendons except the profundus to the small and ring fingers 2 cm proximal to the wrist crease on a broken window. **A.** Seven weeks after repair. Flexor tendon function is recovering, and Tinel's sign is in the palm (asterisk). **B.** Abduction and opposition of the thumb is not possible because the thenar muscles do not function. **C.** Two years, four months postoperative. Comparative views demonstrate excellent thumb opposition. The patient recovered full flexion and extension of the fingers, and near normal sensation in the median distribution. Two-point discrimination is 2 mm.

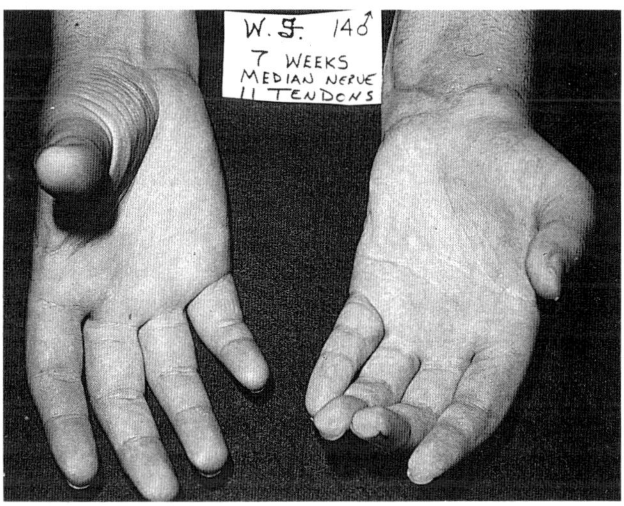

B

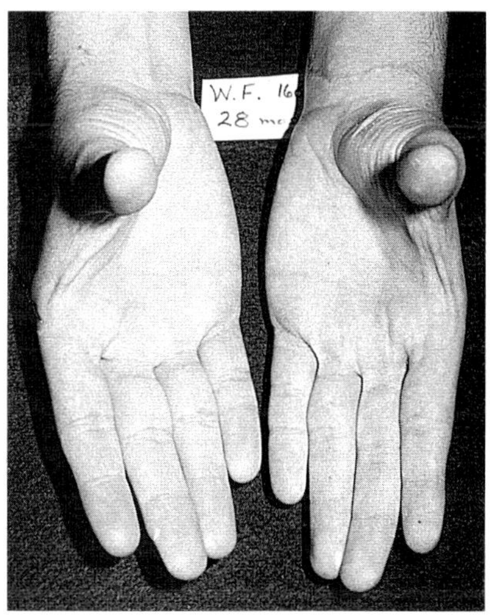

C

recovery of which the nervous system is capable, and although we know that we will frequently not achieve this, it can serve as our goal.

It is possible to use laboratory data and clinical observation to define the ideal nerve repair. The surgeon must be prepared in each case to vary his timing and technique as clinical circumstances dictate to secure the best possible result. The following conditions are important factors in the ideal repair.

1. *The ideal repair should be performed as early as possible.* In a tidy wound, where there has been a sharp transection with no adjacent injury, it may be unnecessary to trim the nerve ends, the topographical appearance might be easily determined, and no tissue loss exists. The small gap which exists is due solely to elastic retraction, and the conditions are ideal for a primary repair; such a nerve should be sutured as soon as conveniently possible (Fig. 14.5).

Under other circumstances, repair may be performed within the first few days of injury; it might still be considered a delayed primary repair, that is, one which is accomplished before significant fibroplasia occurs in the wound. (Kleinert has noted that the period of primary repair ends when the wound can no longer be opened by blunt spreading with a haemostat.) Once scar has formed and the wound must be surgically incised, the repair becomes secondary. Not only does scar exist within the surrounding soft tissue at this point, but it will also be present as part of a neuroma on the nerve end. In secondary repair, one is dealing with a gap that results from a combination of tissue loss and inelasticity of the nerve ends. It is to avoid this circumstance that repair should always be performed at the earliest possible date that is consistent with primary healing of the wound.

2. *The repair must be between viable nerve ends.* It goes without saying that a non-viable nerve segment will be converted to scar tissue and is an unsatisfactory substrate for regenerating axons. Under such circumstances, axon regeneration either does not occur or occurs only in fewer numbers and with great difficulty.

The problem facing clinical surgeons is that one cannot always determine on the day of injury whether nerve ends are viable or not. A nerve may have undergone major trauma at the time of injury but still appear relatively normal to inspection. The temptation is not to resect the ends of such nerves. For this reason, if there has been significant crushing or stretching of nerve ends (as might occur in a blast injury or major fracture), it is better to restore circulation, stabilise fractures, repair tendons and simply join the nerve ends with two sutures to maintain their length, and then return later for an early secondary repair. (The joining of nerve ends by suture is not to aid in future identification but to avoid retraction. This manoeuvre may sometimes permit a direct nerve suture when a graft would otherwise have been required.) It may be surprising when one re-explores such nerves to see the length of nerve that must be resected to overcome intrinsic damage. Re-exploration can be performed as early as six weeks following injury or whenever the wound is otherwise suitable.

3. *There must be a minimum of foreign body.* Wound toilet is essential, and all debris, devitalised tissue, haematoma and otherwise contaminated material should be removed. The objective is two-fold: the avoidance of infection, and healing with the least amount of scar. Many a nerve repair has either not functioned or had its functional potential compromised because of peripheral scarring. Such scarring results in external compression and relative ischaemia. Repairs glide less well and are generally less well-nourished. The quality of the clinical result in such patients can sometimes be improved at a later date by neurolysis, but it is always best to employ those measures which will minimise the amount of scar at the first procedure.

4. *Accurate fascicular identification and alignment* is critical to a successful outcome. In an immediate repair of a tidy injury, alignment may be relatively easy, but it is more difficult in the secondary repair. Where possible, one must try to determine with certainty which fascicles contain motor fibres and which contain sensory fibres. In addition, one must know the destination of sensory fascicles so that crossover or overlap of fascicle ends will not occur (see discussion of awake stimulation, p. 212).

5. *There cannot be excessive tension* as it leads to distraction and a wide scar, as described on p. 206.

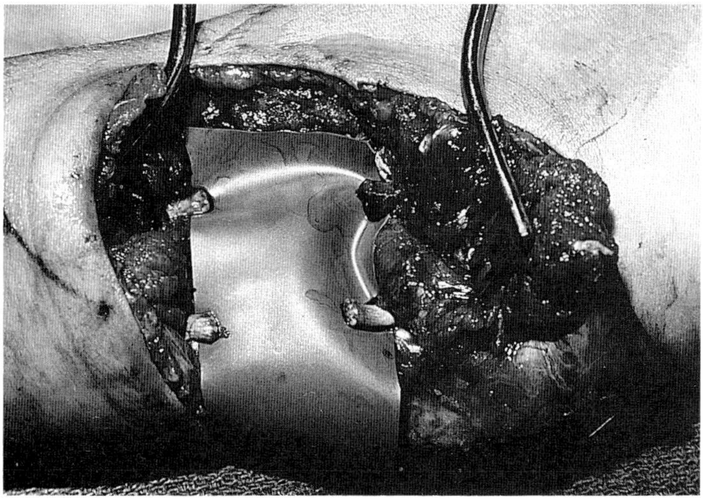

A

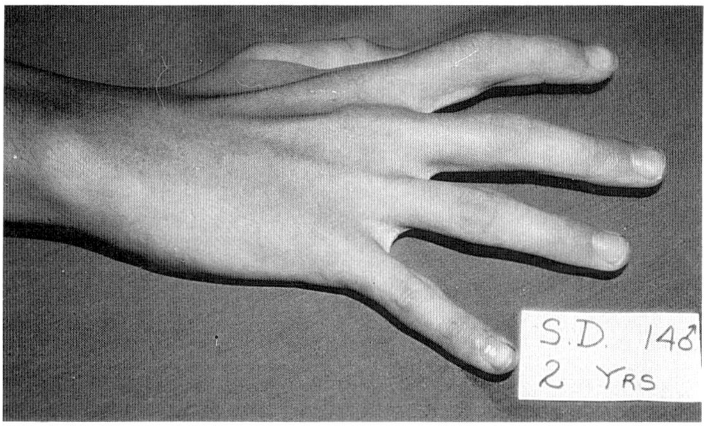

B

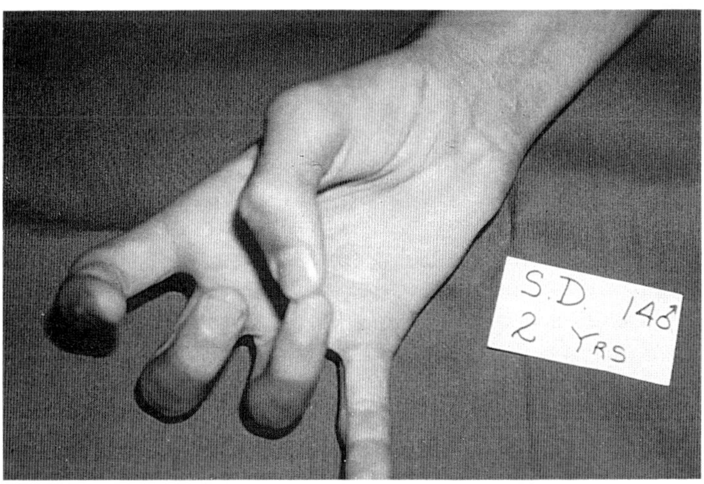

C

Fig. 14.5 This 12-year-old boy was referred 36 hours after a life-threatening laceration of the upper forearm causing haemorrhagic shock. He required transfusion and an operation to control the bleeding. **A.** Proximal forearm wound with transection of all major forearm muscle bellies and some forearm extensor muscles, and ulnar artery. The widely separated median and ulnar nerve ends, lying on a rubber background, can be seen prior to repair. No nerve tissue has been removed and the several centimetre 'gap' is due to the natural elasticity of the nerves. Both nerves, the ulnar artery, and all muscles were repaired. **B.** Two years postoperative. Both the median and ulnar innervated intrinsic muscle groups have recovered, but not to normal strength. A claw deformity was present initially but has disappeared. Bulk is returning to the hypothenar eminence, and the interosseous muscles are functioning. **C.** The thumb is opposing reasonably well, but the abductor pollicis brevis has only minimal function. Two-point discrimination is 5 mm in the median nerve area, and 13 mm in the ulnar nerve. Nerves injured at this level may recover, but a certain amount of muscle atrophy or dropout usually occurs.

6. *There must be no separation or telescoping of ends following suture.* If nerve ends are joined with excessive tension, there is a tendency for them to distract. To overcome this tendency, one may be tempted to take wider bites of external epineurium. This will telescope or overlap the underlying fascicles. Either situation makes axonal bridging into distal fascicles more difficult.

7. *Minimal amounts of suture material must be used.* The purpose of stitches between nerve ends is for maintenance of alignment, not for strength. If a repair can be performed without tension, fine sutures that are non-reactive and few in number can minimise the amount of foreign body that is employed. The use of a splint of epineurium, (author's technique), can be helpful in this regard.

8. *The repair must lie in a well-vascularised bed.* If the repair is performed in tissue that is ischaemic, heavily contaminated, badly traumatised, or otherwise injured, it will eventually become fibrotic and scarred. By its nature, scar lacks elasticity and softens little or not at all with time. It also impairs gliding of the repair (Wilgis & Murphy 1986). Excess scar translates eventually into external compression and poor results.

SURGICAL ANATOMY OF NERVES

Peripheral nerves in the extremities are best approached through the internervous planes. These relatively avascular areas can be dissected with minimal trauma if one understands the surgical approaches. They are clearly outlined in Spinner's monograph (Spinner 1978). The nerves themselves lie in filmy adventitial layers, and can be mobilised for some distance in either direction without significant injury to their blood supply. Surgical mobilisation of nerves adds very little length if one must overcome a gap, but it permits the surgeon to take advantage of the natural elasticity. A segment of nerve might be lengthened by 10% or so by surgical dissection, but this is gained mostly by stretching and should not be considered a primary method for overcoming a deficit of nerve tissue.

The adventitia around a nerve changes almost imperceptibly to blend with the external epineurium surrounding the nerve proper. Dissection in the external epineurium of a previously uninjured nerve is not difficult, but is best accomplished with magnification since there are significant vessels within this layer which can be injured (Lundborg 1979, Miyamoto, Watari & Tsuge 1981). Although dissection can be done bluntly by teasing away adventitia with forceps or by spreading it with scissors, the least traumatic way to dissect external epineurium is with a knife. In such dissection, perineurium is the layer to be identified and preserved. The epineurium can be trimmed off the underlying fascicles with a minimum of damage, so long as crossovers between fascicles are recognised and respected. Magnification is essential to such dissection, and 4–6× is the least acceptable power.

Fascicular anatomy is unique for all levels of each nerve, but the topographical anatomy of fascicles is not subtle. One can see the larger interconnections between fascicles with the naked eye, and magnification makes it easier yet. These interconnections are of two types: the first is filamentous in size, approximately 25–50 μm in diameter. The function of these filaments is not known, but it has been suggested that they may be branches of the sympathetic system. The second are the larger interconnections. These may be as large as the fascicles themselves. These are easily identified, cannot be stripped away from their parent fascicle, and resist dissection. If cut, a stump is easily seen and the damage can be recognised. Axoplasm will produce a characteristic bulge at the cut surface.

To repair or graft fascicles or groups of fascicles, one must dissect away the epifascicular (external) epineurium. As noted above, this can be done with a minimum of trauma, and most microsurgeons can master this technique. The fascicles themselves can then be separated and arranged into groups for grafting or primary union. The interfascicular (or internal) epineurium is usually sparse in amount and need not be excised in most cases.

For many years, neuroanatomists debated the arrangement and significance of the internal topography of peripheral nerves. The monumental works of Sunderland, beginning in 1945, clarified their configuration for the first time (Sunderland 1978). He dissected and serially sectioned the major peripheral nerves in both the upper and lower extremities of a number of human specimens. Unfortunately, there was little practical significance to the work when it was first published, and its value only became apparent when microsurgeons began to work within the nerve. As surgeons reviewed Sunderland's work, many misinterpreted the studies of topographical anatomy and assumed that his descriptions of the changing cross-sectional appearance of nerves from level to level precluded accurate fascicular repair. Additional studies have suggested that this is, in fact, not the case (Jabaley et al 1980). The majority of injuries to nerves occur in their more distal portions, and it appears that fascicles in those regions travel for considerable distances without changing their relationships to each other. This observation has now been corroborated by others (Terzis et al 1984, Chow et al 1985, Williams & Jabaley 1986).

Each nerve consists of fibres originating from more than one level of the spinal cord. These fibres are gradually sorted and arranged in the major plexuses to form peripheral nerves and their branches. Once a specific nerve is formed, the sorting process continues within it as each branch is organised. The branches, once formed, travel within the epineurium for variable distances before reaching their exit point. Thus, a completely formed branch may be found within a nerve, and its components may be localised in a certain quadrant for an even longer distance.

These findings all suggest that there is hope for the nerve surgeon and that the goal of accurate alignment is by no means hopeless, even in secondary repairs. Accurate fascicular alignment remains the goal of peripheral nerve surgery, and the debate should be about how to recognise and maintain such alignment, not about where sutures should be placed (Orgel 1984).

TECHNIQUES OF NERVE REPAIR

For the past century or so, surgeons have been preoccupied with the joining of nerve ends. The principal method for doing this has been with sutures, and considerable research effort has been expended in this area alone and has resulted in a succession of developments, mostly for the better. We have seen suture material evolve from braided natural fibres, such as cotton and silk, to less reactive synthetic monofilament materials, such as nylon and polypropylene. At the same time, the suture gauge has been progressively reduced from 4–0 and 5–0 to 10–0 and 11–0, while needle technology has improved to the point that 50–75 μm needles are now available for nerve suture. Needles have no 'eye' and the material is actually swaged onto the shank of the needle. Metallised suture ends may eventually do away with microsurgical needles altogether. Complementing such material are instruments which have been designed to allow surgeons to manipulate such suture with ease. Optical devices permit easy visualisation by both surgeon and assistant as well as by observers, and video capability promises further improvement. The day may come when the microscopes now in use become the dinosaurs of microsurgery.

In recent years, several different techniques of nerve suture have been advocated. The nomenclature describing these is often unfortunate because it mostly emphasises the wrong things. Several publications have described the advantages and disadvantages of 'epineurial suture or perineurial suture'. These names should probably be discarded and repair methods described on the basis of their objective. Thus, we should know in a repair whether the whole nerve, groups of fascicles, or individual fascicles are aligned, and whether stitches are placed in external or internal epineurium or perineurium (Millesi & Terzis 1983).

Based on this discussion, nerve repair can properly be of two types: whole nerve suture or group fascicular suture (as a practical matter, interfascicular suture is rarely indicated). In whole nerve suture, no attempt is made to isolate and join individual fascicles or bundles. Sutures are placed only in the external (or epifascicular) epineurium, and alignment, as determined by the cross-sectional appearance, is dependent on this suture placement. This technique is most applicable in the most proximal and distal portions of nerves, but for different reasons. In the brachial plexus and most proximal areas of peripheral nerves, fibres destined for all sensory territories and motor branches are widely dispersed through several fascicles. Definitive sorting has not yet occurred and it is more difficult to assign specific function to individual fascicles. On the other hand, digital nerves consist of only 2–4 fascicles. The fascicles comprise a high percentage of the cross-sectional area, and there is relatively little connective tissue. Thus, there seems little to gain by separating fascicles for individual suture; external epineurial suture is usually consistent with satisfactory results.

In many areas, where mixed nerves are present or where specific functional assignment can be made to individual bundles, external epineurial suture alone cannot be relied upon for maintenance of correct alignment; the make-up of the nerve is too complex. In such situations, group fascicular suture or suture of individual fascicles is indicated (Sunderland 1979). The median and ulnar nerve at the wrist, the radial nerve above the elbow, the median nerve in the forearm at the branch point of the anterior interosseous, as well as all the major forearm trunks, are important examples of such a situation. Here, we know that function is well delineated and that there is little chance of functional recovery if incorrect alignment occurs.

In repairing the median nerve at the wrist, for example, one should identify the motor branch with certainty, and suture it separately. The same is true for the terminal branches of the median nerve before they make their exits as common digital nerves. If one can achieve and maintain alignment with sutures in the internal epineurium, this technique is preferred. If placement of sutures in perineurium is necessary to maintain alignment (as it might be in a single large fascicle), they should be used, mindful of the caveats mentioned earlier. In the acute case, identification of topographical landmarks can often be made by visual inspection of the cut ends. In secondary cases, where it is necessary to trim the ends or resect neuromas, electrical stimulation in the awake patient has proven to be a valuable adjunct (Jabaley 1984b).

Direct electrical stimulation of transected nerve ends has been proposed and described in the past by other authors (Hakstian 1968, Gaul 1983) and no claim is made for priority. We do feel that availability of newer drugs and techniques facilitates its application in patients. In our technique (described in detail in Jabaley 1984b), the initial dissection is accomplished and the nerve ends mapped, using light sedation and an intravenous lidocaine anaesthetic (Bier block). We currently use midazolam (Versed®) for sedation, and fentanyl for analgesia because both are extremely potent and short-acting. Before deflating the tourniquet, the *skin only* is infiltrated with a local anaesthetic, usually lignocaine or bupivicaine. After tourniquet deflation, we allow 15 minutes for recovery from ischaemia before stimulation is begun. Although sophisticated systems are available for computerised signal averaging and recording, we have found a simpler system (already available in most operating suites), which relies on patient's perception and verbal response, to be satisfactory for clinical use.

Patients must be counselled in advance if the method is to be effective. We begin with stimulation of the proximal nerve end. The previously-drawn map must be at hand. If the patient reports no feeling when a fascicle is stimulated, it is assumed to be a motor branch and so labelled. In sensory fascicles, the patient will localise sensation to a specific territory, such as the radial or ulnar side of a fingertip, the palm or some other area. In acute cases, the distal end can also be stimulated and motor response noted. In secondary cases, however, this is not possible, and one must dissect motor and sensory branches, beginning at their branch points and proceeding proximally, to determine their nature. If the injury is too far proximal in the nerve for this method to be useful, it is necessary to use the cross-sectional maps of Sunderland and join the appropriate quadrants by one's 'best clinical guess' (Sunderland 1978). Even in this situation, correct quadrantic alignment should improve clinical results.

Some investigators have studied specific clinically important nerves, and corroborated earlier impressions about specific branch locations (Chow et al 1985). Although our series is too small and variable to assign statistical significance, we believe that awake stimulation has allowed us to improve our results. Using a similar approach, Gaul (1983) reports definitely improved results with suture of the median and ulnar nerve.

OTHER METHODS OF NERVE UNION

If one considers the techniques that have been applied in recent years to nerve suture, certain facts are obvious and certain conclusions are inescapable. Authors have advocated smaller and smaller sutures with less and less reactivity and placed in fewer and fewer numbers. If one extrapolates from these observations, it should be obvious that nerve 'suture' eventually will use no sutures. In practice, this is already occurring. In Europe (Egloff & Narakas 1983, Smahel et al 1987), fibrin glue is being investigated both experimentally and clinically and seems to offer promise, in that comparable nerve regeneration can be obtained. The logical advantages of such a technique are: 1) a saving in time; 2) less trauma to individual fascicles and bundles; 3) less foreign body to cause reaction; and 4) less likelihood of telescoping or gap formation between fascicular ends. The disadvantage of fibrin glue techniques is that most presently recommended techniques still advise one or more anchoring stitches of some type. Although there are no reported instances of viral illness transmission, fibrin glue has not been approved for distribution in the United States, and current concerns about hepatitis and the AIDS virus make approval of pooled fibrin unlikely. Whether fibrin glue eventually will prove to be useful in practice remains to be seen, but it is likely that some bonding agent will eventually appear. The concept is basically sound.

Other techniques that are currently being investigated include the use of lasers for 'spot welding' of nerve ends, and tubulation (about which more will be said later). Although these have some practical advantages in the laboratory, they have yet to be employed in patients to any great extent, and may or may not prove useful.

AUTHOR'S TECHNIQUE FOR NERVE SUTURE

As noted earlier, abundant evidence from human and animal studies suggests that a prime deterrant to axon regeneration following nerve suture is excessive tension. The principal advantage of a nerve graft over conventional suturing is the absolute elimination of tension. For this reason, one can assume that the best direct nerve repair is one which most closely mimics nerve grafting and eliminates tension. Several methods have been advocated which use some variant of 'suture at a distance' to avoid tension. One such technique (Tsuge et al 1975), places external epineurial sutures and a single longitudinal 10–0 nylon through the centre of each fascicle. The 10–0 suture is then brought out at a distance and subsequently removed.

The best method for relieving tension in my hands has been with the use of an epineurial splint (Jabaley 1984a). In this technique (Fig. 14.3) we rely on a flap of external epineurium *on the posterior surface only* to stimulate the conditions which exist in nerve grafting. The aim is to approximate the ends, relieve tension, and cause the fascicle ends literally to fall together. A minimum number of microsutures is then required to maintain fascicular alignment. The repair is reliable, and it avoids many of the problems associated with the use of circumferential sutures to keep the repair together. Recent evidence (de Medinaceli & Seaber 1989) has provided a biomechanical basis for this repair (which has been employed on an empirical basis for about 10 years).

GENERAL RECOMMENDATIONS FOR NERVE INJURIES

As a policy statement, one can say that it is unwise to perform nerve suture under any but the best possible circumstances for the particular patient and injury in question. As noted in the description of the ideal repair, we prefer primary nerve suture, but repairs should probably not be performed in the middle of the night unless ideal anaesthesia is available and a full operating team (including a rested surgeon), is on hand to perform the work — a condition which may not always prevail. It appears much wiser to debride and dress the wound or even suture the skin, and perform the surgery electively under the best possible circumstances. If a wound is heavily contaminated and there is a high likelihood of infection, as in soiled wounds resulting from roadside injuries or farm accidents, it is best to debride the wound, perform delayed primary wound closure, and return for an early secondary nerve repair. (In actual practice, many patients are referred with nerve injuries who have had some variant of this treatment anyway, and the first opportunity to repair the nerve is several days after the injury.) Finally, when the wound is untidy and there has been a significant crush, stretch or concussion, it is advisable to repair the other structures and return for an early secondary repair when the amount of devitalised nerve can be determined.

These ground rules apply at all levels, and comment will now be made on injury to nerves at specific levels.

NERVE INJURIES AT SPECIFIC LEVELS

Digital nerve injuries

Transections of digital nerves can usually be satisfactorily repaired with a few sutures in the external epineurium. These usually require relatively low magnifications, although higher magnification is necessary at certain levels, such as the distal trifurcation. Transections about the DIP crease level may be quite challenging, since the nerve divides into three branches: one dorsal, one distal, and one to the volar pulp area. These are all large enough to sew if magnified, and repair at this level is advised on either side of the thumb, the radial side of the index and long fingers and the ulnar side of the small finger. For repairs at the DIP joint and beyond, loupe magnification is inadequate. Secondary repairs by direct suture of digital nerves can usually be accomplished if there has not been too much damage to the nerve ends. One can often gain additional length by mobilisation of the nerve trunks, and short gaps can be overcome by slight flexion of the joint. One should resist the temptation to mobilise digital nerves and flex fingers excessively to accomplish union. A short graft probably functions better and reduces morbidity.

Common digital nerves

These nerves extend proximally from the distal palmar crease to the terminal portions of the median or ulnar nerves. Although primary repairs usually can be accomplished without difficulty, it is very difficult to overcome significant gaps, and nerve grafts are frequently necessary in secondary repairs at this level. The common digital nerves are relatively short, little length can be gained by mobilisation, and there are no joints to flex. Patients should be forewarned of this problem in secondary repairs and advised of the possible necessity for nerve grafts.

Terminal portions of the median and ulnar nerves

These nerves are characterised by complex anatomy but identifiable branches to which specific function can be assigned. They are ideally suited for group fascicular repairs. The motor portions of the median and ulnar nerves can easily be identified by their terminal destination and by their location within the nerve. It is possible to separate the motor branch of the median nerve for approximately 5 cm proximal to its point of exit from the main trunk, and the motor portion of the ulnar nerve for 8–9 cm (Jabaley et al 1980). In neither case are there significant crossing branches. Once isolated, the motor branches can be joined by either individual fascicular or group fascicular suture. Again, it should be stressed that it is not necessary to place sutures in the perineurium, but it is necessary to align the perineurium. Once correct alignment is obtained, it can be held with 1–2 stitches in the interfascicular epineurium.

Median and ulnar nerves in the forearm

Awake stimulation in humans has demonstrated that specific function can be assigned at all levels in the forearm, and that individual groups of fascicles can often be identified and joined. Thus, group fascicular suture can be very helpful in this area. Such branches as the palmar cutaneous branch of the median, and dorsal cutaneous branch of the ulnar nerve should be identified and sutured separately when forearm injuries are treated.

Median and ulnar nerves about the elbow

In the median nerve, both the anterior interosseous and the branches to the flexor-pronator group can be identified at their exit points and within the substance of the nerve itself. They can be dissected to a point above the elbow crease and they should be joined separately. The same is true at a slightly more proximal level of those branches of the ulnar nerve going to the flexor carpi ulnaris and flexor digitorum profundus. These branches may be multiple and smaller, but they should be sutured where possible.

Median and ulnar nerves above the elbow

No significant branches exit from either of these nerves above the elbow (in fact, motor branches of median and ulnar nerves described above, as in the forearm, sometimes exit above the elbow to enter the muscles whose origin is the medial epicondyle), and individual fascicles progressively lose their identity as one proceeds proximally. As one approaches the axilla, it becomes progressively less useful to try to assign function to specific fascicles. Nevertheless, accurate alignment of quadrants is important and should still be attempted. External landmarks, cross-sectional appearance, and the Sunderland maps should all be used in such repairs, because fibres destined for specific branches will consistently occupy a specific quadrant.

Radial nerve on the dorsum of the hand/wrist

The superficial radial nerve branches can be identified at the level of the distal forearm, anatomical snuffbox, and dorsum of the hand. They are similar in size to digital nerves and are not difficult to locate, even in the acute situation. When unrepaired, painful neuromas sometimes result (Dellon & Mackinnon 1986). Repair by external epineurial suture is indicated and may prevent this distressing result. This nerve can be further identified as a single trunk at the forearm level and back to its exit point from the distal radial nerve. Repair is again possible and advantageous. For reasons that are not completely clear, but which may be related to motion and exposure to frequent stimulation, the superficial radial nerve is prone to painful neuromas if unrepaired. The recommended treatment for such problems is nerve repair — immediate if possible, but secondary if not — even if grafting is necessary.

Posterior interosseous nerve

The posterior interosseous nerve is a relatively short, but important, terminal branch of the radial nerve. It travels a complicated course beneath the arcade of Frohse and through the supinator muscle to innervate that muscle and then arborise into several muscular branches. Transection results in motor paralysis of wrist, finger and thumb extensors. Despite its course, repair within the supinator is sometimes possible and should be attempted when otherwise feasible. This is particularly true in stab wounds or other tidy wounds, if recognised early. When successfully accomplished, relatively rapid return of function is possible after posterior interosseous repair because of the short distance to target muscles, and the quality frequently exceeds the function that can be obtained by tendon transfers.

Radial nerve in the upper arm

Repair of the radial nerve in the upper arm has an advantage over the median and ulnar nerve sutures at the same anatomic level: the target organs are much closer. Thus, the motor branches of the radial nerve must only recover to the forearm extensor muscles. For this reason alone, the outlook is significantly better than in the median and ulnar nerves where the intrinsic muscles of the hand and the sensory territories are considerably further removed (Fig. 14.6). In addition, there are other poorly understood features of the radial nerve which seem to make it a better candidate for repair. These may include the relatively high percentage of neural tissue and a simplified fascicular arrangement. For all these reasons, the level of recovery is consistently better than that of the other two major nerves, and one is well justified in undertaking repair of the radial nerve, even at a relatively late date.

NERVE GRAFTING

It can be seen from the preceding section that excessive tension has been one of the major limiting factors in the surgeon's ability to perform satisfactory coaptation of nerve ends. Efforts to overcome

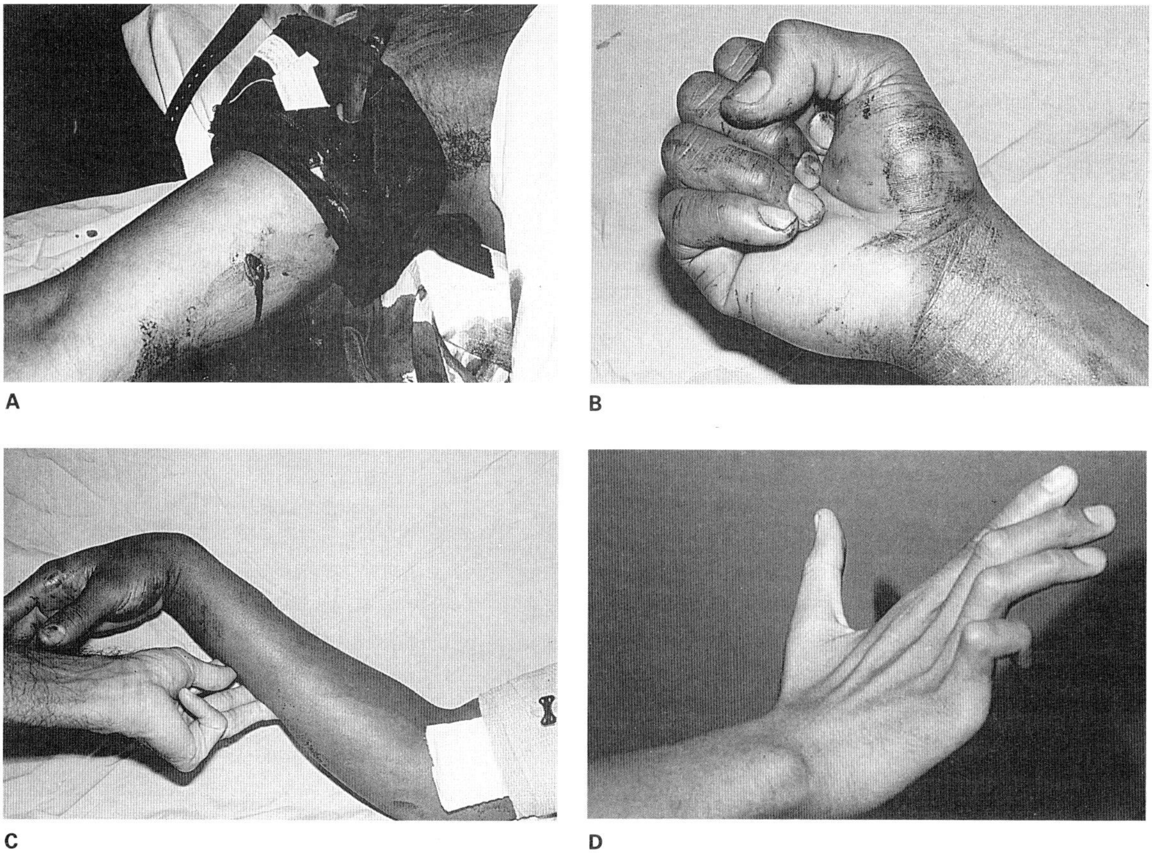

Fig. 14.6 This 19-year-old male arrived in the emergency room in shock after blood loss from a stab wound of the upper arm which transected the axillary vein, the intercostobrachial nerve, the ulnar nerve and the radial nerve. **A.** A tourniquet was applied to staunch the blood loss. **B.** The absence of profundus tendon flexion in the small and ring fingers suggests ulnar nerve transection. Sensory loss was also present. **C.** A wrist drop and inability to extend the fingers signals radial nerve transection. **D.** $3\frac{1}{2}$ years following repair. The radial innervated forearm muscles are now fully recovered and are strong, but intrinsic atrophy is still evident in the hand. Sensation in the ulnar nerve distribution is protective only, and two-point discrimination is greater than 20 mm. Timing and technique of the two nerve repairs was similar, and it is evident that a number of factors influenced the eventual outcome of repair.

tension (some extreme) have included: extensive mobilisation of nerve trunks proximally and distally; use of numerous heavy sutures in the external epineurium; extreme joint flexion; rerouting of nerve ends through extra-anatomic paths; and bulb suture, whereby a neuroma and glioma are sutured together and allowed to stretch the nerve ends so that subsequent neuroma excision and direct suture can subsequently be performed. Although these and other techniques allowed apposition of the nerve ends, recovery was usually disappointing at best.

To circumvent the problems associated with tension on sutured nerve, surgeons turned to grafting. Early attempts used whole nerves as donors. Xenografts were sometimes employed. More recently, allografts, either freeze-dried or irradiated, have been tried. These have resulted in little or no useful function and are not recommended. In the first two-thirds of the 20th century, nerve grafting was not widely accepted as a solution and was viewed with skepticism by most surgeons.

With the advent of clinical microsurgery, interest in peripheral nerve problems increased in the 1960s. Important among these investigators were Millesi, Meissl and Berger. Their presentation at the American Society for Surgery of the Hand in 1970 and subsequent publication can truly be described as seminal (Millesi, Meissl & Berger 1972). Although the work had been previously published in the European literature, this date marks the renewal of interest and understanding of modern-day nerve grafting in the English literature. Although widely practised and now generally accepted, the fundamental principles have changed little in the two decades since they were first espoused.

The 'gap' versus the deficit

Thoughtful surgeons will recognise that at least two factors are operative in producing excessive tension. The overall distance between two nerve ends is often referred to as a 'gap', but in reality this visible distance may be comprised of a number of factors. Firstly, nerves normally are elastic, and there is a natural tendency for the ends to retract when a trunk is transected. This produces a gap, but no deficit in nerve stock. If a transected nerve is allowed to retract and to remain in that position for any length of time, natural shortening and fibrosis of the epineurium occurs and it may become impossible to return it to its natural length. This circumstance may be minimally improved by dissection outside the nerve and mobilisation of the trunk. When extraneural fibrosis occurs after an injury, and surgery is then superimposed, the process of shortening is magnified and its relief becomes even more difficult. All these factors contribute to the production of an enlarging gap, but none of them create a deficit of nerve tissue.

When injury occurs, other factors, separate and apart from those just described, may result in an actual deficiency of nerve substance. These factors also must be recognised and dealt with. Firstly, the injury itself may destroy nerve tissue. Furthermore, as noted earlier, when a significant degree of crush or stretch occurs, nerve tissue which is still present may have been rendered non-viable and may be unsatisfactory for regeneration. In such instances, nerve damage may extend for considerable distance along a nerve trunk. Unfortunately, this may not be apparent on inspection and cannot be appreciated when evaluating an injury in the early stages. Nevertheless, the combination of loss of nerve tissue and subsequent devitalisation of remaining tissue are two contributors to a nerve tissue deficit.

If a nerve is transected, allowed to retract, and then remains unrepaired, the process of degeneration includes the formation of a neuroma on the proximal end, and a glioma on the distal end. These processes involve a portion of the fascicle ends themselves, and further contribute to the creation of a deficit. Finally, if one returns secondarily to such a wound to perform a repair, the neuroma and nerve ends must be resected back to viable, healthy-looking fascicles, and this resection adds further to the deficit.

One can see, therefore, that the two sets of factors which produce a deficit and a gap are distinct in nature, but both contribute to the overall problem: the formation of a variable distance between nerve ends which must be overcome. When this cannot be satisfactorily accomplished by direct suture, one must turn to alternative methods.

When to graft?

A carefully performed nerve suture between viable ends, provided it can be accomplished with acceptable tension, is always preferable to a graft. A nerve graft (like any graft) must first be vascularised to survive and function. It necessarily entails two suture lines. There is a greater likelihood of malrotation and incorrect apposition of nerve ends, and accurate fascicular alignment is difficult. Regenerating axons must find their way across two junctures instead of one. Finally, such factors as graft length, additional operating time, donor site deficit and other factors take their toll. *Nevertheless, all of the disadvantages of a nerve graft, theoretical and real, are more than offset by its major advantage: a nerve graft allows a tension-free union of nerve ends.*

Surgeons must ask (and then answer) the question: how much tension is too much? A simple answer in millimeters cannot be given because it varies with each nerve, with each level, and with the size of each extremity. Still, in all, a simple rule suggests that if nerve ends can be joined with microsurgical suture without placing the joint in extreme flexion, tension is not excessive. This may sometimes mean that gaps of only a few millimeters in a digital nerve must be grafted, while those greater than 2–3 cm in the forearm may be sutured.

The surgeon must always make the final judgment in each case, but it is obvious that tension which can be relieved by joint flexion, for example, but which will come into play when the joints are eventually extended, will still detract from functional results. For this reason, joint flexion alone cannot adequately solve the tension problem. Similarly, if flexion is of such a degree that residual stiffness will retard the patient's use of the part, then such tension should be avoided.

If the decision is made to graft a nerve (Fig. 14.8), the technique has been well described and certain principles should be emphasised. The donor nerve(s) must be an autograft. In most instances, cutaneous nerves from remote sites have been employed, although one may sometimes use nerve from the injured extremity (Table 14.1).

Table 14.1 Potential donor nerves for grafting

1. Lateral antebrachial cutaneous nerve of the forearm
2. Medial antebrachial cutaneous nerve of the forearm
3. Posterior interosseous nerve (sensory portion)
4. Sural nerve
5. Lateral femoral cutaneous nerve
6. Saphenous nerve
7. Dorsal cutaneous branch of ulnar nerve*
8. Superficial radial nerve*
9. Any nerve from an amputated part

* If already injured

The graft must lie in a well-vascularised bed between two viable ends. The graft should be placed while all joints are in full extension. The length of the graft segments should be slightly greater than the length of the gap itself to allow for an unexpected stretch, or any shortening which might occur with fibrosis secondary to healing. Since the graft is inserted with no tension, one relies on a fibrin bond and as few sutures as possible to secure the union. The suture material should be a minimally-reactive monofilament, non-absorbable synthetic. The part should be immobilised for 10–14 days to allow early collagen formation for strength (but not so long as to result in secondary joint stiffness and tendon adhesion which might otherwise retard the rehabilitation). Efforts should be made to assure as much gliding as possible of the graft and its junctures.

One should anticipate that recovery following nerve grafting will be slow and that sometimes years are required to reach it (Fig. 14.7). For more proximal grafts in the arm, one should anticipate a follow-up period of 4–5 years before making a final judgment about success or failure. We have seen patients where progress in both motor and sensory function could be documented for this long a period. The results of nerve grafting can be materially enhanced by therapy and re-education techniques designed to maximise function in remaining uninjured structures and to teach the patient to use whatever regeneration occurs as a result of the grafting (Dellon 1981).

SPECIFIC NERVES AND GRAFTS

As noted above, several potential donor nerves are available, and one can frequently select a donor whose diameter and fascicular composition most nearly approximates the nerve being grafted. Other considerations in donor nerve selection include: sensory deficit in donor area; length of graft available; ease of harvesting; skin scarring; and general patient acceptance.

The diameter of *digital nerves* varies, depending on the side and the digit involved. Graft choices include: a digital nerve from an otherwise damaged or unsalvageable finger (when available); the lateral or medial antibrachial cutaneous nerves of the forearm; the sural nerve; the lateral femoral cutaneous nerve; the terminal portions of the posterior interosseous nerve; or the dorsal cutaneous branch of the ulnar nerve. We have used all these donors with success. Other cutaneous nerves can theoretically be employed as well.

Digital nerves usually require only one bundle of whatever donor is used. The graft can be inserted in antegrade or retrograde fashion. Research on this point to date is sparse, but it suggests that there is little difference between the two. The advantage of a retrograde graft is that there is little likelihood that regenerating fibers will escape through any branches which might be present. Antegrade grafts afford whatever advantages might accrue from regeneration in a natural direction. As with repairs, grafting of digital nerves can be

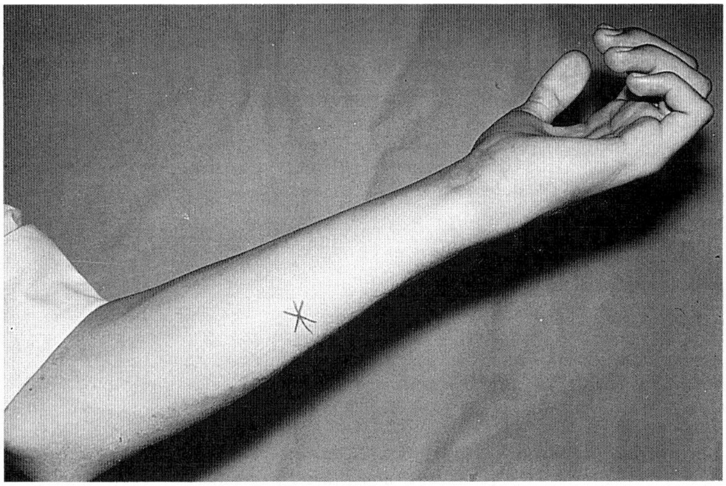

A

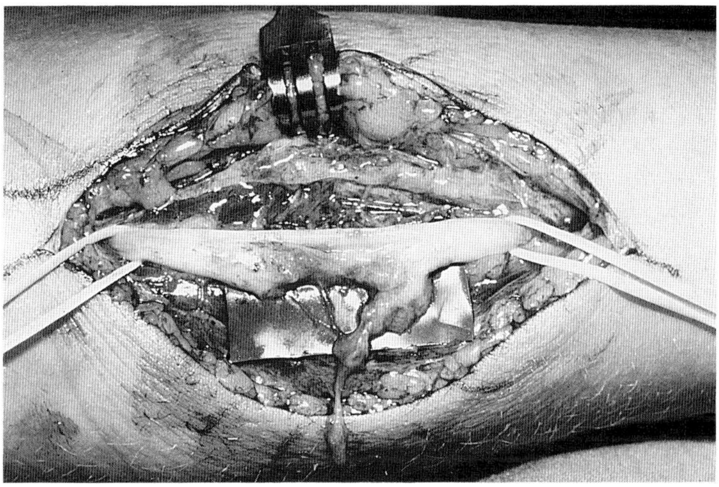

B

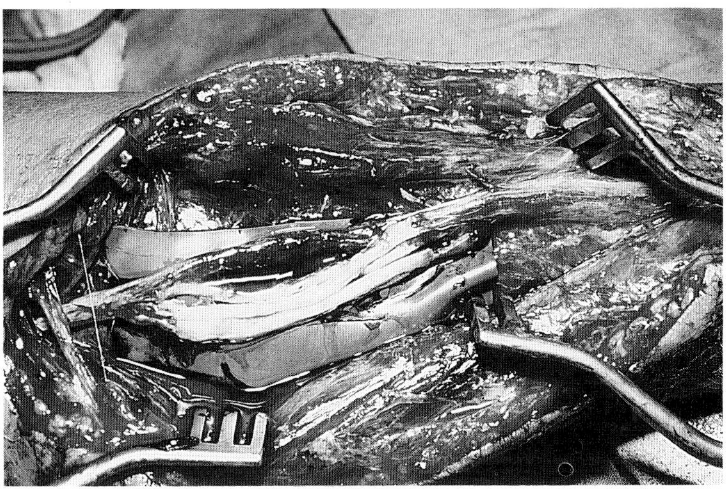

C

Fig. 14.7 This 16-year-old physician's son was seen six months after a closed fracture of the mid-ulna and radius. He developed a secondary partial ulnar nerve palsy after the injury and did not improve with time. **A.** Six months after injury, Tinel's sign is present in the mid-forearm. There is intrinsic muscle wasting and function is minimal. Sensation is present but diminished. **B.** At exploration, the ulnarmost portion of the nerve was irreparably imbedded in the fracture callous, but the radial portion was uninvolved. An awake stimulation (see text for details) confirmed that the damaged fascicles did not conduct, and they were resected. The resulting defect was grafted. The remainder of the nerve conducted well and was left intact. **C.** Three interfascicular nerve grafts, each approximately 6 cm long, were placed between the damaged portions. The uninjured fascicles of the ulnar nerve were left undisturbed. (Note the swelling which occurs with tourniquet deflation.)

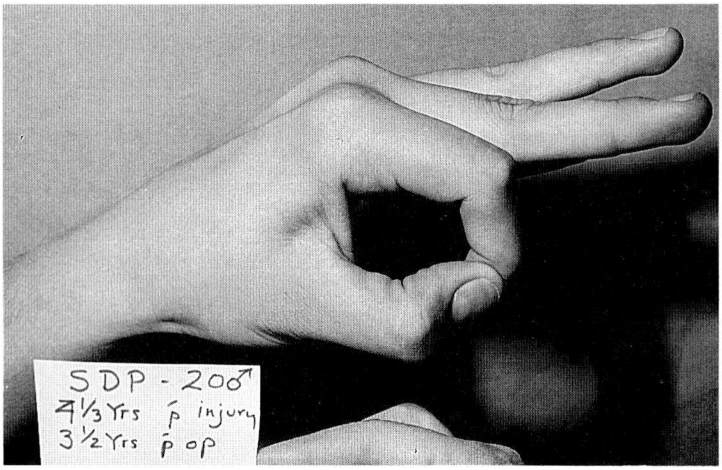

D

Fig. 14.7 (**cont**) **D.** Froment's sign is absent and the 1st dorsal interosseous now functions and has reasonably good bulk. There is no claw, and finger flexion is initiated at the MP joints, indicating return of lumbrical function. Two-point discrimination is 4–6 mm.

secured by epifascicular sutures, and there seems no advantage to isolation of individual components of the recipient nerve except in the terminal portion of such nerves as the ulnar digital nerve of the thumb.

The *common digital nerves* frequently require grafting in secondary cases. They are short, they lie over no joints, and little length is gained by mobilisation. One is frequently in the situation of dissecting and suturing beneath the superficial volar arch. Distally, one usually must graft to two proper digital nerves, and proximally to a single stump. Nevertheless, results of grafting common digital nerves can be excellent. The distance to the target area is short, and cutaneous territories are well-defined.

When one reaches the *proximal palm and wrist area*, a different situation pertains. Here, nerve function becomes more complex and the cross-sectional anatomy is mixed. Both sensory and motor components are present and these must be identified and isolated for separate grafting. Nerves at this level and more proximal are prime candidates for the technique of interfascicular grafting. Here, the surgeon must use one or more of several techniques to positively identify bundles and relate them to specific function. Once done, each specific component must be joined by a graft of like calibre. Depending on the length of the gap in question, one or more donor nerves must be used to obtain enough sections of graft. In selecting donor sites, it is wise not to jeopardise other functioning nerves in an already partially innervated extremity, if possible. Fortunately, patients tolerate loss of skin sensation on such areas as the lateral dorsal surface of the foot or the distal forearm satisfactorily and will willingly pay this price, *so long as they have been warned in advance*.

Major nerves in the *forearm and upper arm* require major dissections and longer grafts. Usually, one (or sometimes both) sural nerves are required. Awake stimulation is sometimes helpful in planning alignment. Additional information can be obtained by the distal dissection of known branches or the separation of identifiable segments, such as the dorsal cutaneous branch of the ulnar nerve. Finally, known branches usually occupy at least a predictable quadrant, and this may hold for a several centimetre distance. If in doubt, one can at least make an educated guess about such localisations. Sometimes, in desperate situations, one may have to rely on parts of all these techniques.

Grafting of a major forearm or upper arm nerve usually requires 4–6 separate grafts, and it is well to emphasise the amount of donor nerve required to the patient. For major grafting, I prefer not to take donor nerves from the injured extremity, since this adds to the loss of sensation already present.

Preparation of the nerve ends

Practically all nerve grafting is performed as a

secondary procedure. It is assumed in the following description that a neuroma and glioma are present.

One begins by opening the epifascicular epineurium of the proximal nerve stump at a level proximal to the neuroma. A T-shaped incision works satisfactorily and facilitates subsequent removal of epineurium. Fascicular bundles are individually identified and traced distally toward the neuroma. At the level where it becomes abnormal, each fascicle or bundle is transected. In this manner, the neuroma is gradually excised and one is left with several bundles, each cut at slightly different levels and from which the epifascicular epineurium has been freed. The process is then repeated on the distal stump, removing the glioma. One now has proximal and distal bundles and fascicles, separated by a gap, which can be measured.

At this point, the surgeon must make a map of the proximal and distal nerve ends. This should be done while arranging individual bundles of fascicles for suturing. The maps are then studied, and appropriate bundles chosen for matching.

Based on the length of the gap and the maps of the nerve ends, one then determines how many sections of graft will be required and what their length should be. This offers a guide as to what donor nerve(s) should be obtained. Once the donor nerve has been harvested, actual placement of graft lengths can commence.

One may either pre-cut each graft, or determine graft length after one union to a stump has been made. If one does not pre-cut the grafts, the full-length donor nerve is laid in place and one end secured to a nerve trunk. The opposite end is then measured and cut precisely to length. Either technique is acceptable. The graft should be slightly longer than the gap with all joints extended, so as to avoid tension.

Each graft is secured by one or two sutures, placed 180° from each other. For this purpose, I use 11–0 or sometimes 10–0 nylon suture. When the first graft is inserted, a single suture may serve as a pivotal point and allow the graft to rotate 180° so that alignment and apposition cannot be reliably maintained (Fig. 14.8). At least two sutures, 180° apart, are required to avoid this situation. When several grafts are used, it is gratifying to see that subsequent ones can often be maintained with even a single suture. This entire process is aided by the natural tissue fibrin which causes the ends literally to 'stick together.'

When grafting has been completed, wounds can be closed, usually in layers but sometimes with skin sutures only. In such areas as the carpal canal, a technique should be used to assure that as much subcutaneous tissue as possible covers the grafts, so that they are not immediately beneath the dermis of the skin. The extremity is then splinted in a comfortable position and motion is begun in 12–14 days.

As data accumulates, it is becoming apparent that longitudinal excursion of nerves is a factor to be considered (Wilgis & Murphy 1986). It is probably useful that reconstructed nerves, whether by suture or by graft, be mobilised to whatever extent is consistent with safe healing, in order that the repair not be bound by scar to a single location. Even while the extremity is splinted, patients should be encouraged to flex and extend the fingers, thereby minimising the likelihood of adhesions between the tendons and nerves.

OUTLOOK FOR THE FUTURE

The final chapter of nerve repair, whether by direct union or by graft, remains to be written. Major strides in technical surgery have occurred in recent years and have clearly influenced results for the better. Nevertheless, we are now at the point where significant shortcomings in function sometimes remain that are not likely to be overcome by further technical advances. We must now make a concentrated effort to understand better the process of nerve degeneration and regeneration, and to seek those approaches which will allow us to modify it for the better. Toward this end, research is ongoing and will surely have eventual effect at three levels: the cell body, the site of nerve union, and peripheral motor and sensory targets.

Cell body

An elusive dream of surgeons has been, and remains, that some degree of control might be ex-

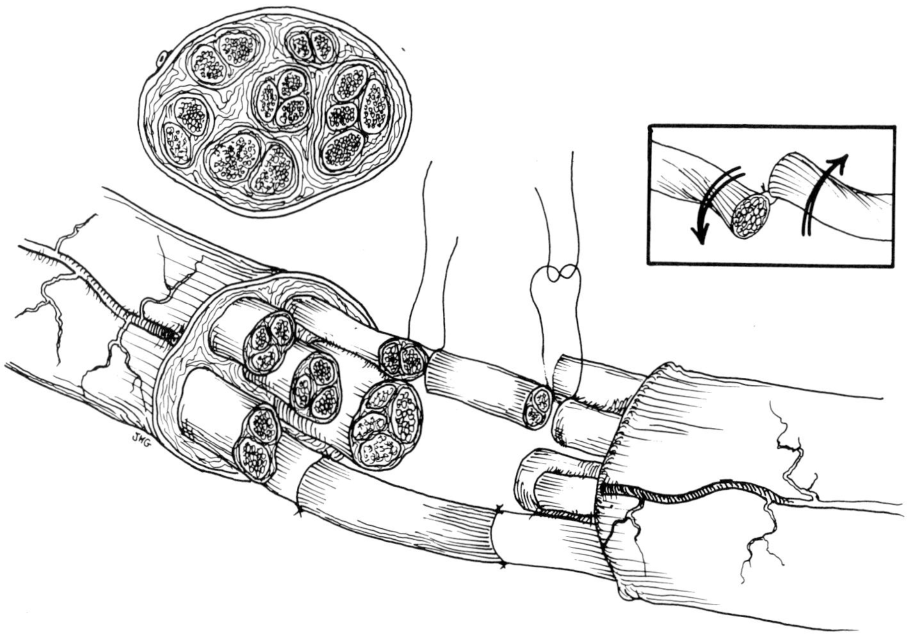

NERVE GRAFT

Fig. 14.8 Interfascicular nerve graft, technique of Millesi and associates. (See text for details). A nerve graft guarantees a tension-free union and this is its major advantage. A minimal number of sutures are required, but two may be necessary at either end to prevent 180° rotation of the graft and recipient nerve.

ercised in areas remote from the injury. Toward this end, a number of techniques and compounds are under investigation with the hope that one or more of them might prevent cell death and affect the metabolic rate of regeneration. Such an effect could hasten the speed of recovery and would clearly be valuable. For example, the galactosides are of interest and may well prove useful. Electrical stimulation of nerve repairs has been attempted and has not as yet been shown to be of value, but the microelectronic revolution may change this.

Level of nerve juncture

Alternate techniques of bonding nerve ends are being explored, and repair devices which obviate this whole concept are also being studied. Fibrin glue has generated considerable interest but has potential problems still. The hope of a biological glue which is ultimately absorbed, is non-reactive, and which will join ends may someday be in the offing. Tension-sparing devices, such as suture at a distance, also have been employed. The laser is being studied, but remains a research tool at this point.

The technique of tubulation is attractive and is currently receiving considerable attention. The use of autogenous tubes as a laboratory tool for nerve repair is not new and was introduced by Weiss in 1944. It was repopularised in the 1970s, and several investigators have explored a variety of autogenous and synthetic materials as nerve conduits. Among them have been blood vessels, mesothelium, perineurium, epineurium, and synthetics such as polyethylene and polyglycolic acid. Some of these will doubtless find their way into clinical use, but it remains to be seen whether they can be transferred to the clinical setting and produce functional results comparable to those which have been obtained in the laboratory.

Nerve growth factor has been available for many years, and has held the interest of those looking for a method to improve axon regeneration. To date, it has not been found clinically valuable. More recently, however, other neuronotrophic factors have been identified and are currently being explored in the laboratory. Laminin is a substance which has been shown to be active, and laminin-containing gel has been introduced into biodegradable tubes to serve as a substrate for regenerating nerve fibres. Other such factors may have a role in guiding regenerating nerve fibres and, specifically, in assisting them in the choice of a motor or sensory conduit. Agents which might provide a better substrate for regenerating axons, which might speed their advance or lessen their resistance would be clearly valuable. (Seckel 1990).

Distal receptors

Target areas, both motor and sensory, undergo progressive degeneration and atrophy following nerve injury. During the obligatory time of regeneration, any factors which could retard or avoid this effect would obviously be useful. Two approaches are being considered and may show promise: electrical stimulation and pharmacological agents.

Electrical stimulation has long been an obvious method to retard muscle atrophy. From a practical standpoint, it has been useless because of the size and crude nature of available devices. More recently, the age of microelectronics has encouraged a new look at this area, and stimulators are now being employed on a clinical basis. Early impressions suggest that atrophy is minimised and that final results are enhanced. It is likely that nerve surgery units in the future will include such devices in their armamentarium.

From a pharmacological standpoint, the drug leupeptin has shown some promise in retarding Wallerian degeneration in animals and allowing faster growth of regenerating axons. Animal studies have been encouraging and it is likely that approval will permit clinical trials in humans soon. Leupeptin (or a similar drug) may well find a role in the management of clinical problems.

Lastly, a variety of pharmacological agents have been employed at the site of nerve bonding, in an effort to provide a more favourable milieu in which regeneration might occur. This has been accomplished in two ways: when nerve ends are physically bound to each other, the materials are simply placed about the nerve juncture; when tubulation techniques are used, the agents have actually been placed in the tubule, whether synthetic or biological. As with all other areas of nerve research, the actual value of such techniques in the treatment of real injuries in human patients remains to be seen. The potential for abuse and exploitation is great because evaluation of results is difficult.

At the time of writing, it is fair to summarise by saying that rejoining of transected nerve ends by direct suture or grafts is, and is likely to remain the cornerstone of treatment for the immediate future. At the same time, it is obvious that we have pushed the technical aspects of repair about as far as we can. The hope for further progress lies in our willingness to entertain and pursue new approaches.

REFERENCES

Chou J A, VanBeek A L, Meyer D L, Johnson M C 1985 Surgical significance of the motor fascicular group of the ulnar nerve in the forearm. Journal of Hand Surgery 10A: 867–872

Dellon A L 1981 Evaluation of sensibility and reeducation of sensation in the hand. Williams and Wilkins, Baltimore, p 203–246

Dellon A L, Mackinnon S E 1986 Radial sensory nerve entrapment in the forearm. Journal of Hand Surgery 11A: 199–205

deMedinaceli L D, Seaber A V 1989 Experimental nerve reconnection: importance of initial repair. Microsurgery 10: 56–70

Egloff D V, Narakas A 1983 Anastomoses nerveuses par fibrinocollage. Annales de Chirurgie de la Main 2: 101

Gaul J S Jr 1983 Electrical stimulation as an adjunct to nerve repair. Journal of Hand Surgery 8: 289–296

Hakstian R W 1968 Funicular orientation by direct stimulation. Journal of Bone and Joint Surgery 50A: 1178

Jabaley M E, Wallace W H, Heckler F R 1980 Internal topography of major nerves of the forearm and hand: a current review. Journal of Hand Surgery 5: 1–18

Jabaley M E 1981 Current concepts of nerve repair. Clinics in Plastic Surgery 8: 33–44

Jabaley M E 1984a Technical aspects of peripheral nerve repair. Journal of Hand Surgery 9B: 14–19

Jabaley M E 1984b Electrical stimulation in the awake patient. Bulletin of the Hospital for Joint Diseases 44: 248–259

Lundborg G 1979 The intrinsic vascularization of human peripheral nerves: structural and functional aspects. Journal of Hand Surgery 4: 34–41

Millesi H, Meissl G, Berger A 1972 The interfascicular nerve grafting of the median and ulnar nerves. Journal of Bone & Joint Surgery 54A: 727–750
Millesi H, Terzis J K 1983 Problems of terminology in peripheral nerve surgery: committee report of the International Society of Reconstructive Microsurgery. Microsurgery 4: 51–56
Millesi H 1986 The nerve gap: theory and clinical practice. Hand Clinics 2: 651–663
Miyamoto Y, Watari, Tsuge K 1981 Effects of tension on interneural microcirculation in end to end neurorrhaphy. In: Gorio A, Millesi H, Mingrino S (eds) Posttraumatic peripheral nerve regeneration. Raven Press, New York, p 81
Orgel M G 1984 Epineurial versus perineurial repair of peripheral nerves. Clinics in Plastic Surgery 11: 101–104
Russell R C 1986 Transmission and scanning electron microscopy of peripheral nerves. Hand Clinics 2: 665–676
Seckel B R 1990 Enhancement of peripheral nerve regeneration. Muscle and Nerve 13: 785–801
Smahel J, Meyer V E, Bachem U 1987 Glueing of peripheral nerves with fibrin: experimental studies. Journal of Reconstructive Microsurgery 3: 211–218
Spinner M 1978 Injuries to the major branches of peripheral nerves of the forearm. Section VII. W B Saunders, Philadelphia, p 66
Sunderland S 1978 Nerves and nerve injuries, 2nd edn. Churchill Livingstone, Edinburgh
Sunderland S 1979 The pros and cons of funicular nerve repair. Journal of Hand Surgery 4: 201–211
Terzis J K, Feeker B L, Sismour E N 1984 A computerized study of the intraneural organization of the median nerve (abstract). Journal of Hand Surgery 9A: 605
Tsuge K, Ikuta Y, Sakaeu M 1975 A new technique for nerve suture. Plastic and Reconstructive Surgery 56: 496–500
Wilgis E F S, Murphy R 1986 The significance of longitudinal excursion in peripheral nerves. Hand Clinics 2: 761–766
Williams H B, Jabaley M E 1986 The importance of internal anatomy of the peripheral nerves to nerve repair in the forearm and hand. Hand Clinics 2: 689–707

G. Brunelli and F. Brunelli

15 Direct muscular neurotisation

In our everyday emergency or planned surgery, there are cases in which muscles or group of muscles are paralysed, either because the terminal branches of the motor nerves are avulsed from the muscle itself or because the neural parts of the muscles (where the terminal branches of the nerves end in the motor end-plates) are destroyed. Such lesions cannot be cured by means of conventional nerve surgery. Patients with these kinds of lesions can only be treated by means of palliative operations, such as tendon transfers, joint fusions, etc., occasionally with poor results.

In the earlier 20th century, Heineke (1914), Erlacher (1915), Steindler (1915) and Elsberg (1917) had undertaken research and attempted clinically directly to implant nerves into denervated muscles, but with inconsistent results.

Aitken (1950), Guth and Zalewski (1963), Katz and Miledi (1964) and Gutman and Hanzlikova (1967) performed physiological studies, laying a nerve on the surface of a denervated muscle. Based on knowledge currently available, research was started at the beginning of the 1970s to investigate the possibility of re-innervating muscles by means of the direct implantation of a nerve into the muscle tissue (the remnants of the avulsed muscles) (Brunelli et al 1976). The achievement of useful clinical results by means of such an operation seemed to most surgeons to be impossible. Nevertheless, this is what is done now, with a large percentage of good results.

The research on animals lasted eight years and was done first on rabbits and then on rats using different techniques; the details of these have been progressively modified in order to obtain the best results.

BIOLOGICAL BASIS AND RESEARCH

The above mentioned physiological experiments had shown that by laying a nerve on the surface of a denervated muscle, and stimulating this nerve some days later, weak contraction of the muscular fibres neighbouring the nerve was obtained. This was not the case with normally innervated muscles, and seemed to demonstrate that new synapses (motor end-plates) had formed between the nerve and the denervated muscle fibres.

The explanation given for this phenomenon was that a denervated muscle fibre is sensitive to acetylcholine all over its surface and can accept a new innervation at ectopic sites, whereas a normally innervated muscle does not accept additional new innervation, as its sensitivity to acetylcholine is localised at the motor end-plates (Lomo & Slater 1980).

Motor end-plates which form in 'aneural' zones (i.e. where normally no motor end-plates exist) are functional adaptations of the nerve endings and of the muscle membrane when in contact with each other.

In the early 1970s, we undertook research in rabbits, removing the distal part of the tibial nerve, with its intramuscular branches, and implanting the peroneal nerve into the proximal part of the lateral head of the gastrocnemius muscle (Fig. 15.1). This part of the muscle is an 'aneural' zone and normally does not have motor end-plates.

The first experimental model (in rabbits, from 1970 to 1973) consisted of the removal of 2 cm of the tibial nerve, and stripping its terminal branches in order to denervate the gastrocnemius

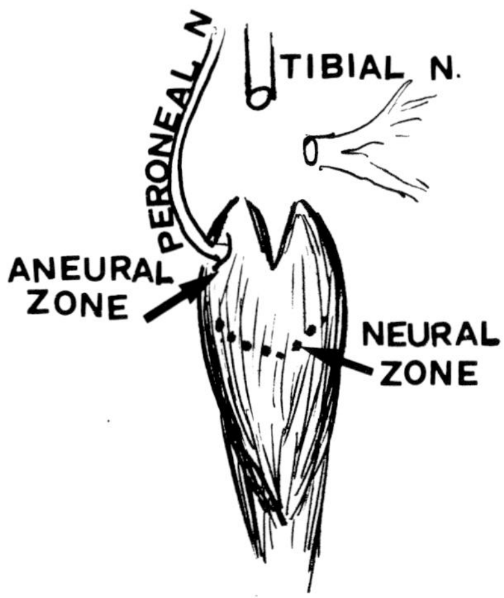

Fig. 15.1 Scheme of the first experimental model in rabbits removing the distal part of the tibial nerve with its branches, and inserting the peroneal nerve into the lateral part of the gastrocnemius ('aneural' zone).

muscle. The peroneal nerve was then severed and implanted into the proximal end of the lateral head of the gastrocnemius. The proximal part of the muscle had previously been examined histologically and found to be almost completely lacking in motor end-plates ('aneural' zone).

Twenty-one rabbits were operated upon using this technique; they were sacrificed at 1 or 2 months. At the moment of sacrifice, the transplanted peroneal nerve was electrically stimulated. Contraction of the muscle was demonstrated. The distal ends of the transplanted nerves were then identified and removed.

Several one-millimetre nerve segments were resected and prepared for transmission electron microscopic examination by means of Carnowski solution, osmium oxide and epon* inclusion. Other segments were frozen with liquid nitrogen, fixed in formalin and then stained by means of 1% ammonium sulphide with a few drops of $CuSO_4$ 0.1 mol, in order to detect cholinesterase, and therefore to demonstrate motor end-plates. The electron microscope showed the formation of functional adaptation of the branches to the muscle, and of the muscle surface to the arriving axons. This new neuromuscular junction was like a normal motor end-plate (Figs 15.2 and 15.3). These experiments were published in 1976 (Brunelli et al 1976).

A larger series of animals (40 rats) was operated upon between 1973 and 1978 using an improved technique, removing the epineurium of the peroneal nerve for a distance of 1 cm and dividing the nerve into several fasciculi or subfascicular units (as many as possible, using the operating microscope) (Fig. 15.4).

These small nerve units were then implanted into the muscle through small slits atraumatically made in the muscle surface; the implantation sites were spread as widely and deeply as possible in order to increase the supply of the new innervation to the largest possible mass of muscle, and to raise the number of neurotised muscular fibres. If the slit bled, the nerve division was not implanted into it, as scar formation around the axons would have been likely. Instead, a new slit was made close to the original slit (Brunelli 1982, Brunelli & Monini 1985). The nerve was anchored to the muscular fascia by means of a 6–0 suture passed through the epineurium and the muscle fascia, and the fine nerve divisions were sutured to the muscle with 10–0 or 11–0 nylon (Fig. 15.5).

Histological examination by light microscopy revealed a great quantity of newly formed motor end-plates in all cases. The number of motor end-plates in different microscopic fields depended upon the distance from the site of nerve implantation. It was also evident that the muscular fibres on which new motor end-plates had formed had regained normal appearance, whereas the non-re-innervated fibres showed typically dystrophic appearances (Figs 15.6, 15.7 and 15.8).

Electrical stimulation of the peroneal nerve transplanted into the triceps muscle demonstrated good functional re-innervation of the muscle, even after one month.

Transmission electron microscopy showed that the synaptic contacts between the implanted nerve and the previously denervated muscular fibres had the typical structure of normal motor end-plates. Bare axon branches, rich in pre-synaptic vesicles, were in direct contact with the cell membrane of muscular fibres, which had undergone the typical folding of motor synapses. Other typical findings were post-synaptic vesicles, many mitochondria in

* Epon is a plastic material used in anatomy to prepare specimens for transmission electron microscopy

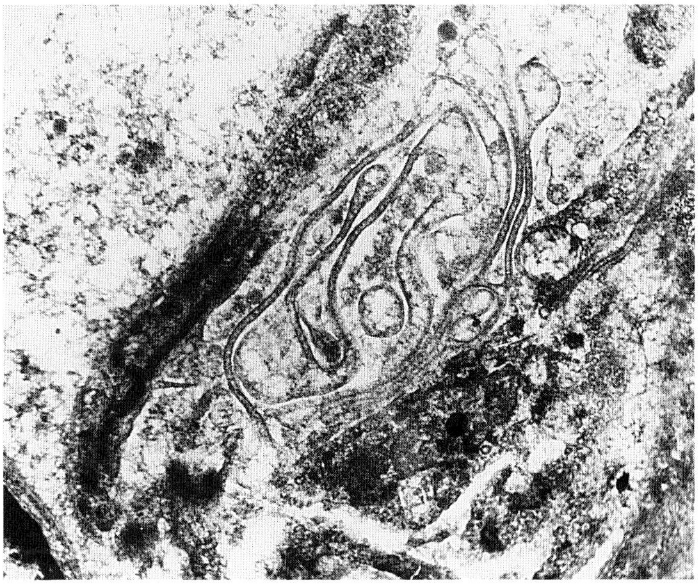

Fig. 15.2 Electron microscopic appearance of philopods* coming from the implanted nerve and searching for denervated muscle fibres.

* A philopod is a kind of sprout of the distal part of the axon which searches for the muscle.

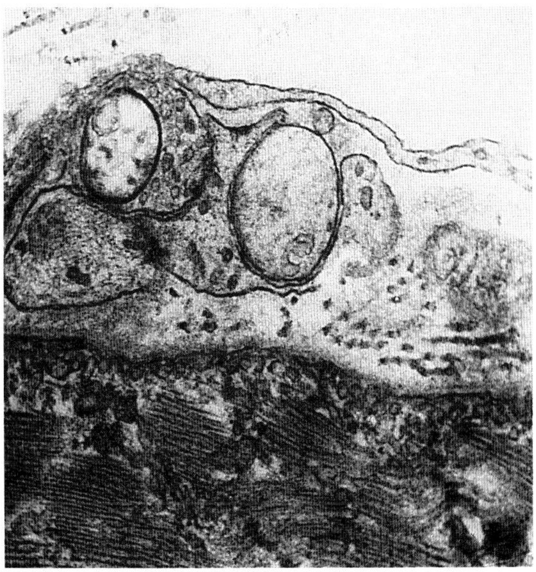

Fig. 15.3 Electron microscopic appearance of a newly-formed motor end-plate which shows normal features.

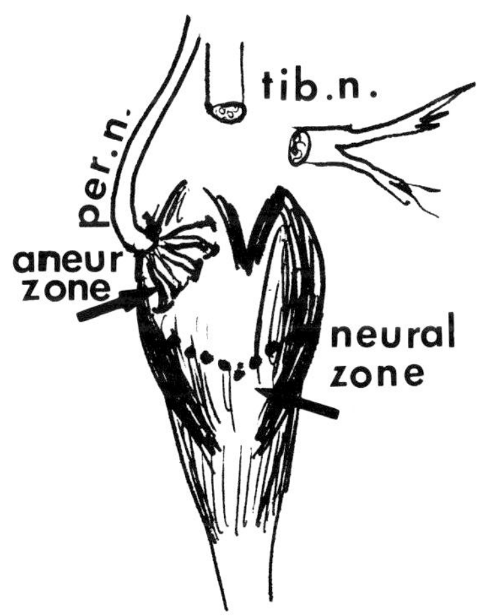

Fig. 15.4 Scheme of the second series of operations in rats. Notice that the end of the nerve is split into many parts.

the muscle, and the presence of a simple layer of Schwann cells above the axon branches (on the side opposite the synaptic contact), while no connective tissue element, not even thin fibrils, lay between the axon branches and the muscle (Fig. 15.9).

In further research (which is still in progress) we tried to investigate if the different types of fibre of the motor nerve, implanted into the muscle, are also able to regrow.

The same surgical technique was used, but the nerve specimens were stained by the Koelle Tsuge method, which stains brown-yellow the motor fibres due to their acetylcholine contents. We saw that some of the fibres of the nerve entering the muscle were not stained, even if stained normally

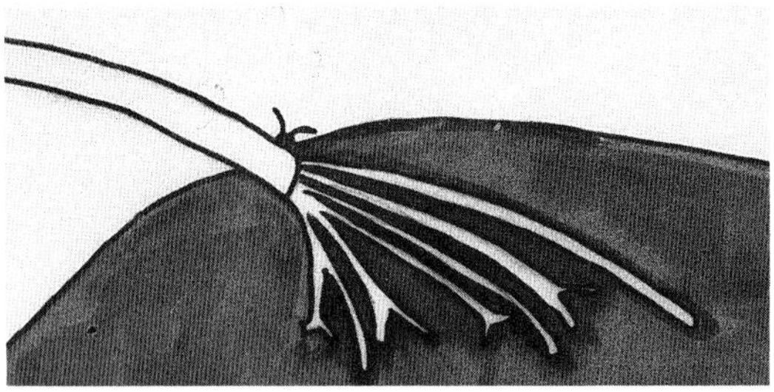

Fig. 15.5 Scheme of the anchorage of the epineurium to the muscle fascia.

with haematoxylin and eosin. This is an indirect demonstration that both afferent and efferent fibres of motor nerves regenerate after this operation (Fig. 15.10).

These results seem to demonstrate:

1. The formation of new motor end-plates by the axon sprouts
2. The morphological normality of these new synapses
3. The great improvement in technique and of results by use of microsurgery.

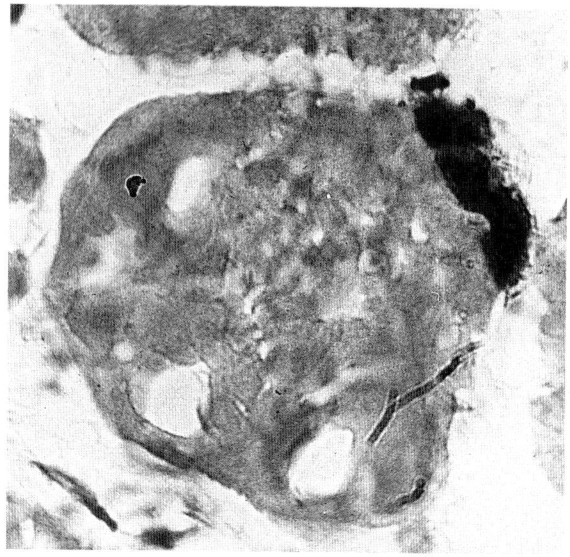

Fig. 15.7 Muscular fibres at the beginning of re-innervation.

Therefore, after the completion of the first research (1973), we were encouraged to use the same technique clinically in those cases which presented with very severe lesions of the neuromuscular

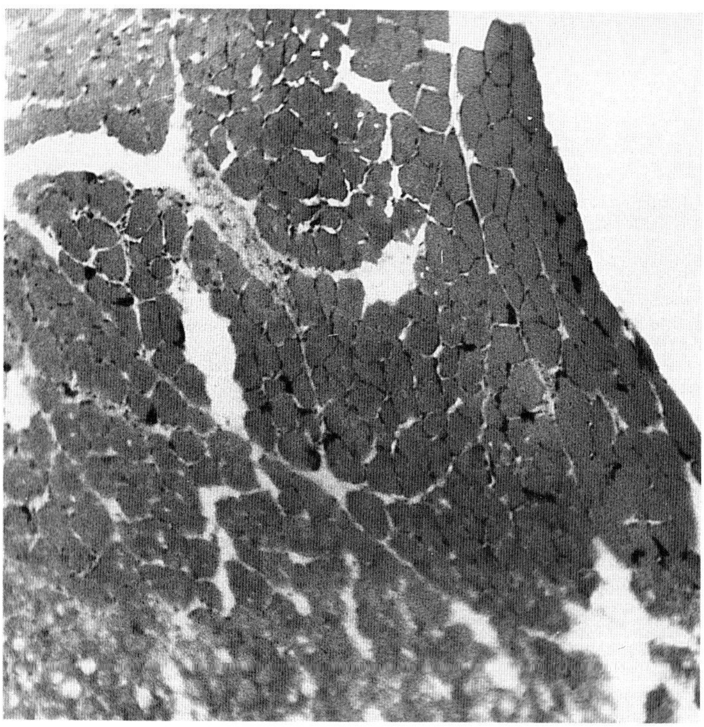

Fig. 15.6 Light microscopic view of a muscle, part of which has been re-innervated and shows motor end-plates and no atrophy, while the surrounding denervated fibres show denervation dystrophy.

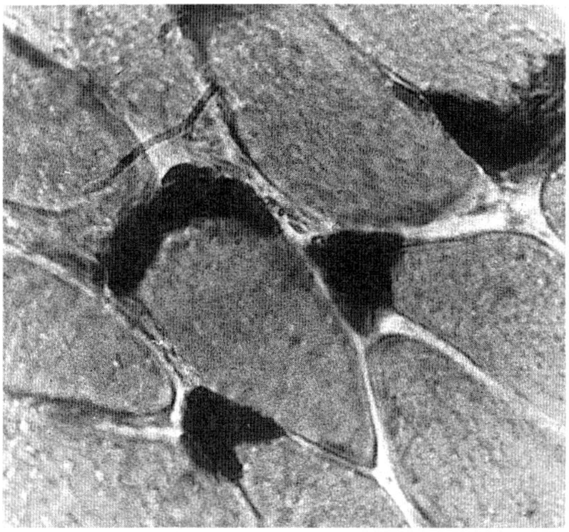

Fig. 15.8 After complete re-innervation, the muscle fibres appear completely normal.

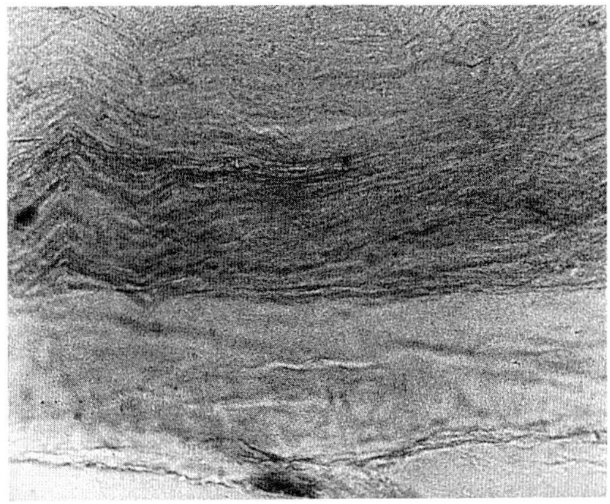

Fig. 15.10 Nerve fibres stained by the Koelle Tsuge cholinesterase method. Those fibres of the motor nerve not stained are interpreted as being afferent.

junction, i.e. where the nerve was avulsed from the muscle or the neural part of the muscle was destroyed, leaving a denervated distal part of the muscle. In fact, in cases like these, no classical technique was available to restore the innervation.

CLINICAL CASES, TECHNIQUE AND RESULTS

The original nerve was always dissected proximally from scar up to normal nerve tissue, and then lengthened by nerve graft to the remnants of the denervated muscle.

The distal ends of the grafts were divided into as many thin slips as possible, and introduced (by means of the experimentally developed technique) into the muscle through many slits made atraumatically in the sound distal part of the damaged muscle. The epineurium was sutured to the muscle fascia, and all the divisions of the grafts sewn to the muscle with 11–0 nylon (Figs 15.11 and 15.12).

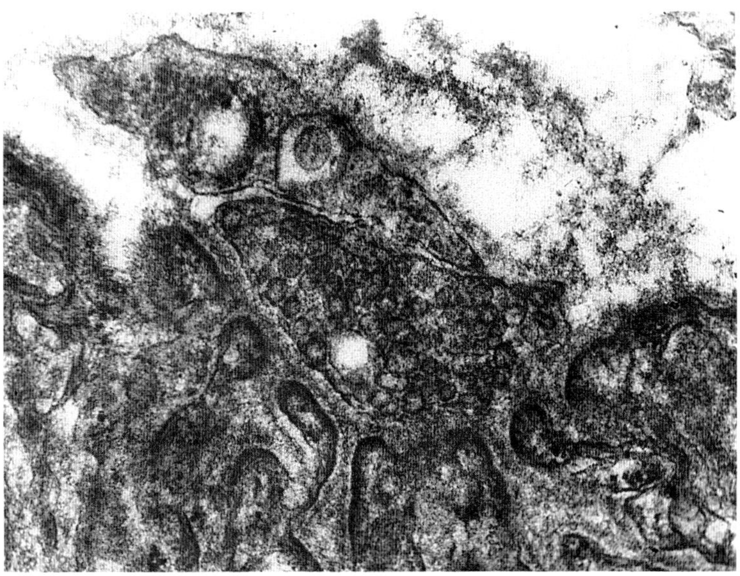

Fig. 15.9 The features of a newly-formed motor end-plate after complete re-innervation.

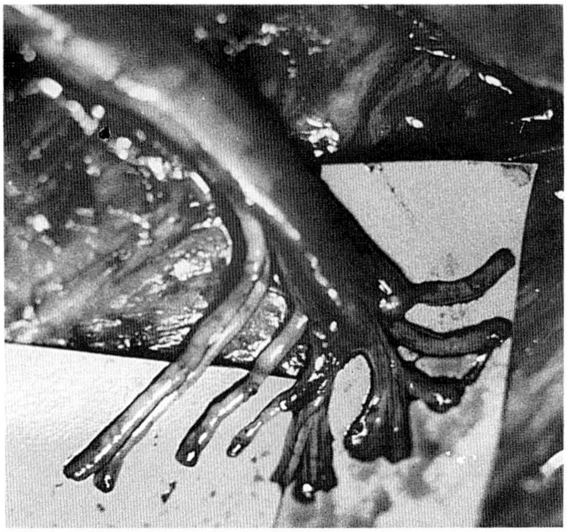

Fig. 15.11 Example of how a sural nerve graft is divided into many filaments.

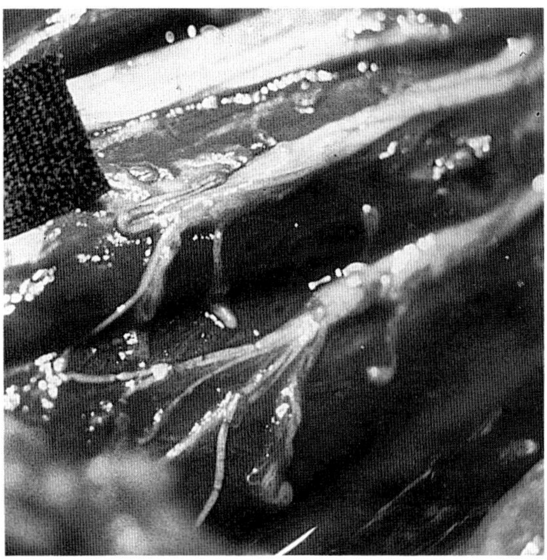

Fig. 15.12 Example of the insertion of the filaments into a muscle.

The re-innervated muscle was kept at rest for 15 days, then passive movement (distension), electrotherapy and massage were allowed. Post-operative treatment also included local radiation therapy and steroid administration to reduce scar formation, and gangliosyde administration.

We have operated upon 39 clinical cases (in 13 years) in which there was no possibility of identifying the distal stump of the damaged nerve, mainly because of traumatic avulsion of the neural part of the muscle, including the distal portion of the motor nerve. This was done:

— 11 times for damaged extensor muscles in the forearm with total palsy of extension of the wrist and digits (Figs 15.13 and 15.14)
— 10 times to extensor muscles in the leg with destruction of the neural part and total palsy of foot extension (Fig. 15.15)
— 5 times for iatrogenic denervation of the trapezius muscle (Fig. 15.16)

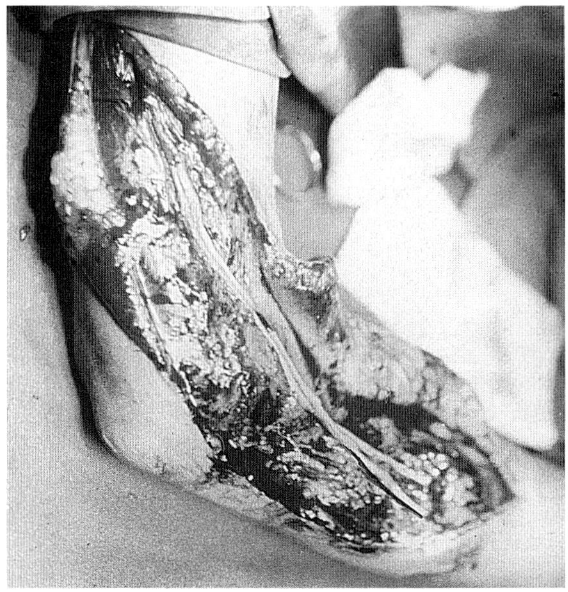

Fig. 15.13 Direct neurotisation of a small distal part of the extensor muscles of the forearm, the proximal part of which had been avulsed by a boat screw one year previously, by means of two sural nerve grafts 22 cm long.

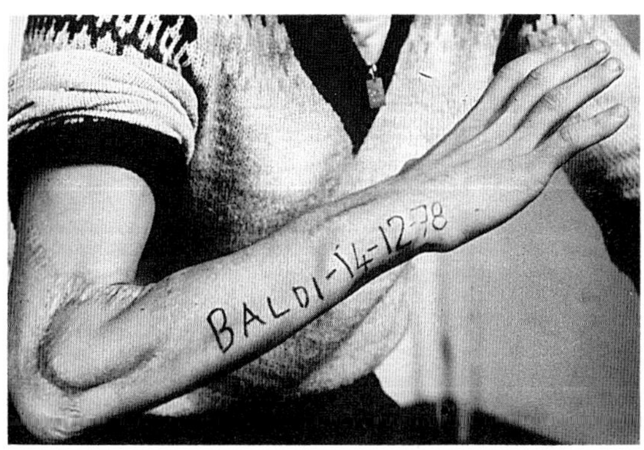

Fig. 15.14 Result two years later.

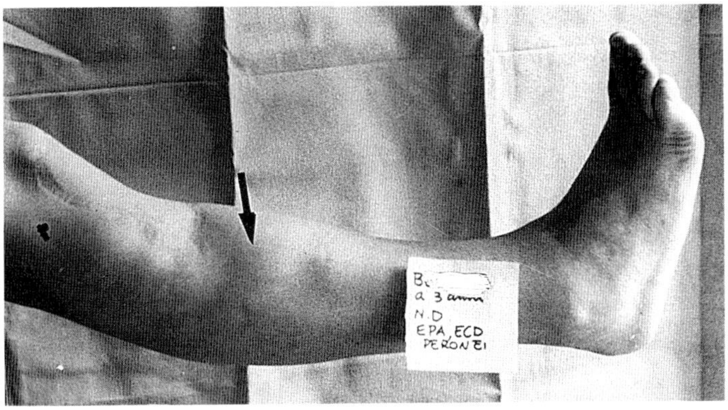

Fig. 15.15 Example of a very good result after direct muscular neurotisation of the remnants of the extensor muscles of the leg, the proximal neural part of which had been avulsed.

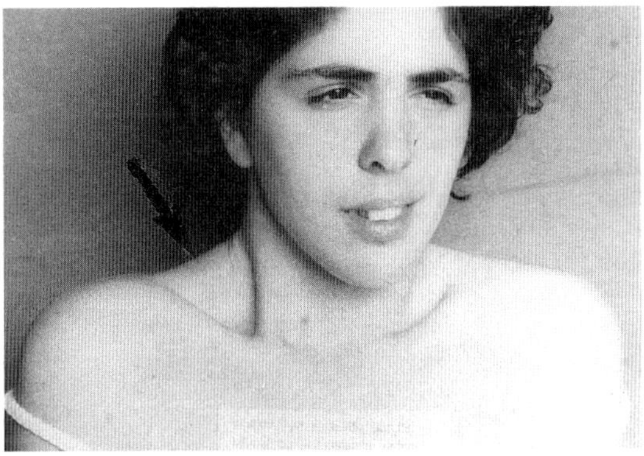

Fig. 15.16 Result of direct muscular neurotisation of an iatrogenic denervation of the trapezius.

—3 times for denervation of the thenar muscles (Figs 15.17 and 15.18)
—5 times for deltoid denervation, due to avulsion of the C5 & 6 roots of the branchial plexus in 3 cases, and in 2 cases due to avulsion of the muscular branches of the axillary nerve (Figs 15.19, 15.20 and 15.21)
—Twice for avulsion of the musculocutaneous nerve from the biceps muscle (Figs 15.22 and 15.23).
—Once for denervation of extensor pollicis longus
—Twice for denervation of the tongue (bilateral lesion).

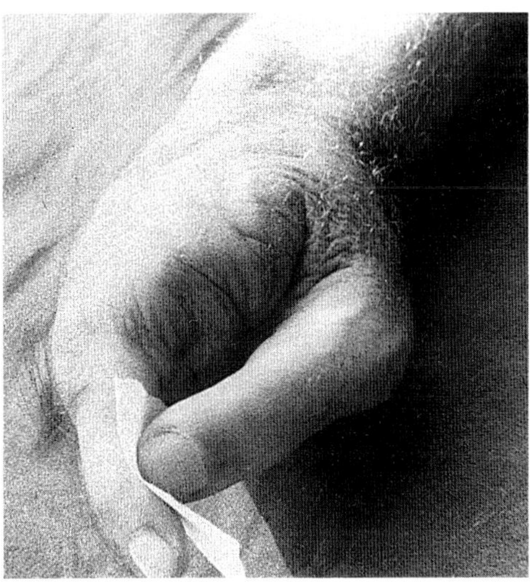

Fig. 15.17

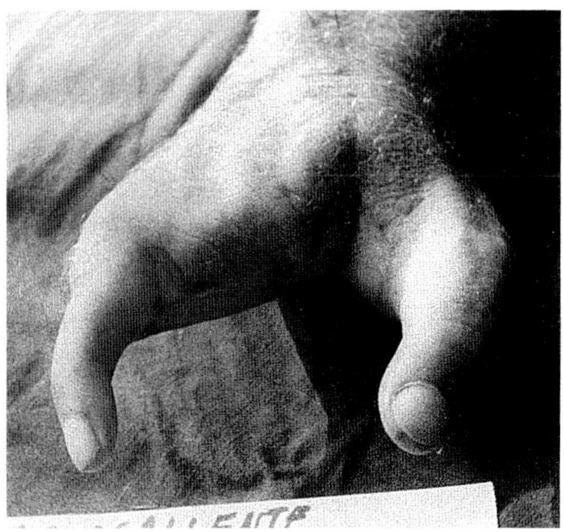

Fig. 15.18

Figs 15.17 and 15.18 Result of direct neurotisation of thenar muscles

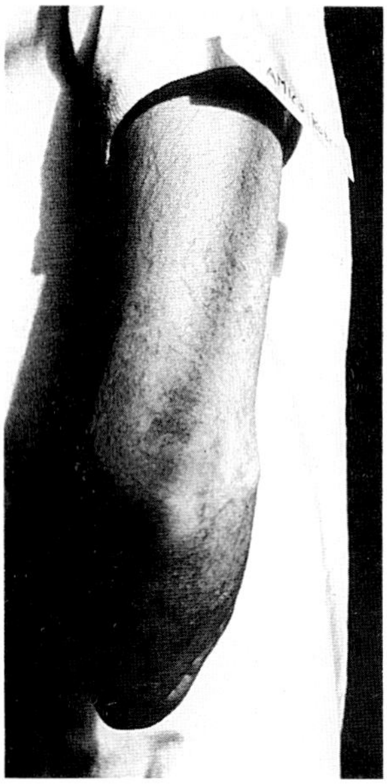

Fig. 15.19 Young man with avulsion of C5, C6 & C7 roots and amputation of the forearm.

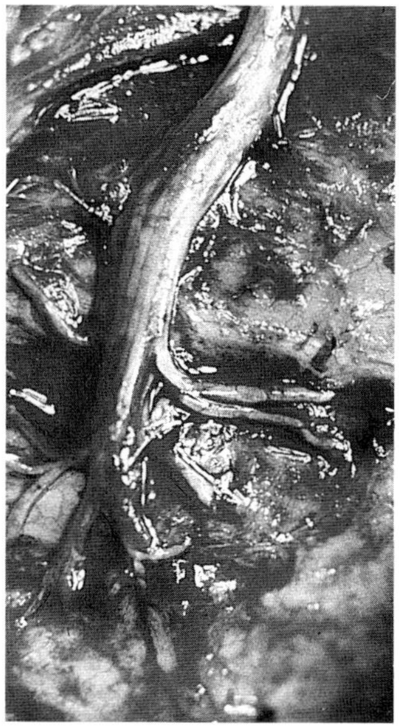

Fig. 15.20 The ulnar nerve, in good condition, but useless because of the amputation, was used to directly innervate the deltoid muscle.

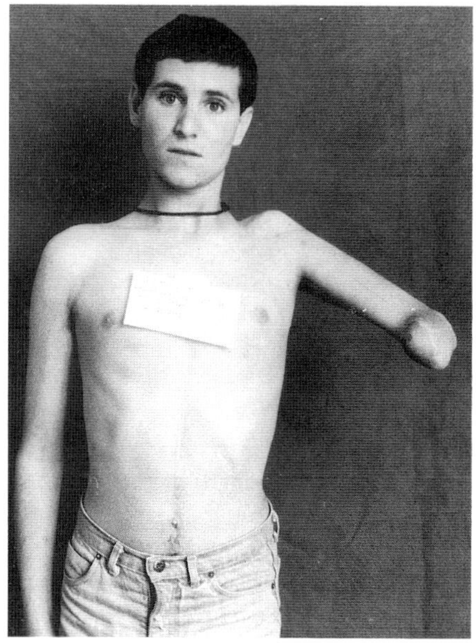

Fig. 15.21 Good function of the deltoid which allows the young man to wear a useful prosthesis.

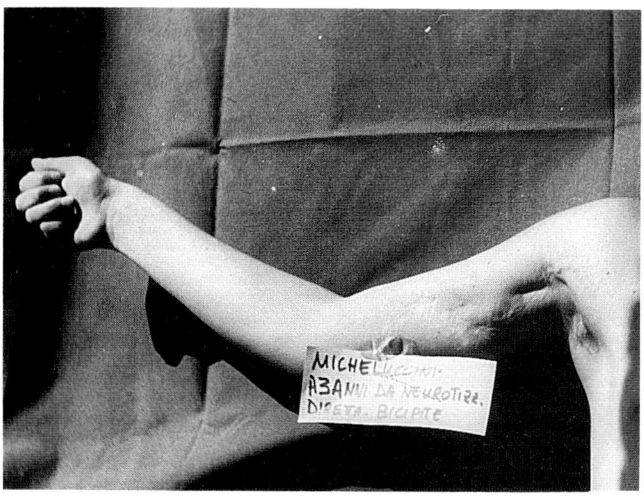

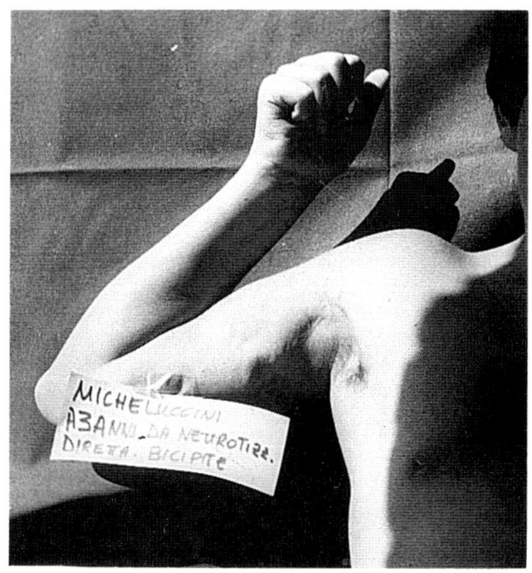

Figs 15.22 and 15.23 Very good result of a direct neurotisation of the biceps muscle after musculocutaneous nerve avulsion.

Results are shown in Table 15.1 (see also Figs 15.12 to 15.23).

There were 34 very good and good results out of 39 operated cases. This operation was accepted by several other surgeons after seeing our first results.

Their results are shown in Table 15.2

DISCUSSION

The explanation for these results is difficult to ascertain. We would have expected some improvement, but not such a great percentage of very good and good results.

Table 15.1 Results of the direct neurotisation of severely damaged muscles: ('very good' is when the muscle or majority of muscles score M5; 'good' is M4; 'fair', M3+; 'poor', M3 or less).

Muscle	*No. of cases*	*Very good*	*Good*	*Fair*	*Poor*
Extensor muscles in forearm	11	9	1	1	
Extensor muscles in leg	10	9	1		
Trapezius muscles	5	3	1	1	
Biceps muscles	2	2			
Thenar muscles	3	2	1		
Extensor pollicis longus	1		1		
Deltoid mucles	5	1	2	1	1
Tongue muscles (hypoglossal)	2		1		1
Totals	39	26	8	3	2

Table 15.2 Results of other surgeons carrying out direct neurotisation of severely damaged muscles; (written answers to a survey made in 1983)

Surgeon	*No. of cases*	*Very good or good*	*Fair*	*Poor*
Alnot (Paris)	3		2	1
Bufalini (Florence)	1		1	
Foucher (Strasbourg)	3	2		1
Landi (Modena)	4	2	1	1
Millesi (Wein)	2	2		
Morelli (Legnano)	1		1	
Palazzi (Barcelona)	4	2	1	1
Strauch (New York)	1	1		
Freilinger, Holle & Frey (Wein)	16	13	1	2
Comtet (Lyon)	8	4	3	1
Celli (Modena)	4	1	1	2
Verbal communication from the same or other surgeons after 1983	27	18	6	3
Totals	74	45	17	12

Perhaps, by using a nerve graft which is inserted directly into the muscle, we use a nerve which undergoes Wallerian degeneration, but which is reinhabited by axons before the endoneural tubes narrow.

Furthermore, in nerve grafts, there is not the Schwann cell proliferation (and diminution of size) that occurs in the distal vascularised part of a severed nerve after some months.

Another tentative explanation is that, perhaps, by inserting the thin branches of the nerve graft directly into the muscle, we put them into an isomorphic medium which is better than having to pass a second nerve-to-nerve suture line.

CONCLUSIONS

Whatever the explanation may be, the results have been very good and exciting. We are thus convinced that this technique should be used more and more frequently in the future, provided that it is based upon strict indications.

INDICATIONS

1. The impossibility of making a traditional nerve repair (either direct nerve suture or nerve graft) because of lack of the distal nerve or because of destruction of the neural part of one muscle or a group of muscles
2. Good condition (and vascularity) of the remnants of the muscle
3. The patient's general condition is suitable for the operation.

SUMMARY

The technique of directly neurotising a muscle severely damaged by the avulsion of the terminal branches of its nerve, or by the destruction of its neural zone, is presented.

The clinical series follows the presentation of the research in different experimental animals and using different surgical models.

Our series of 39 cases, with 34 good and very good results, and 5 fair and poor results, is presented, together with 74 more cases from other series.

The conclusion is that this method, provided strict indications are applied, is a valuable operation to be used more and more frequently.

REFERENCES

Aitken J T 1950 Growth of nerve implants in voluntary muscle. Journal of Anatomy 84: 38

Brunelli G, Brunelli Monini L, Antonucci A, Maraldi N 1976 Neurotizzazione in zona aneurale di muscoli denervati. Policlinico Sezione Chirurgica 83: 611–616

Brunelli G 1982 Direct neurotization of severely damaged muscles. Journal of Hand Surgery 7: 572–579

Brunelli G, Monini L 1985 Direct muscular neurotization. Journal of Hand Surgery 10A: 993–997

Elsberg C A 1917 Experiments on motor nerve regeneration and the direct neurotization of paralysed muscles by their own and by foreign nerves. Science 45: 318

Erlacher P 1915 Direct and muscular neurotization of paralysed muscles. American Journal of Orthopaedic Surgery 13: 22

Gutmann E, Hanzlikova V 1967 Effects of accessory nerve supply to muscle achieved by implantation into muscle during regeneration of its nerve. Physiol Bohemoslav 16: 244

Guth L, Zalewski A A 1963 Disposition of cholinesterase following implantation of nerve into innervated and denervated muscle. Experimental Neurology 7: 316

Heineke D 1914 Die Directe enipflazung des nerven in den muskel. Zentralblutt fur Chirurgie (Leipzig) 41: 465

Katz B, Miledi R 1964 The development of acetylcholine sensitivity in nerve free segments of skeletal muscle. Journal of Physiology 170: 389

Lomo T, Slater C R 1980 Acetylcholine sensitivity of developing junctions in adult rat soleus muscle. Journal of Physiology 303: 173

Steindler A 1915 The method of direct neurotization of paralysed muscles. American Journal of Orthopaedic Surgery 13: 13

J. Michon

16 Neurolysis

Neurolysis is a technique which can be used in many different pathological or traumatic conditions, but always in non-acute situations after a detailed clinical and electrophysiological assessment, i.e. for a specific indication and within a narrow range of expected lesions.

Firstly, we shall review the circumstances of the usual pathology, basically the compression syndromes; then we shall consider the most important indications and techniques in the field of trauma, where problems tend to be more complex, since the demarcation line between the need for neurolysis or repair, by suture or graft, is sometimes unclear.

BASIC TECHNIQUE

The first step in a neurolysis is to detect by a suitable method the nerve trunk involved, and to eliminate any element of external pressure, such as the anatomical factors in spontaneous compressions, or cicatrix in the case of trauma. The evolution of microsurgical techniques has made it possible to add to this classical external neurolysis a method of internal pressure relief by incision, or excision, of the epineurium, whose fibrosis can eventually result in increased endoneural pressure. In severe or old lesions, this prevents the re-establishment of conduction in cases of neurapraxia, or axonal regrowth in cases of axonotmesis.

In most cases, epineurotomy or epineurectomy eliminates the constriction of the compressed nerve trunk, and the surgeon can see how the size of the fasciculi becomes normal within a few minutes, right in front of his eyes. In some especially severe cases, however, the constriction persists, due to fibrosis of the intraneural interfascicular connective tissue which opposes re-expansion. This is where intraneural dissection or fascicular separation is indicated. This requires the use of the operating microscope, so as to avoid damaging the healthy neural tissue, i.e. the perineurium and its axonal contents, and so as to preserve the fine fascicular connections through which interfascicular exchanges take place, as well as the blood vessels. At this stage, it may be justified to release the tourniquet to facilitate preservation of the blood supply.

This dissection within the nerve trunk must be done with great care, and extend, both in length and in depth, only so far as to allow the nerve elements to expand, without isolating them too much, thus causing their devascularisation.

In the most severe cases of constriction, the perineurium itself may have reacted and will remain shrunken. In these cases, the size of the fasciculi will not change during the operation, and there is no better technique, to date, to deal with this situation. It is essential to respect the perineurium, even if shrunken, or the fibres which it protects may degenerate. In such conditions, neurolysis can improve the painful symptoms, but the functional prognosis must remain reserved, since we do not know the state of the axons, and only an electromyographic study carried out a few months later will clarify the situation.

NEUROLYSIS IN COMPRESSION SYNDROMES

The tunnel syndromes are by far the most common causes of the symptoms of pain and peripheral deficit which justify resorting to surgical pressure relief by neurolysis. The carpal tunnel is the most frequently involved.

This paper is not meant to be an exhaustive study of these various syndromes with their respective symptomatology and anatomy; we merely wish to stress the importance of intraneural decompression as an essential complement to the release of the responsible ligament, muscle or tendon.

Experience gathered over more than ten years has shown that the quality of the recovery, as defined by the electrophysiological measurements of conduction speed and distal latency, was considerably improved by endoneural neurolysis in stages 2 and 3. Especially in stage 2, there is a rate of nearly 60% of return to near-normal measurements, whereas external decompression alone achieved less than 30% in our previous series. In stage 1, the fibrosis seems to be spontaneously reversible in many cases, and it is therefore less easy to provide figures. As for stage 4, the involvement of the intrafascicular structures probably explains the absence of functional response to treatment, because the axonal structures have degenerated. As far as motor function is concerned, when drawing up a prognosis, we must also bear in mind the degree and duration of the muscular atrophy, upon which irreversibility depends.

In practice, it is not necessary to touch the epineurium if the history of the case goes back less than one year, and if distal latency is less than 5 ms; but it is our personal tactic to make at least one longitudinal incision into the epineural sheath. More often, we make several parallel incisions, refusing to allow a constricted nerve to persist. Although this concept is very subjective, many years of practice have not revealed that it is contradicted.

At the more advanced stages, we excise the epineurium along the whole front surface of the nerve, which in more than half the cases is enough to restore normal size, thus making it unnecessary to proceed further. But if the fasciculi remain shrunken and condensed, they must be gently separated by sliding in and separating the blades of fine scissors, or by working very carefully with a microsurgery scalpel. This in-depth dissection is stopped as soon as normal-sized elements are encountered, as happens more frequently as we move away from the site of the compression. Although we are utterly convinced of the value of this technique, we also think that excessive zeal would do more harm than abstention, and that our awareness of the fragility of the endoneural structures, and of their vascularisation, must prevail in all circumstances.

Right through the operation on the nerve, it is, indeed, the degree of the constriction, the density and resistance of the fibrosis, and the reaction of the fasciculi to release which must guide our action, and put a stop to it when necessary. In this respect, nothing can replace surgical experience and the observation of many patients over a long time.

NEUROLYSIS IN TRAUMATIC CONDITIONS

Greater problems are met with in trauma when it comes to prognosis and indications, as well as the surgical technique. Even with the help of electrophysiological methods, it is not always possible to distinguish, beyond any doubt, whether a deficit is purely due to compression, or to a complete or partial anatomical interruption. The first surgical stage of locating the nerve must also provide the diagnosis of the lesion, and determine the final technical decision. Indeed, up to this stage, there is an open choice between neurolysis, and suture or graft, including a possible combination of these procedures. From the outset, a distinction must be made between nerve lesions due to closed trauma (contusions, crushes, fractures and subluxations) and those accompanying open wounds, either accidental or surgical. In the case of open lesions, the condition of the nerve has usually been recognised as either intact or contused in continuity, thus justifying neurolysis if spontaneous recovery fails to occur within the expected period, or, on the contrary, more or less completely interrupted and requiring secondary repair. Even if this initial condition is unknown, in the great majority of cases, the date when the first paralytic symptoms appeared makes it possible to conclude that there is scar compression, provided that its onset has been late and, especially, progressive; immediate and non-regressive paralysis is usually due to section of a nerve.

In case of closed lesions, doubt is greater; this is because the pathology may include temporary bruising and compression which will resolve spontaneously, as well as more serious trauma and compression which persists, with no chance of recovery unless the block is surgically released. It may be added that in fractures, for example, a nerve may have been cut by a bone fragment, or that the nerve lesion may be ischaemic, as in Volkmann's syndrome.

Electromyography provides important information for making the diagnosis of the degree of nerve damage after the third week. It specifies whether the case involves neurapraxia or axonotmesis. However, one single examination on a given date does not enable us to make an accurate prognosis; neurapraxia, which is usually benign, can last indefinitely if compression is permanent, whereas axonotmesis with total blockage can recover fully without requiring an operation, provided that bruising (even if intensive) has only lasted an instant. After a first assessment, it is therefore often necessary to make the patient wait for two or three months, so as to be in a position to estimate whether the evolution of his lesion is favourable or unfavourable, and then make a decision, based on full knowledge of the facts.

The decision must thus be made between the third and the fourth months at the latest. There is no advantage to be gained by waiting any longer, as otherwise muscular atrophy will progress to an irreversible stage, especially if the intrinsic muscles, which are particularly fragile, are concerned. In case of continuing doubt, a cautious surgical exploration provides a better prospect for recovery than a long waiting period, which may unfavourably affect the eventual result.

Technique in trauma

First and foremost, preparation must be made with a view to possible repair by suture or graft; this involves considerable longitudinal exposure, especially if other structures are also involved. It is usually preferable to avoid re-opening the primary scar if it is directly over the path of the nerve, but instead to circumscribe the critical area, thus raising a large flap. This reduces the risk of subsequent scar compression.

The nerve itself must be exposed in healthy tissue proximal and distal to the lesion before entering the scarred area, where the nerve may run an abnormal course, especially in cases of fracture or lesion caused by avulsion. The nerve segment affected by the trauma can then be gradually freed from any extrinsic compressive element, and all fibrous tissue, which could subsequently reproduce the situation, is excised.

Once external neurolysis has been achieved in this way, it is necessary to examine the nerve itself. This is because its external appearance and consistency on palpation are very variable and are not always conclusive in indicating the functional value of the content of the nerve, which may be partially or totally disrupted.

Total section is usually followed by retraction of the two ends with the formation of the characteristic appearance of a proximal neuroma and a distal glioma, which may or may not be connected by a band of fibrous tissue. This situation is obvious, and requires suturing or nerve grafting according to the length of the defect, and to the tension required to close the gap after excising scar. This is the only case where longitudinal endoneural dissection is not essential, other than for specific technical indications in the field of repair which are outside the scope of our present article.

In some total functional interruptions due to violent crushing or traction, epineural continuity is maintained. In the case of traction, the internal ruptures can be at multiple levels, especially near the brachial plexus. These sub-epineural ruptures take the form of indurated swellings, which are more or less obvious on inspection, but very easy to palpate a few weeks after injury.

Although such internal ruptures justify resection and repair, the same appearance of indurated swelling can be caused by less severe lesions, especially compressive epineural fibrosis, which may

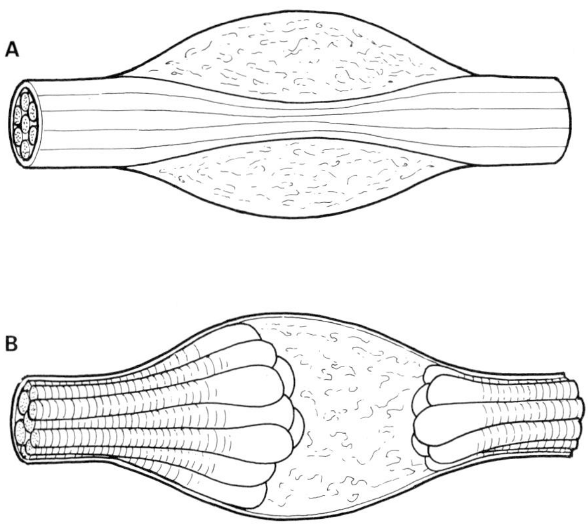

Fig. 16.1 Elongated indurated swelling of a nerve trunk may correspond to: **A.** compressive fibrous epineurial thickening, **B.** complete or partial sub-epineural rupture.

also be associated with partial rupture of one or more fascicular groups (Fig. 16.1).

The only safe method of detecting the various fascicular components is internal microscopic exploration, identifying those which are intact and those which are interrupted and will require repair.

This endoneurolysis must be carried out systematically from 1 cm proximal to the scar. A superficial group of fascicles is isolated and followed into the fibrous block step by step, guided by the characteristic appearance of the perineurium.

If there is interruption, the fascicle ends by tapering or in a neuromatous swelling in the fibrous block. Any element which is in continuity is isolated, whereas every interrupted fascicle is cut in the healthy area and repaired by perineural suturing later on.

Once all the fascicular groups of the proximal end have been identified in this way, the distal ends of the interrupted fasciculi remain attached to the scar tissue and they too are dissected. This is done from the lower end, one after another, whereby their topographical correspondence with those of the proximal end must be identified as accurately as possible. This, too, is outside the scope of the present chapter, because it involves a repair whose technical choices and methods are covered in another chapter of this volume.

The appearance of fusiform narrowing, which is characteristic of simple scar compression, is treated in the same manner as a tunnel syndrome.

A more localised narrowing can be due either to compression by external scar (Fig. 16.2), or to a scarred partial wound (Fig. 16.3). Here, too, it is microsurgical longitudinal dissection which leads to a precise diagnosis and suitable therapy.

Where there is a partial severance, dissection has to be particularly delicate within the scar, because of the risk of damaging intact elements, and

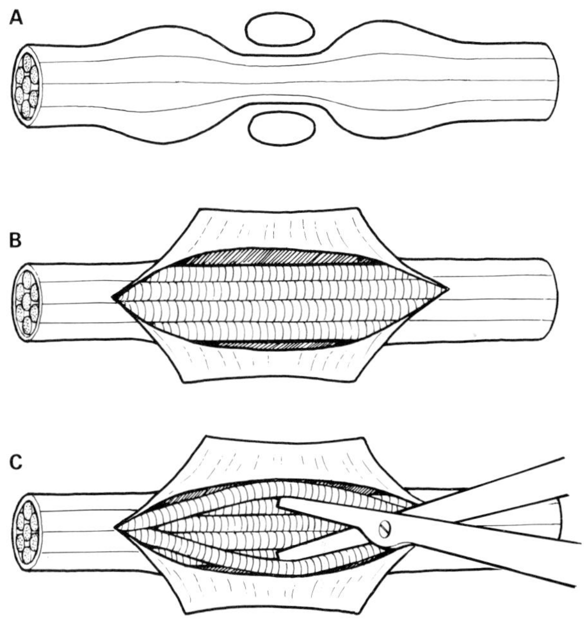

Fig. 16.2 A localised narrowing is: **A.** most likely to be due to compression, calling for **B.** epineurectomy, **C.** under certain circumstances, fascicular dissection and neurolysis.

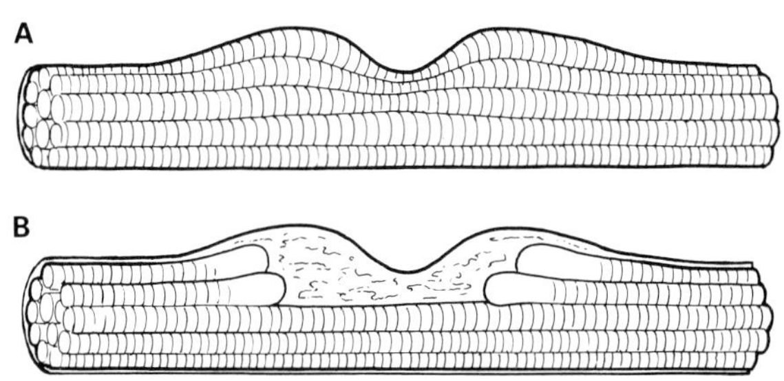

Fig. 16.3 A localised indentation may be a sign of: **A.** simple compression (prolonged neurapraxia), **B.** partial or, rarely, total, rupture.

the repair of interrupted fasciculi requires grafts in most cases. However, in emergency cases, the damage is obvious and very easily repaired by direct suturing without danger to the intact parts. Primary repair is therefore clearly favoured, especially since, at that time, topographical alignment is easy.

The results of neurolysis in trauma are still unpredictable in some cases, since often we do not know the condition of the axons under an apparently intact perineurium; nor are we certain of the post-surgical evolution of the perineural scar, which may result in compression, not to mention the effect of surgical exploration upon the vascularity.

However, overall, if the surgical technique is applied cautiously and with the help of the microscope, it is possible to avoid deterioration from the presurgical condition, and obtain, in the great majority of cases, a full functional recovery, although, in some cases, only a more limited recovery. Failures still occur in cases of severe initial injury at multiple levels or very proximally, such as traction injuries of the brachial plexus.

CONCLUSION

The microsurgical techniques applied to peripheral nerve lesions have provided neurolysis with new precision and flexibility, making it possible to treat endoneural compression, and increasing its efficiency in the treatment of both tunnel syndromes and post-traumatic compression.

In the latter group, a more reliable diagnosis of the lesion is the key to specifying more precisely the indications for neurolysis or repair by suture or grafts.

C. R. Rayner

17 Microsurgery in the treatment of congenital hand deformities

INTRODUCTION

The surgical correction of congenital hand abnormalities differs from post-traumatic reconstruction in one fundamental way. Post-traumatic reconstruction can attempt either to restore to the patient the part that has been lost, or to re-establish familiar patterns of function that the patient has developed. The two may not be quite the same; for example, a big toe transfer may reconstruct a thumb-like digit whereas an opposition post can restore pinch grip even though it does not look particularly like a natural thumb. In the congenitally deformed hand with absence of parts, there is no pre-existing pattern of function and it is unlikely that a digit which is added to the anatomy of the hand can induce anatomical cortical representation in the brain. (It is, perhaps, this consideration that has led some workers to recommend corrective hand surgery at as early a stage in infancy as is technically feasible). It follows, therefore, that the treatment should be designed to maximise the existing function in the hand, and to set up a mechanism that allows the patient to adapt what nature has provided.

There are two conceptual errors that surgeons must be aware of. Firstly, one should not think that surgical transfer introduces new function into the hand. For example, a big toe transfer will not bring with it the power of flexion; that power has to be obtained from existing power in the upper limb. Secondly, the surgeon must put aside the normally valid notion that appearance and function are most perfected when they are united in an anatomically normal hand. This is the Holy Grail of hand reconstruction and is perhaps validly fought for in the post-injured hand. When dealing with congenital deformities however, this concept becomes an inhibition on the surgeon's psychology and may interfere with planning the design of surgery. Major congenital abnormalities of the hand are so infinitely variable, especially as they increase in severity, that any one patient will present some unique problems. The surgeon must be sufficiently free intellectually to plan operative procedures that are specifically appropriate to the particular patient. If one regards microsurgical reconstruction in congenital conditions simply as an extension of replant surgical technique or post-traumatic toe transfer, then one runs the risk of creating a surgical illusion; something that resembles a hand without proper function, as useful as a teapot that won't pour tea. Add to that the lost opportunity and the donor site morbidity, and the patient may have had a serious disservice done to him. For example, the resting position of the normal thumb may be a totally inappropriate position for a toe-transfer to a congenitally abnormal hand (vide infra).

General considerations

The practice of microsurgery makes one more critically aware of the relationship between vessel size, the tissue perfusion of vascularised grafts and the blood supply required for grafts to stabilise and heal (and, in the case of bone, to consolidate). The vascularised bone grafts contained in the radial forearm flap consolidate well when used to reconstruct the mandible. The block of bone has only a tenuous capillary circulation to the periosteum, so that it must be supposed that this circulation becomes enhanced by inflammatory changes or the demands of its new environment. It is sometimes possible to move small segments of bone within the hand based on pre-capillary-sized vessels contained within soft tissue pedicles that transgress normal anatomical boundaries. Such small vessels can just be visualised with the naked eye, but much more precisely so with magnification. It is presumed that vasodilatation occurs to enhance the flow to the segment to facilitate healing.

Microsurgical techniques are thus used in three ways in the treatment of congenital hand anomalies: one, to repair or join nerves and blood vessels; two, as a means of improving the quality of fine dissection, as in separating nerves or vessels from pathological surroundings; three, as a tool to critically evaluate the pre-capillary perfusion of tissues.

Technique is the servant of design. In some ways, it is possible to become obsessed with the fact that microsurgical techniques can make it possible to create digit-like structures. It must be remembered, however, that the microsurgical procedure is only part of an overall plan. In children, this plan must take into account the effect of growth and the significant softening of scar that may occur later in life. This softening may make an initially stable digit into an unstable one after some years. The writer has one overriding guiding principle when planning operations for congenital deformities: *to magnify existing function in the hand.* The corollary of this is that nothing should be done to encumber the hand or to reduce potential function by sacrificing existing structures in the hope of enhancing the function of structures added to the hand. The early result may flatter the surgeon's efforts, but the result may deteriorate later.

Evaluation of the deformity

If one accepts the premise that microsurgery enhances the range of possibilities for treating congenital hand deformities by providing a quicker means of achieving the objectives of traditional techniques as well as creating new ones, then what information is sought pre-operatively that might influence the choice of procedure?

The family background must be supportive and able to accept a change in appearance of the hand. A video is made of the child at play in a non-staged environment. Based on analysis of this, the surgeon may decide to reinforce or create one or two main features of hand function: key pinch, tripod grip, for example. The patient and family must never be allowed to think that a sophisticated or wide range of functions is to be gained. From observation of what the child can do, the surgeon imagines what structures added to the hand (or modified from within it) can allow this existing movement to be applied more usefully by the patient. If there is really nothing of potential value in the hand, then no digital transfer from the foot would be of any value. The emphasis placed on enhancing existing function in the hand puts the value of radiological investigation into perspective. Ectopic bones may be capable of realignment, and 'good' epiphyses can be redeployed. Standard X-rays are sufficient. I no longer undertake routine arteriography. Chesney and Schenk have shown experimentally that the contrast medium may predispose to small vessel occlusion many weeks later (Chesney 1985). Furthermore, there are many vascular anomalies that are difficult to interpret on X-ray. Instead, at operation, the main forearm vessels are temporarily clipped off to check the circulation to the hand. An appropriate artery can then be chosen for microvascular anastomosis. Whatever the cause of congenital abnormalities, the 'final common pathway' in their development may be failure of vascular development (Rayner 1986a). It is, therefore, essential to try the effect of occluding the arteries at operation, and this makes the value of arteriography insignificant.

CASE HISTORIES

In this section, the case histories have been selected to illustrate the place of microsurgical procedures as part of the overall treatment plan for the particular patient.

Case 1 (Fig. 17.1)

This girl presented for treatment at the age of 7

years. She was observed to have a positive range of movement towards the ulnar border of the hand from the thumb resting position. The excursion of the thumb tip was approximately 1.5 cm. The single digit was used as a proprioceptor and for pushing. The wrist was normally placed with approximately 15° of movement in both dorsal and palmar directions, i.e. a 30° range. A digital fixed post was constructed from a segment of big toe. This consisted of a free neurovascular island flap wrapped around a free bone graft (non-vascularised) (Fig. 17.1). The child never developed any cleft grip function, and appeared to lose some movement from the thumb. She did, however, develop useful sensation in the new digit and used it as a 'knitting needle' by wrapping soft objects around it. Subsequently, the post was moved towards the ulnar border of the hand, a silastic joint inserted to the base and the cleft between the two digits was deepened. The thumb flexor was reinforced by wrist extensor transfer. Eighteen months later, no new function had been evolved. Although the cleft was wider, the child did not find it useful, as no significant grip pressure could be exerted on objects placed in it. The width of the gap, the poor range of thumb movement and the poor power all combined to result in a poor functional result. The addition of one finger-like structure to the hand was not considered by anybody to have significantly improved the appearance of the hand. The best result for this child would now be the use of a powered hand with a cosmetic glove. The residual thumb movement could be a motor for this.

Some of the lessons from this case are as follows. Do nothing that reduces existing movement. Cosmetic improvement requires the hand to be nearly anatomically perfect; this may be far in excess of the requirements for simple functional improvement. The emotional background of this child was also unfavourable. Partial absorption of the free bone graft occurred. In all subsequent cases, a soft tissue connection between the blood supply and the bone fragments has been preserved.

Case 2

The child in Figure 17.2A illustrates some of the features that it is desirable to establish in a hand when trying to create a functioning cleft. This child is able to obtain pulp-to-pulp pinch, and the cleft itself is square in shape. Pulp pinch would tend to force objects into the cleft. This child did not require surgical correction. The effect of having a V-shaped cleft with lateral pinch grip is shown in Figure 17.2B. The forces tend to drive objects out of the cleft.

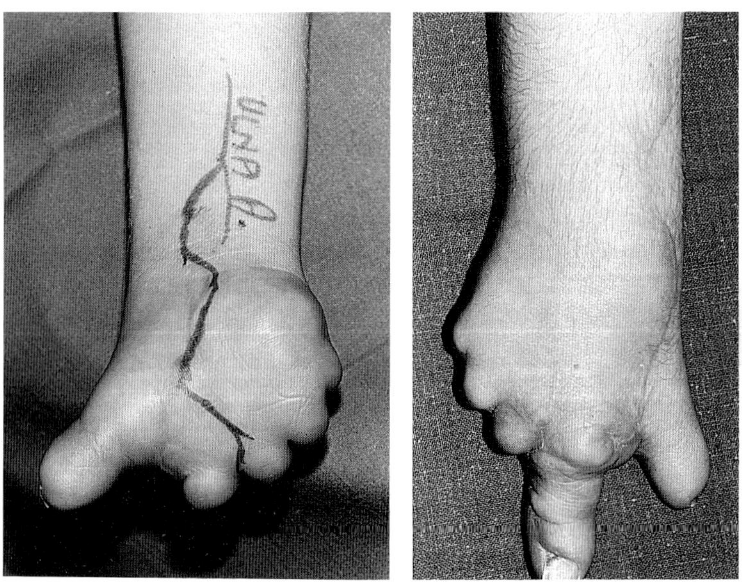

Fig. 17.1 Case 1. A child with absent fingers before and after digital reconstruction with an island flap wrapped around a bone graft.

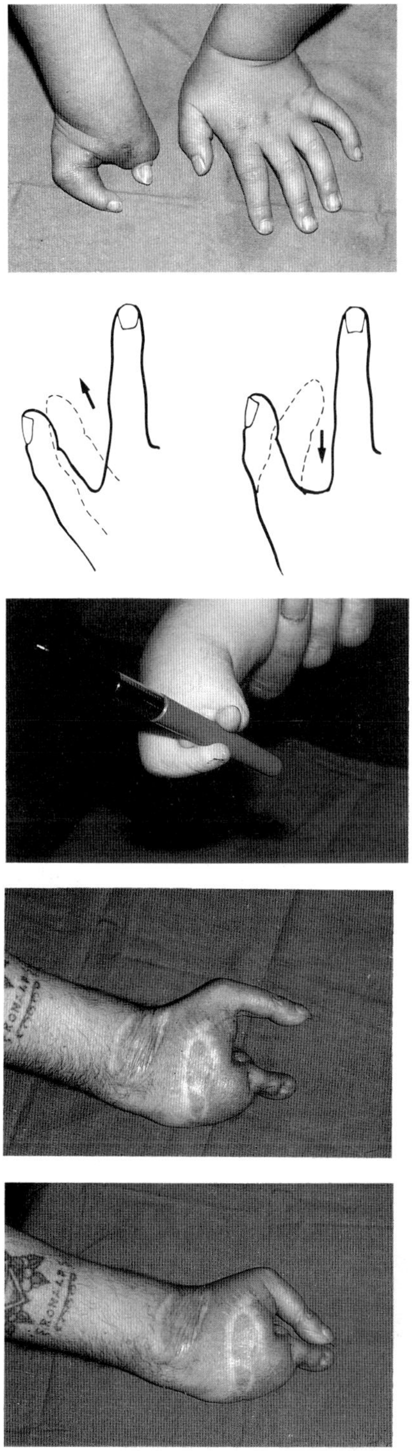
A
B
C
D
E

Fig. 17.2 A. Child with open cleft. **B.** A V-shaped cleft forces objects out of the grasp; a square cleft forces objects into it. **C.** Cleft holding a pen. **D., E.** Post-traumatic reconstruction of the hand in a patient who lost 4 digits.

Case 3

Figure 17.3 shows a child who was able to obtain pulp-to-pulp pinch between the vestigial thumb and transversely lying little finger. The size of the gap between the two was small. At 3 years of age, the cleft was enlarged. The result at 6 weeks post-operatively can be seen in Figure 17.3. Despite the apparent severity of the deformity in early infancy, the child appeared to favour the affected hand for grasping. The simple deepening of the cleft and its square shape magnified the hand's function.

Case 4 (Fig. 17.4)

This patient sustained a traumatic amputation of her fingers in early infancy, and presented at the age of 16 years complaining of lack of stability of grip between thumb and index finger remnant. A lateral segment of great toe pulp and distal phalanx was transferred to the middle finger positions, and excellent stable grasp was obtained. This segment was tailored in size to match the length of residual index finger. The great toe defect was closed by syndactylising the great toe to the second toe to create a cosmetically acceptable foot (Fig 17.5).

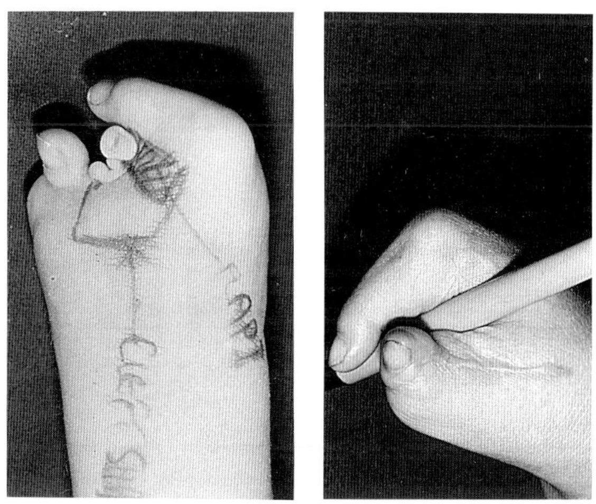

Fig. 17.3 Case 3. A child with pulp-to-pulp pinch enhanced by cleft deepening.

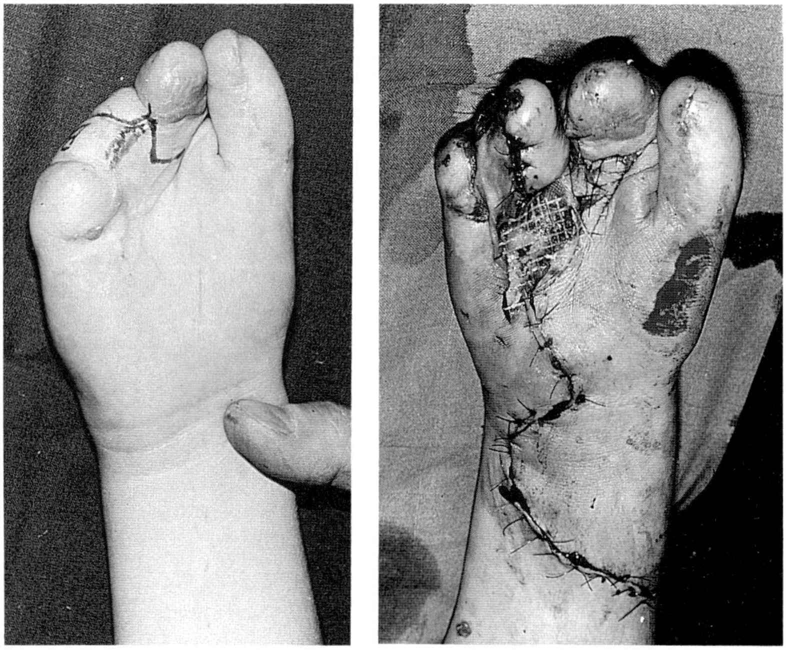

Fig. 17.4 Case 4. A small segment of great toe used to elongate the middle finger.

Although not a congenital case, this patient illustrates certain guiding principles. Firstly, the size of the reconstructed part should be in proportion to the existing parts on the hand. Secondly, three-point fixation gives more stable grasp in two positions: one, pulp-to-pulp pinch; and two, when grasping spherical objects such as a small canister. Thirdly, the donor site defect can be improved by fusing the great and second toes together.

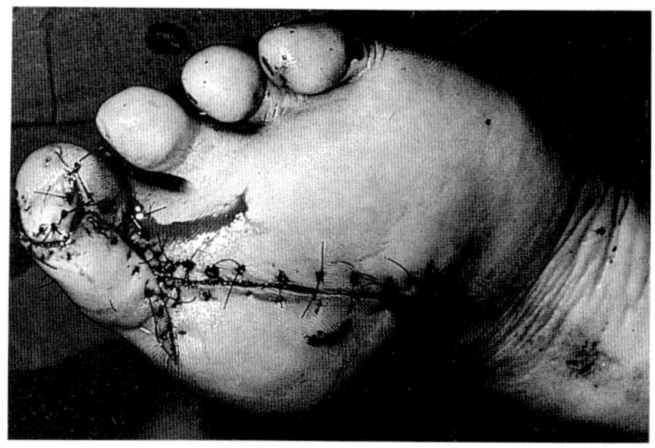

Fig. 17.5 Case 4. Reconstruction of the great toe by syndactylising it to the second toe.

Case 5

A 3-year-old girl with a normal right hand and a four-fingered left hand. Pollicisation was refused, and in any case the index finger was abnormal and showed no sign of rotating into an opposed position. A big toe transfer was undertaken. As a preliminary procedure, the bulk of the big toe was reduced by excision of a longitudinal central segment. Two years later, the new thumb is still larger than the normal. The child has excellent function for dressing, play, etc., but has some regrets about the limitation of choice of fashionable footwear. The reason for the parents' insistence on free toe transfer was cultural. It is said that free toe transfer to a four-fingered unilateral hand deformity is not indicated. Seven years after the transfer, the parents report that the patient has not experienced any adverse comments on the appearance of the hand. Social and cultural considerations must be allowed to influence the design of hand reconstructions. The pre-transfer reduction of toe bulk was not considered by the surgeon to have achieved its aim in debulking the great toe. At present, one only moves precisely the amount of toe required.

Case 6

Just as pollicisation should be considered before toe transfer, so should 'digitisation'. Figure 17.6 shows a child with a good potential grasp between thumb and little finger. Using the same dissection technique as for pollicisation, the 'index' remnant was moved ulnarwards and 'stacked' on top of the adjacent vestigial finger. This had the effect of deepening the thumb web and providing a third digit of comparable length to the others (Fig. 17.7).
Stable three-point fixation was achieved.

Case 7

A 10-year-old boy had a single digit on the radial aspect of his hand. This had a resting position at 90° to the axis of the forearm (Fig. 17.8). Active extension over a short (15°) range was present and powerful. The digit was repositioned on the ulnar border of the hand (reverse pollicisation) to take advantage of its line of movement, and an opposition post fashioned for it from a segment of great toe (Fig. 17.9). A useful cleft grip developed. It is justifiable to reposition part of the hand provided a functional loss does not occur.

Case 8

Transverse aplasia of the hand (Fig. 17.10). On examination, the hypothenar eminence was seen to be well developed and mobile. Figure 17.10 shows the appearance of the hand after elongation with the Matev distraction technique. Figure 17.11 shows the appearance of the hand after great toe transfer to construct a thumb. The central area of the hand has been excised to create a cleft. The hypothenar eminence is the power for cleft grip. It achieves this by longitudinal rotation on the axis of the fifth metacarpal. The hand functions like a mini-Krukenberg reconstruction, and the possibility of using a custom-made powered hand exists. Elongation of a moving part and the creation of a cleft have created some useful function in an otherwise non-manipulative hand.

Case 9

Almost identical to Case 8 except that two extra digits were fashioned from toe segments to give a three-digit hand. Disrupted home circumstances with lack of support from the family were associated with failure to use or exhibit the hand. This is an example of technical success associated with complete failure to achieve the objectives of surgery. It is impossible to overstate the importance of environmental factors on the results. Surgery at the time of family breakdown is likely to be unsuccessful.

Case 10 (Fig. 17.12)

Bilateral mitten hands with absent thumbs. The

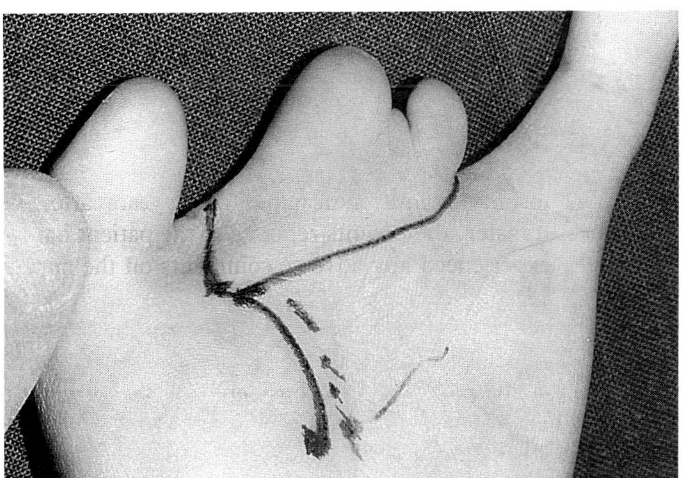

Fig. 17.6 Case 6. Vestigial digits.

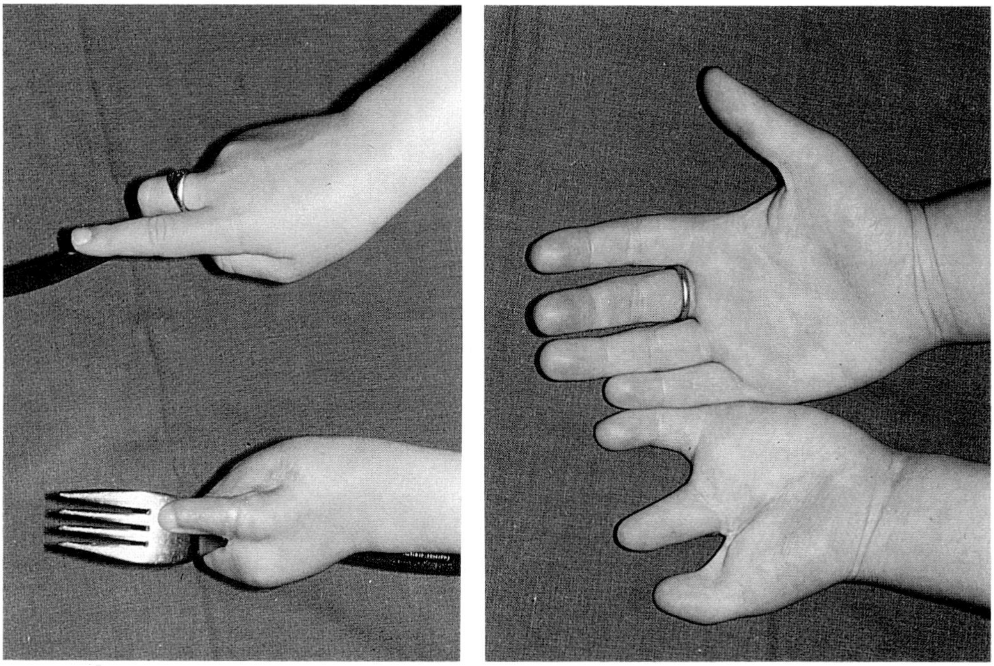

Fig. 17.7 Case 6. Two vestigial digits 'stacked' to give one longer digit and a deeper thumb cleft.

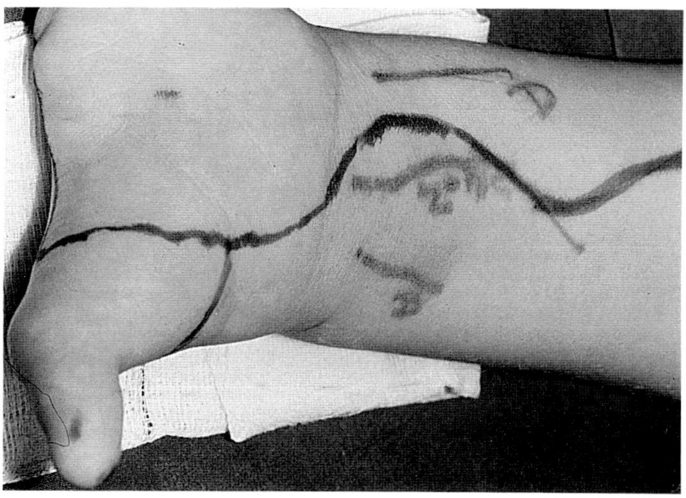

Fig. 17.8 Case 7. Preoperative view.

left thumb was reconstructed by fusion of the two abnormal toes (Fig. 17.13). The right thumb was constructed from the hypoplastic great toe (Fig. 17.14). At the first operation (the right thumb), the syndactyly was not separated and the motor tendons were connected to the 'anatomical' muscles in the forearm (FPL and EPL). No useful movement developed. At the time of left thumb reconstruction, the tendons were inserted into the functioning finger motors and the right thumb tendons revised accordingly. Figure 17.14 shows the result after the separation of the right hand

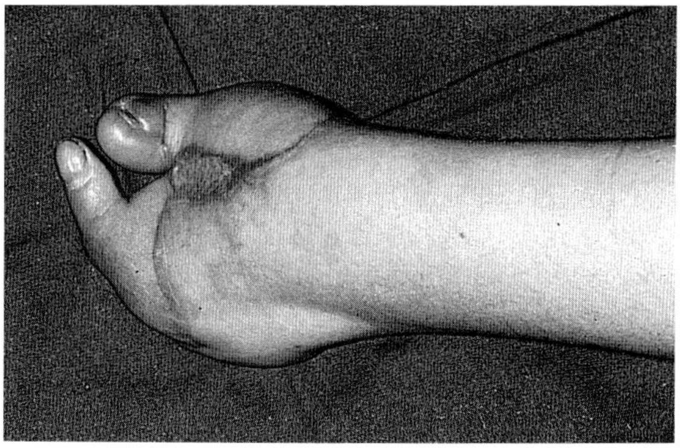

Fig. 17.9 Case 7. The single digit has been moved by 'reverse pollicisation' to the opposite border of the hand, and an opposition post fashioned from a great toe segment.

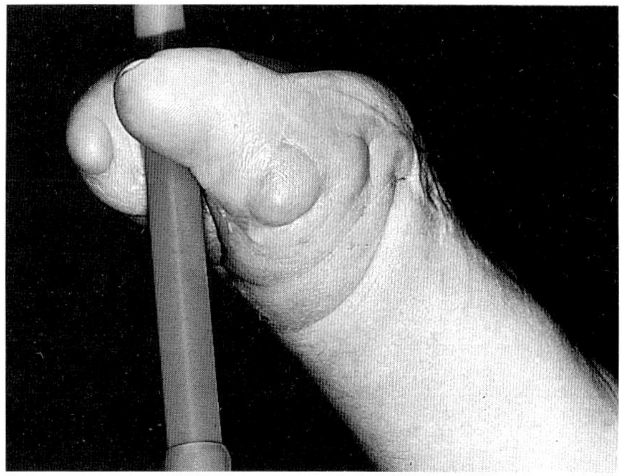

Fig. 17.11 Case 8. After great toe transfer.

syndactyly. At this time, the flexor tendons were tightened to leave the thumb and index fingers resting in pulp-to-pulp apposition.

Case 11 (Fig. 17.15)

A unilateral mitten hand. A one-stage great toe transfer and separation of syndactyly was undertaken. The motors of the new thumb were primarily joined to the existing finger motors. Figure 17.15 shows the result at one year. This case illustrates the principle of sharing the existing function rather than trying to join the graft to anatomical 'thumb' motors in the forearm.

Case 12

Similar to Cases 9 and 10. A segment of great toe, including distal and part of the proximal phalanges but sparing the first metacarpophalangeal joint,

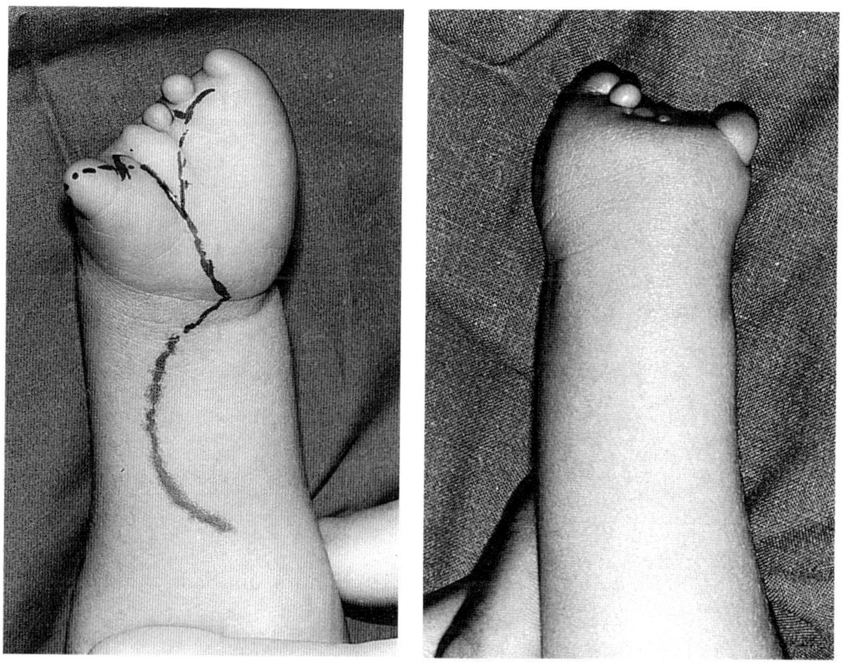

A B

Fig. 17.10 Case 8. Transverse aplasia of the hand, (**A**) before and (**B**) after elongation of the ulnar border.

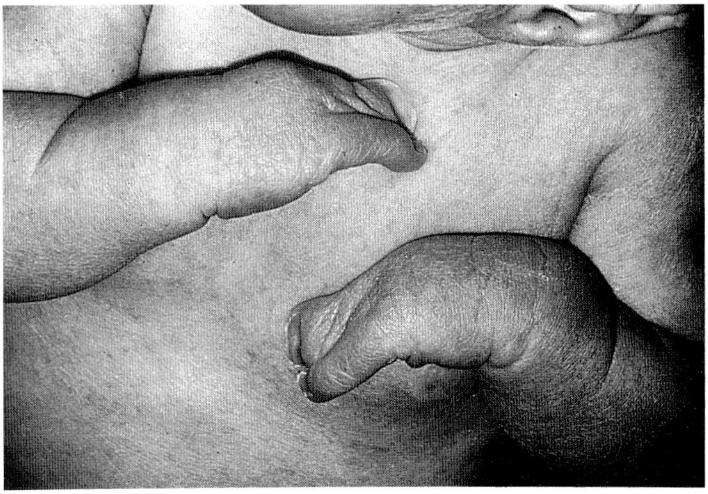

Fig. 17.12 Case 10. A child with absent thumbs, syndactyly and deformed right leg and foot.

was transferred to create a thumb. The fingers were separated at the single-stage operation. The great and second toes were syndactylised.

DISCUSSION

General

Initially, the clinical use of microsurgical techniques seemed to offer a means of converting toes into fingers or thumbs. It seemed that the anatomical integrity of the grafted digit should be capable of conversion to finger/thumb-like action by connecting its parts to the appropriate anatomical structures in the hand or forearm. Thus, in cases of congenital absence of the thumb, it may be possible to identify the flexor pollicis longus muscle belly in the forearm, and connect the toe's flexor to it. However, if that muscle has developed between two fixed points and never enjoyed any excursion, then it may never function as an effective contractile unit. Similarly, in the early days

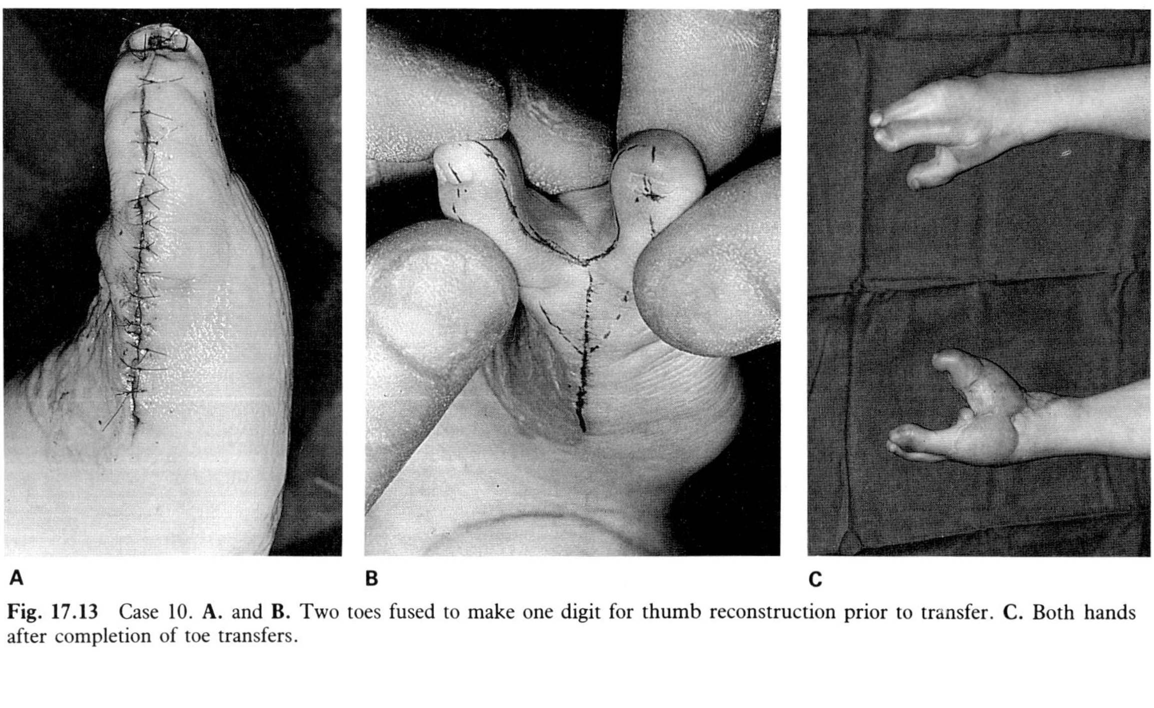

A B C

Fig. 17.13 Case 10. **A.** and **B.** Two toes fused to make one digit for thumb reconstruction prior to transfer. **C.** Both hands after completion of toe transfers.

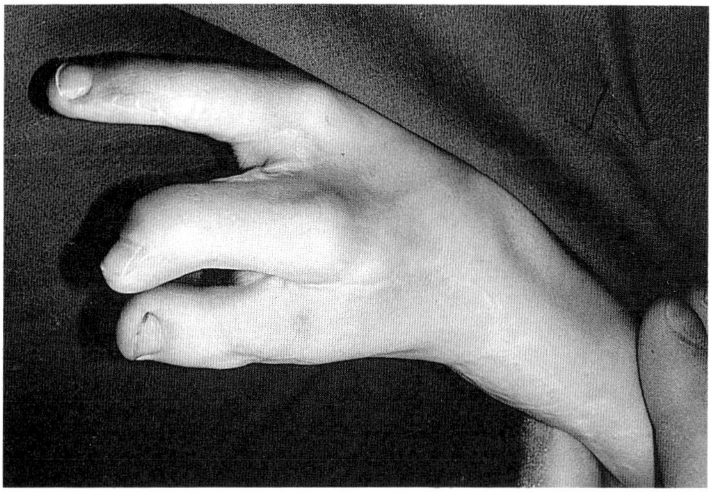

Fig. 17.14 Case 10. The final view of the right hand after separation of syndactyly. Note the resting pulp apposition.

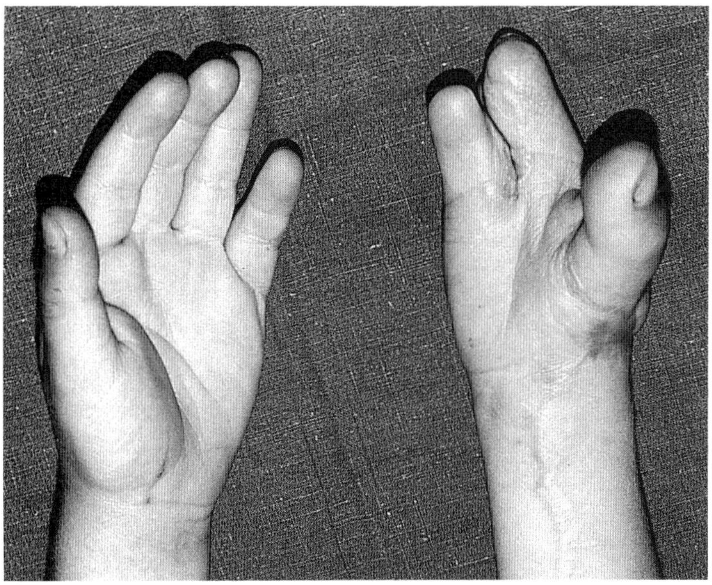

Fig. 17.15 Case 11. One year after single-stage correction with whole great toe transfer.

of microsurgery, the creation of a thumb would seem to require the presence of two thumb joints — namely, an interphalangeal joint and a metacarpophalangeal joint. However, whilst simple flexion and extension may be achieved at one joint, the sequential or coordinated movements at two joints are infinitely more complex and beyond the control of available motors. Furthermore, differential functional stabilisation at either one of two joints during a complex range of movements is also a requirement, and this too is beyond the range of available functioning motors in an abnormal hand. The idea of maintaining the anatomy of the transferred toe to allow its conversion to a functioning hand digit would also preclude any reduction in its size. The reconstructed digit could therefore be of correct shape but disproportionately large. When altering the appearance of a congenitally abnormal hand one must try very hard not to create any grotesque new feature. For all these reasons, the simple transfer of a toe to a congenitally abnormal hand can be seen to be too simplistic. Also, the technical ability to accomplish this feat may cause one to overlook the possible use of some microsurgical techniques to transfer parts from within the hand or the forearm itself.

The present role of microsurgery in the treatment of congenital hand deformities represents an evolution from the original idea of whole great toe transfer, through whole second or whole second and third toe transfers, to a situation where transfers are tailored more precisely to the requirements of a particular part of the hand. Second toe transfer certainly gets round the size problem of a great toe transfer, but has a tendency to flexion deformity with the multiple joints involved; they can look remarkably like hammer toes on the hand. Combined second and third toe transfers are severely mutilating to the foot and have the same flexion problems when in place on the hand. Nevertheless, the size of the second toe pulp and the flexion deformity can lead to a form of gratifying pulp-to-pulp precision grip in post-traumatic hand reconstructions.

The author's present approach to microsurgical, reconstruction

Although, in practice, children do not appear to suffer significant functional problems in the foot after removal of the whole great toe, including the metatarsophalangeal joint, some doubts must remain about the long-term outcome. Because of these doubts, and associated with the realisation that the whole toe is usually surplus to requirements, the practice of whole great toe transfer has now been abandoned. Resection of the whole toe included the head of the metatarsal. Outside of athletic pursuits, this weight-bearing area of the foot is probably more important than the toe itself. The concept of segmental toe transfers to include only one joint means that it is possible to spare this part of the metatarsus. Furthermore, if only a longitudinal segment of the great toe is taken, then the remnant can be effectively splinted by syndactylising it to the second toe. Thus, the great toe becomes a 'bank' to draw on for the smaller parts required for hand reconstruction. In longitudinal resections of the great toe, the flexor and extensor tendons can also be split longitudinally to maintain some tone across the residual interphalangeal joint. Cosmetically, the reconstructed big toe is unremarkable, and a four-toed foot scarcely registers as abnormal to the uninitiated observer.

The fate of the transferred hemi-joint requires some consideration. As only half of the interphalangeal joint is included in the transfer, it follows that there will be a tendency for instability on one side of the new joint in the hand. To some extent, the degree of angulation that develops depends on the way that the new digit is stressed and functions. If lateral pinch grip is the aim, then the intact collateral ligament should face the cleft if possible. Scarring is inevitable in the section lines of the bone and may reduce the angulation. The same peri-articular scarring will limit the 'normal' range of movement of the joint. No attempt has been made as yet to construct a new collateral ligament at the site of bone transection. As already indicated, the range of movement that can be expected to develop in the new digit is limited by the availability of suitable motors — if function is to be shared with the pre-existing digits, then the excursion of the tendons in the new digit must necessarily be limited. In practice, wherever possible, the new digit is placed in resting contact with one of the original digits, and any movement is therefore restricted but is converted into power. Relatively little movement is therefore required of the new joint.

Associated with the question of joint function is the development of bone growth. Firstly, it must be said that no bone resorption occurs as it does with free bone grafts. Secondly, whole vascularised joints do undoubtedly grow. Thirdly, in the longest follow-up in this personal series (8 years), vascularised segmental grafts appear to keep pace with the original donor toe, which does not appear significantly smaller than its untouched opposite number. On X-ray, the bone shape may be bizarre, however. Fourthly, if the graft is functioning well, then the pre-existing structures adapt to it and there is thus, theoretically, some compensation for disproportionate growth. It is, in fact, the writer's belief that a longitudinally resected epiphysis will continue to grow provided its blood supply is intact. If present practice is to take precisely the amount of toe required to match the size of the existing hand structures, then it must not be forgotten that large amounts of additional skin may be required on the hand to supplement the positioning of the new digit, for example, a web space may need to be created, or a cleft lined. A dorsal skin flap from the foot can be combined with a segmental toe transfer. The donor site on the dorsum may have delayed healing, but its long-term function has not been impaired and the dorsal scarring is accepted.

In the same way as the choice of tendon-to-muscle repair of graft to hand has changed from the original concept of re-establishing 'normal' anatomy to the idea of uniting graft tendon to what actually functions in the hand, so too has the concept of nerve repair. In the writer's earliest cases, the graft digital nerve was united to the median nerve at the wrist. However, this nerve may peter out in the proximal palm and may never have had any end-organ connections. In an already abnormal hand, the surgeon should avoid damage to those cutaneous areas of the hand that are already well innervated. In two cases, sensation did not develop satisfactorily, and the digital nerve was rejoined to a forearm sensory nerve. As a baby develops in utero, it is subjected to cutaneous stimulation, and this probably induces cortical representation. At the time of operation in this series (3 years of age or more), one would have to postulate that the joining of the graft digital nerve to the blind-ending forearm recipient nerve could result in the induction of cortical representation for the new digit. Possibly, such a mechanism exists in neonates or babies up to a few months old, but it would appear to be unlikely after the age chosen for operation by this writer (vide infra timing of operation). Thus, present practice is to select a forearm cutaneous nerve for the nerve repair. The well-known adaptive capabilities of young children can quickly convert this familiar forearm sensation into 'hand' sensation. Case 10, the child with bilateral thumb reconstructions, could, after 2 years, accurately identify her 'thumbs' without directly looking at them, as well as identify passive positioning of them by an observer. Case 11 has an identical but unilateral deformity. He recognises his reconstructed digit as 'thumb' but, interestingly, said it was 'different' from his normal thumb. He too had good proprioception, and did not suffer from any functional confusion when using both hands simultaneously. The elective toe transfers are human models for 'ideal' nerve repair. Initially, fascicular repair was practised, but this has now been abandoned for simple end-to-end tension-free apposition by one or two epineural (10–0) sutures. Two-point discrimination is not a meaningful test after toe transfer in congenital hand anomalies. Such a subjective test produces a variable response in children. In practice, the lack of secondary injury, the ability to identify with the graft and the practice of normal childhood activities give the most useful assessment of the results.

Rayner (1986), in attempting to evaluate the long-term results of toe transfers (in excess of 3 years), has concluded that the best areas of improvement are, in order of benefit: 1) additional sensation to the hand; 2) improved cosmesis; 3) tripod grip; 4) a means of balancing objects in the hand; 5) pinch grip. Initially, one was impressed with the conversion in style of grip in these patients. However, in all children, as growth and softening of the digits occurred, then the stability of the new digit diminished. This is due to the resolution of oedema, scarring and stiffness, and the effect of tissue remodelling. Even when the digits have been placed in pulp-to-pulp apposition, some softening occurs and the children tend to perform rather delicate balancing manoeuvres and to return to the preoperative hand usage patterns. Obviously, significant functional gains do result. The main surprise in the long-term follow-up is the importance that becomes attached to improved appearance and sensation — a part that 'belongs' to the patient. The writer's present preference when trying to plan the range of movement in a toe transfer is therefore to consider ways of obtaining a fixed position for the graft with a limited range of movement at a single joint. To see a patient performing a delicate balancing act with a weak moving reconstructed digit confirms the subtlety of sensation in the new digit, and confirms that the use of a forearm sensory nerve is a reasonable choice.

If 'cosmesis' is suggested as the second most important area of benefit, then it must also be said that it is the first area for error. The separation of syndactyly and the provision of a thumb undoubtedly enhance the hand's appearance in every case. However, relative gigantism of one part of the hand may not produce a social problem until school age. It may not then be a simple matter to reduce the bulk of the part. Segmental toe transfer gets round this problem. If, however, the deformity is more complex, then the patient may simply be exchanging one deformity for another. It is a common experience among hand surgeons that, in later childhood and early teenage life, patients become very reluctant to allow any change in the hand's appearance. If, therefore, a radical change in hand appearance is the only way in which extra functional advantage can be gained, it must be achieved before the patient's body image is firmly fixed. At that time, the decision rests with the parents and their reaction may be purely subjective. It requires considerable imagination and intelligence on the part of a lay person, let alone an emotionally involved family member, to visualise the effect of a complex change. If the family background is weak, then the altered appearance of the hand may be met with the same reaction as the original lesion excited at birth. The child may then be forced to conceal the hand or, at best, may not be given positive encouragement to develop its use. The surgeon who is excited by the technical possibilities must guard against this situation and, despite all pressures, should advise against surgery if such a background is identified.

The timing of microsurgical correction of hand anomalies is not really related to technical considerations. There is little difference and difficulty between operating on a baby of 3 months or 3 years of age. The crucial question is, therefore, whether or not there is a developmental gain from operating as soon after birth as is practicable. If so, does this gain outweigh the other advantages, including operative safety, of delaying surgery until later in childhood? The writer's present policy is to wait until about the age of 3 years. By this time, significant features relating to the child's general development will be apparent. At this age, a normally intelligent child may be asking why he cannot do certain things or has not got a thumb. Children of this age positively ask for a part to be given to them. This implies a high level of motivation and can also be used as a basis to obtain the child's postoperative cooperation with positioning, splinting, etc. The patterns of hand function are established and can be used as the basis of the functional aspects of the reconstructed design. This may appear to 'beg the question' as to whether earlier surgery at, say, the age of 6 months would not have resulted in different hand patterns emerging. If it is believed that forearm muscles with failed development and nerves without peripheral function can be induced to function by being stimulated by new connections shortly after birth, then earlier operation could be justified. This approach, however, adds an experimental dimension (neurological induction) to the surgery, which is hard to justify unless the results are superior to later surgery. At such an early age, social development, intelligence and motivation cannot enter into the equation. If the hoped for functional development does not occur, the possibility for a modification by further surgery still exists, but at the price of a further (unnecessary) operation. For all these reasons, 3 years of age is the author's choice, and the long-term results of other workers of operating at an earlier age are awaited with interest.

Some guidelines for the design of microsurgical procedures in congenital hand surgery

1. Magnify existing function
2. Make clefts square
3. Place digits in pulp-to-pulp apposition (not in the middle of the range of motion of the transferred digit)
4. Connect graft motor tendons to existing functional muscles
5. Connect nerves to recipient nerves responsible for existing tactile awareness
6. Rearrange existing structures and design free vascularised grafts to serve these.

SUMMARY

In the reconstruction of congenital hand anomalies, a surgeon should use microsurgical techniques to supplement the possibilities that already exist within the hand.

REFERENCES

Chesney B 1985 Personal communication

Matev I B 1969 Reconstruction of the thumb through gradual lengthening of the first metacarpal with the soft tissues. Ortopedia I Traumatologia (Sophia) 6: 11–14

Rayner C R 1986a Congenital abnormalities of the hand. Surgery 100: 696–698

Rayner C R 1986b The long term results of toe to hand transfer (in preparation)

E. F. Shaw Wilgis

18 Microsurgery in vascular disease

The advancement of microsurgical procedures in the late 1960s and 1970s led to improvements in the treatment of vascular and ischaemic conditions within the hand. In addition to the repair of traumatic injuries, the direct reconstruction of occlusive disorders of the arterial system in the hand and wrist became commonplace. The indirect approach to ischaemic conditions of the hand with pharmacological and surgical manipulation of the sympathetic nervous system has improved the quality of life for many patients with vasospastic disorders. This chapter will elucidate the diagnostic manoeuvres for localisation of these lesions, and the protocols for treatment of these conditions.

DIAGNOSIS

Physical examination of the vascular system includes careful examination of pulses at various levels in the extremity. Although most of these pulses can be easily palpated, a non-invasive listening device such as the Doppler ultrasonic flow detector can be a useful tool. The usual arterial pressure must be reduced by 10% before an observer can note an appreciable difference in the strength of the radial pulse. It is important to record systolic pressures in the upper arm and forearm, and to compare them with systolic pressures recorded in the contralateral extremity. In our experience, the most constant measurement of circulation is the digital brachial index, which gives the pressure of the digit expressed as a fraction of the brachial pressure. If the digital brachial index in the affected digit studied is below 0.85, this is considered an abnormal ratio and will lead the examining physician to further testing and/or treatment. The digital brachial index is obtained by pulse volume recording. This method produces a quantitative reproducible segmental plethysmographic recording of the volume changes within a given segment of an extremity or digit. The system consists of an occlusion cuff, which is placed around the extremity proximal to the segment being tested, and a recording cuff. The recording cuff transmits the pressure changes to an electronic package which, in turn, records the data on hard copy paper for the clinician to read. This device can be effectively used on the digits. The digital perfusion pressure is measured in millimeters of mercury, and then compared to the brachial pressure to produce the digital brachial index.

After the baseline study has been obtained, the vascular system can be manipulated through various exercises, both positional and stressful. Quantitative recording can be made after cold stress and recovery from cold stress. This plethysmographic testing technique has also been found useful during surgery and following arterial repair. The cuffs can be sterilised for intraoperative use. The testing can also be done in the evaluation of vasospastic disorders which will be described later in this chapter.

Direct visualisation of the arterial tree can be obtained in a number of ways. Radionuclide imaging has been found useful in the evaluation of occlusive and vasospastic disorders. Koman et al (1982) have reported over 90% correlation between the test results provided by dynamic radionuclide imaging and those provided by contrast angiography. This author has found radionuclide imaging most useful as a screening test when the symptomatology is obscure, and for following arterial reconstruction. The details of this technique have been described by Wilgis et al (1974) and Maurer et al (1983).

The contrast angiogram has long been used as the method for evaluating the vascular status of an extremity. The contrast angiogram can either be administered as a dose of contrast material directly into the arterial tree, or a venous injection can be given and then traced through the arterial tree with computer enhanced and assisted visualisation. The digital subtraction angiogram allows diagnostic evaluation of patients with suspected vascular disease to be performed in an outpatient setting with minimal risk. This new imaging modality links the image processing capabilities of a computer with the high quality image intensifier fluoroscopy unit. Thanks to this new technology, digital radiography can utilise a much smaller concentration of iodinated contrast agents, making it possible to visualise arterial anatomy from bolus intravenous injection. This technique eliminates many of the risks associated with contrast angiography, such as arterial puncture and catheterisation.

DIRECT MICROSURGICAL APPROACH FOR OCCLUSIVE DISEASE

Thrombosis of the vascular tree at the wrist level and in the palm and digits has been successfully treated by microsurgical reconstruction.

Thrombosis of the ulnar artery at the wrist secondary to blunt trauma was first described by VonRosen (1933). Further studies have confirmed a relatively high incidence of this problem among labourers. Multiple methods of treatment have been used, including conservative management, use of vasodilators, local and regional sympathectomy, ligation and excision of the thrombosed segment and arterial reconstruction. All of these methods have some merit, but none has given 100% satisfactory results. Koman and Urbaniak (1981) reviewed 28 cases of ulnar artery thrombosis of the wrist and presented a guide to treatment. Successful management of an artery such as the ulnar artery thrombosed at the wrist depends on an appropriate diagnosis. Examination should include radio-isotope scanning techniques and pulse volume recordings to determine whether the thrombosed ulnar artery is dominant. If there is any diminution of the flow to the digits normally supplied by the affected vessel, excision of the thrombosed segment and arterial reconstruction should be seriously considered. Once the preoperative pulse volume recordings are done, and operation is deemed necessary, we routinely perform intraoperative pulse volume recordings. These are done after the patient has been anaesthetised by either regional or general route. The tourniquet is then inflated and the vessel exposed. The thrombosed segment is excised. The tourniquet is then released and repeat pulse volume recordings are done. If the circulation to the digit is, in fact, improved and equal to the other digits, then no further surgery is done. If, however, the circulation of the ring and little finger or another digit is not equal to the other digits, then further reconstruction, including vein grafting, should be done. The most common measurement of circulation used is the digital brachial index, which is the pressure of the digit expressed as a fraction of the brachial pressure. If the digital brachial index in the affected digit studied is below 0.85, further reconstruction should be done, in our opinion.

Thrombosis of the smaller vessels, if recognised early, can be treated by thrombectomy and/or excision of the thrombosed segment and replacement with vein graft or direct anastomosis. However, rarely is one given the opportunity to perform this early, because diagnosis is usually delayed and the artery has undergone secondary changes with fibrosis.

It should be emphasised, however, that the patient with generalised atherosclerotic occlusive vascular disease who experiences symptoms of obliterative disease of the upper extremity has a systemic problem. Significant lower extremity or coronary occlusive disease could preclude treatment of the upper extremity disorder. The clinician must be cognisant of all the areas that may be involved, and not be led into treating just one segment of a generalised disease problem unless there is a potential loss of limb or tissue.

INDIRECT APPROACH TO VASOSPASTIC DISEASE

The upper extremity is prey to a vast array of vasospastic disorders that produce a spectrum of symptoms whose complexity evades definitive diagnosis. The symptom complex usually consists of intermittent episodes of ischaemia, often digital, in which the patient notices whiteness and bluish discoloration in the presence of cold, and redness after rewarming. Pain or numbness or both may be present to a mild degree and can be severe. The symptoms are frequently triggered by exposure to cold, and are therefore aggravated by cold weather. However, they can arise even in warm weather if the patient puts his hands in cold water, handles ice cubes or works in a refrigerated room. Moisture in a cold environment seems to potentiate the effects of the cold, and worsens the symptoms. Emotional stress and anxiety have frequently been reported to precipitate the condition. The entire symptom complex can also be initiated by connective tissue diseases, demonstrable arterial diseases, certain neurological diseases such as carpal tunnel syndrome, blood disorders, chemical intoxication and trauma. This group of symptoms, however vague, has come to be referred to as Raynaud's phenomenon. The differentiation between Raynaud's phenomenon and Raynaud's disease is confusing and conflicting. I feel that this classification and categorisation is clumsy and confusing and should be discarded. All of these conditions should be referred to as vasospastic disorders.

Blood flow through the digital vessel exists in a very dynamic state. The velocity of blood flow is dependent on several factors: the pressure, the diameter of the digital artery itself, and the presence of any constricting elements within the vessel. In dealing with these patients, it must be assumed that, with a normal pressure and a normal intravascular endothelial state, the important variable which could be addressed is the diameter of the vessel itself. Inasmuch as the diameter of the vessel is controlled by the sympathetic nerve causing relaxation of the muscle within the arterial wall, manipulation of the sympathetic nerves pharmacologically or surgically becomes a realistic alternative.

Catecholamine substances such as noradrenaline, (norephinephrine) are produced in the body of the adrenal cortex as well as the cell body of the sympathetic nerves. Circulating humoral catecholamines produced in the adrenal glands can cause constriction of the muscles within the arterial walls and, therefore, spasm. This spasm is frequently induced by fear, pain, anxiety and heavy metals. It can be influenced by biofeedback and pharmacological agents. Noradrenaline is also produced and stored in the sympathetic nerve endings, and released by the arrival of an impulse. Noradrenaline is continuously manufactured in the cell body of these axons and transported down the post-ganglionic axons to the terminals, which are located at the myoneural junctions in the vessel wall. Noradrenaline is released at the nerve level and also through the adrenal cortex, and acts on the myoneural junction following an impulse of the sympathetic nerve. It is therefore reasonable to expect that if we can interrupt the myoneural reflex or the sympathetic nerve impulse by either surgical or pharmacological means, we can effectively diminish or eliminate the release of noradrenaline at the myoneural junction in the vessel wall, thereby eliminating spasm and dilatation of the arterial muscle and therefore increasing the diameter of the artery. With a larger diameter of the artery and normal pressure, the volume of blood flow reaching the target end organ in the digit will, in fact, increase.

Conservative medical management consisting of avoidance of cold and tobacco is adequate for the majority of patients with mild to moderate symptoms. Generally, favourable results have been obtained from drug therapy in patients with severe, frequent or prolonged vasospastic attacks. The current preference for oral medication is nifedipine, 10 mg t.i.d. This drug has been more effective with fewer side-effects than guanethidine, which was formerly used. Patience and meticulous attention to the fundamental principles of conservative management, including tobacco abstinence, gentle cleansing and debridement of ulcer, leads to gratifying results in most patients. Injection of reserpine in a regional fashion to achieve a regional sympathectomy has been of benefit in a number of resistant patients. Long-term results of proximal sympathectomy performed in the upper limb have been discouraging, in general, while reports of digital sympathectomy have been encouraging. Only patients who have had a thorough diagnostic evaluation and who have failed at conventional methods of treatment are considered as candidates for sympathectomy in the hand. Thus, only about 10% of patients presenting with these symptoms are candidates for surgical treatment. Proximal vessel disease is ruled out by the surgeon with non-invasive techniques or by digital subtraction angiography of the aortic arch, subclavian and brachial vessels. Aneurysm and constriction of the subclavian artery can give rise to peripheral embolisation and chronic digital ischaemia; and correction of the proximal disease is absolutely necessary prior to any local treatment in the hand. Pulse volume recordings, radio-isotope scanning and Doppler evaluation are all done. Pulse volume recordings with digital perfusion pressures measured in the resting state and then under cold stress constitutes the principle evaluation. Cold stress involves immersing the hand in water at 12°C. In a normal hand, cold stress produces significant alteration in the resting pulse volume recording, which rebounds to normal or even greater than normal at 5 minutes following cold stress. The critical measurement is the digital brachial index; a normal digital brachial pressure index is 0.9 to 1. If a tracing taken following the cold stress does not show that the perfusion pressure has returned to the normal state, this is considered an abnormal test. The next step is to block the peripheral sympathetic nerve by injecting 2 ml of 0.5% xylocaine into the distal palm. This effectively stops the conduction of the digital nerve and its sympathetic contributions to the digital vessels. The patient is then subjected again to resting, cold stress and 5-minutes-post-cold-stress pulse volume recordings. If there is a significant improvement in both the cold stress and post-cold-stress tracing, this is a positive test, and these patients are then considered candidates for sympathectomy. We would then try to duplicate surgically what has been accomplished pharmacologically to improve the circulation of the digits. However, there must be a significant improvement in the cold stress test following digital blockade of the sympathetic nerves for the patient to be considered as a surgical candidate.

In summary, the indications for digital sympathectomy are: 1) disabling symptoms; 2) tip ulcerations; 3) failure of conventional pharmacological treatment; and 4) excellent response to digital block anaesthesia with elimination of vasospasm on cold stimulus. Patients with either primary or secondary vasospastic disorders have been considered for this operation. Far more patients are turned down for this surgery after thorough evaluation than actually have it done.

Digital sympathectomy requires: isolation of the terminal branches of the sympathetic nerves which travel with the peripheral nerves; dividing these terminal branches; and then stripping the adventitia from the common digital and proper digital arteries. This procedure is done with the aid of an operating microscope. The procedure, if done on one finger, can be done under local anaesthesia on an outpatient basis with tourniquet control. If done on more than one finger, the necessity of regional anaesthesia for the tourniquet pain must be considered. The neurovascular bundles are exposed from the distal palm and the interdigital web to the proximal interphalangeal joint. The digital nerve is identified and gently retracted from the digital artery. As the digital nerve and digital artery are separated, the communication between these two structures can be seen. All connections between the nerve and the vessel are divided by sharp dissection. We always identify four sympathetic branches travelling from the digital nerve to the vessel, and remove these branches. There is usually one branch arising from the posterior branch of the digital nerve supplying the dorsal aspect of the digital artery.

Then, using jeweller's forceps and some sharp dissection, the loose adventitia surrounding the common digital artery and proper digital artery is removed in a circumferential fashion for an area of 2 cm. This effectively removes all the terminal sympathetic branches, including those travelling in a longitudinal fashion from the vessel. It must be emphasised that the vessel is not to be damaged and the media and intima must be left untouched, or thrombosis will occur. The goal is to assure that there is a greater inflow of blood to the digit, especially the cross-connecting vessels at the level of the proximal interphalangeal joints. If a thrombosis is encountered distal to the proximal interphalangeal joint, the digital artery should be resected, as reported by Zook et al (1978). In two cases, local thrombectomy of the proper digital artery had been done.

Many times, there is not an immediate response due to the strong circulating humoral component of noradrenaline that may still be present. However, a response is observable several hours after the operation; by the following day, the finger is usually warm, and there is a temperature difference of as much as 6°C between the treated and untreated digits. There is some numbness and tingling reported in the digit, which we feel is due to the temporary neurapraxia of the digital nerve secondary to manipulation. In our patients, ulcers have usually healed within two weeks, and the pain has been alleviated. There have been only two patients who have had wound healing problems, and both of these had the diagnosis of scleroderma. Otherwise, there have been no complications and all working patients have returned to work.

Patients with scleroderma have had the poorest responses, while young patients with vasculitis and primary vasospastic disorders have had the best responses. The post-frostbite patients have had excellent responses. In the initial report of 18 digital sympathectomies in 10 patients, surgery was beneficial in 17 of the 18 digits with no recurrence of symptoms reported following treatment. These patients have now been followed for a period of five years, and the results are essentially the same. An additional group of 12 patients has been followed for a period of four years. Because of the vigorous preoperative testing, 10 of these 12 patients have had beneficial results. Both patients who did not obtain satisfactory results also have the diagnosis of scleroderma. A third category of patients has recently been evaluated. These are 15 patients with secondary vasospastic disorders who have been treated with nifedipine, and have experienced failure and breakthrough with recurrence of tip ulceration and pain. 80% of these patients, all of whom responded to the postoperative testing, experienced dramatic relief following surgery.

SUMMARY

In summary, the microsurgical approach to vascular problems and diseases in the hand and upper limb can be used for direct repair of occlusive disorders and for the indirect approach to vasospastic disorders of the digits.

REFERENCES

Allen E V, Brown G E 1932 Raynaud's disease: a critical review of minimal requisites for diagnosis. American Journal of Medical Sciences 183: 187

Barker N W, Hines F H Jr 1944 Arterial occlusion in the hands and fingers associated with repeated occupational trauma. Mayo Clinic Proceedings 19: 345

Darling R D, Raines J K, Brener B J, Austin W G 1972 Quantitative segmental pulse volume recorder: a clinical tool. Surgery 72: 873

Egloff D V, Mifsud R P, Verdan C 1982 Superselective digital sympathectomy in Raynaud's phenomenon. The Hand 15: 110

Flatt A E 1980 Digital artery sympathectomy. Journal of Hand Surgery 5: 550

Koman L A, Urbaniak J R 1981 Ulnar artery insufficiency — a guide to treatment. Proceedings of the American Society for Surgery of the Hand, Journal of Hand Surgery 6: 16

Koman L A, Nunley J A, Urbaniak J R, Wilkinson R H 1982 Upper extremity radionuclide imaging. Journal of Hand Surgery 7: 412

Maurer A H, Holder L E, Espinola D, Rupani H, Wilgis E F S 1983 Three phase radionuclide scintigraphy of the hand. Radiology 146: 761

Morgan R, Riesman N, Wilgis E F S 1983 Anatomic localization of sympathetic nerves in the hand. Journal of Hand Surgery 8: 283

Pick J 1970 The autonomic nervous system. J B Lippincott, Philadelphia

VonRosen S 1933 Ein fall von thrombose in der arteria ulnaris nach einwirkung von stumpfen gewalt. Acta Chirurgica Scandinavica, Supplementum 73: 500

Wilgis E F S, Jezic D, Stonesifer G L, Classen J N 1974 The evaluation of small vessel flow. Journal of Bone and Joint Surgery 6: 1199

Wilgis E F S 1981 The evaluation and treatment of chronic digital ischemia. Annals of Surgery 193: 693

Wilgis E F S 1983 Vascular injuries and diseases of the upper limb. Little Brown, Boston

Zook E G, Kleinert H E, VanBeek A L 1978 Treatment of the ischemic finger secondary to digital artery occlusion. Plastic and Reconstructive Surgery 62: 229

R. A. Chase and J. M. Rosen

19 Microsurgery: the future

In no area of medical science is Shakespeare's oft-quoted, 'What is past is prologue' more fitting than it is in the young and growing specialty of microsurgery. New applications for surgical manipulation under magnification are burgeoning. Simultaneously, technical improvements in the art of microsurgery, and engineering advances in instrumentation, promise spectacular new dimensions in what may be achieved in the years ahead.

At the turn of the century Alexis Carrel (Carrel 1902, 1908) showed the technique for anastomosing large blood vessels. This precipitated the birth of vascular surgery. In 1960, Jacobson and Suarez (1960) from the University of Vermont reported their work applying vascular repair techniques to very small blood vessels using an operating microscope.

Microsurgery has now marked the 25th anniversary of its application to upper limb reconstruction. If one were able to look 25 years into the future and read a chapter on microsurgery commemorating its 50th anniversary, what would be found?

The goal of this chapter is to provide a look at some of the possible future prospects for microsurgery and their application in upper limb reconstruction.

NEW TECHNOLOGICAL REFINEMENTS

Firstly, let us consider some of the developing technology that may influence the future trajectory of microsurgery as a field. Today's operating microscope is enormously improved over versions of just a few years ago. Improving reliability and more precise controls will certainly continue to develop.

Voice control of focus, zoom, field location and light will, in all likelihood, be refined and more standardised in the years ahead. It is unlikely that within the next 25 years the microsurgeon will be replaced by an artificially intelligent robot; however, the electronic computer and the robotic manipulator will become more and more important to the microsurgeon in his daily practice.

The emerging technology in stereovideo will make it possible precisely to manipulate micro-instruments while viewing the magnified field in stereo on a videoscreen with a clarity and magnification superior to that obtained by peering through the diploscope oculars. Such images would be subject to various adjustments in colour, light intensity, specific high-lighting, etc.

Another step away will be micro-manipulators controlled by an operator who is away from the field of surgery. Such devices could add steadiness and predictability to the procedures being performed. Once the manipulator is perfected, the surgeon may be remote from the site of surgery, even at a distant geographic location. Electronic gloves might be worn by the surgeon, to provide detailed data about the surgeon's hand position and motions to the computer. This would allow the computer to place the surgeon's hand within a virtual image environment, to operate and control the motions of an artificial robotic manipulator. The motions of the robot's manipulator could be scaled, so that a macro-motion of the surgeon's hand would be transformed into a micro-motion for the robotic hand. The surgeon's tremor could be dampened by the computer controlling the interface between the surgeon and the manipulator. The surgeon might also feel what the robot's hand feels via sensors in the robotic endpiece.

One of the goals of the North American Space Program is the development of such a tele-operational system. In the case of the space programme, it would allow an operator in a space ship or on the ground to command a robot in space (Fig. 19.1). The computer system would generate a virtual image environment for the operator that would simulate the real environment within which the robot operates. This would require both input and output devices for the operator. For visual feedback, the operator would wear a helmet that presents a 3-D image of the environment that the robot's videocameras are seeing. The operator's head movements would be tracked with the helmet-mounted sensor, and signals would then move the robotic head in precisely the same planes and directions. The environment that such an operator would see would appear three-dimensional and real. Bi-directional controls and feedback would be transmitted between the robot and the operator in both the visual and auditory domains.

These futuristic and developmental initiatives being carried out for the space programme may have direct application to future initiatives in microsurgery.

NEW MICROSURGERY INITIATIVES

Nerve repair

Of the structures that upper limb surgeons are called upon to repair, the peripheral nerves present the major unsolved problem. Some of the reasons

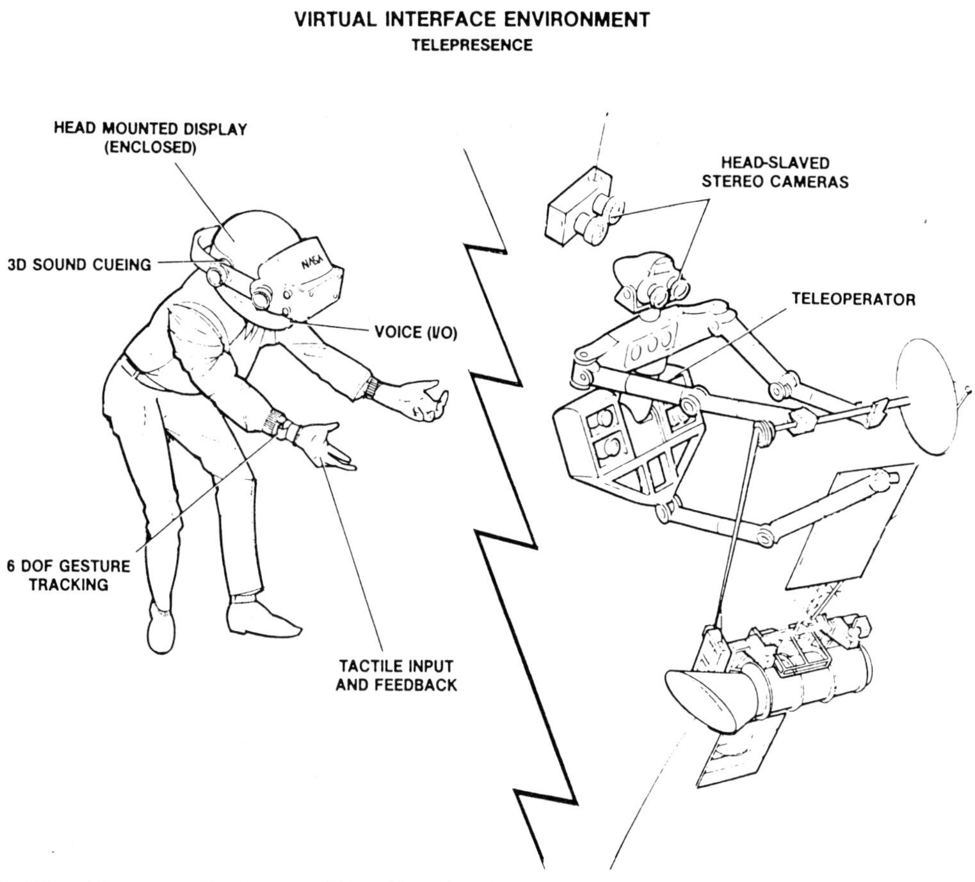

Fig. 19.1 Virtual Interactive Environment Helmet/Dataglove System.

that peripheral nerve repair often produces unsatisfactory functional results are clear. It is exciting to speculate about future solutions to these problems. Today's level of success in nerve repair lies in the accuracy with which the proximal and distal ends of a severed nerve are coapted. The more precise the repair, the more likely it is that a significant number of axons will grow down the proper distal pathways from the proximal cut end of the nerve. Through microsurgery, it is possible to repair structures as small as a single fascicle 1 mm in diameter. Single axons are but 20 μm or less in diameter. Axon-to-axon repair is beyond the capability of microsurgeons at present. In fact, there is little evidence to support the contention that such axon-to-axon repair would produce superior results. Surgery done prior to the era of repair under magnification, generally had consisted of repair of the nerve's epineurium with gross orientation of the cut nerve ends. With the introduction of microsurgery, the surgeon has been able to re-approximate the perineum around groups of axons. Even with such repair, the chances of proximal sprouting axons growing down their original channels are slim indeed. Growth of axons down channels previously occupied by other axons may still be perfectly functional. This is true only if proximal motor axons grow down distal motor channels to peripheral motor end plates and proximal sensory nerves grow distal to join peripheral sensory end organs. Although such axons grow down 'wrong' channels, functional readjustments for this seem to occur in the central nervous system. There is a specific, critical representation map for both the sensory and motor cortex. Such mapping makes it possible for the brain to exercise control of the hand as it carries out its complex tasks. After nerve repair, some sensory impulses may return to the brain at a site at variance with normal cortical representation. The patient may, for example, interpret a touch in the index finger as being a touch on the long or ring finger in the early period after nerve repair. Such misrepresentation, in fact, is incontrovertible evidence that axons have grown from the repair site to the distal sensory end organs, albeit different end organs than those previously innervated by the same axons. As time passes, this perceptive misrepresentation disappears, and is replaced by normal perception of the peripheral stimulus. Experimental work suggests that there is, in fact, a change in the actual central cortical map following such readjustment. Where major disparities exist, particularly in the motor system, it may be possible in the future to shift the impulses passing down a repaired peripheral nerve to the proper distal site.

Expansion of nerve function

Integrated circuits within silicon microchips have excited the interest of biological scientists. One of the potential uses of such chips is to interface peripheral nerve axons and the silicon chip directly. A paper by Llinas and co-workers (Llinas et al 1973) proposed growing squid axons through multiple perforations within such a chip. This would have allowed interfacing between axons and the microelectronics within the chip. In 1976, Loeb and co-workers did further mathematical modelling of nerve chip systems (Loeb et al 1977). Edell (1980, 1986) demonstrated the growth of rabbit axons through micropores within a chip from which he was able to record impulses from the axons to electrodes on the surface of the microchip. The possibility of interfacing elements of the peripheral nervous system with a silicon chip has become a reality. Rosen and Grosser (1987) have shown that a properly designed and fabricated implantable microchip can both record and stimulate elements within a peripheral nerve. If such a chip were implanted between the coapted ends of a nerve repair, for example, the silicon chip might act as a micro-switchboard to transfer signals from proximal axons to the counterpart axons distally. Such a silicon chip could be fabricated by placing thousands of holes in the chip through which axons might grow. Such a chip could be mounted in a nerve coupler that would hold it fixed securely between the two ends of the severed nerve (Fig. 19.2). The chip would be a multi-layered one: the proximal layer would be the first contact with the proximal end of the axon; while the distal layer would interface with the distal axons at the nerve site. The microelectronics of the chip could switch impulses passing in either direction to the proper proximal and distal channels. Such a chip would block mis-

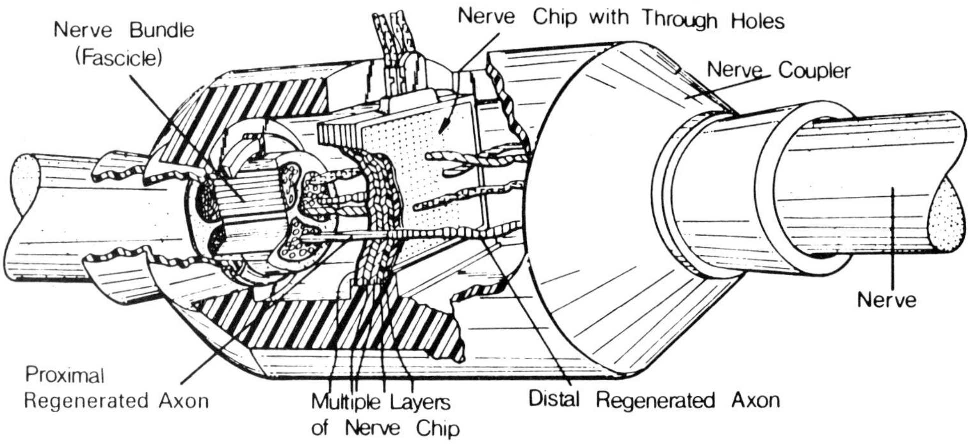

Fig. 19.2 Artist's concept of nerve chip in nerve coupler for nerve repair.

communication and redirect them to the appropriate site.

Such technology might have numerous applications in upper limb nerve reconstruction. It could be applied as noted above to simple nerve repairs. It could serve a similar purpose in relationship to nerve grafts. Such an electronic device might serve as an interface between an amputee and his prosthesis, making it a bioprosthetic functioning arm and hand. Impulses might be bled off in upper limb peripheral nerves, to then be electronically augmented for use in stimulating lower limb muscles in quadriplegic patients.

The amputation neuromas present in the residual limb after amputation are untapped sources of impulses that might very well be processed for use in the prosthesis. Both motor and sensory components of such nerves might well be found to be useful in operation of bioprosthetic devices (see Microsurgery and future prostheses).

Replantation and transplantation

Replantation of amputated parts has become more and more refined with the passage of time. Reliable repairs of smaller and smaller vessels mean replantation of composite parts at more distal sites. In the future, we expect that the distal extreme for such successful revascularisation will reach the point where more distal amputations would be likely to survive if replaced as free composite grafts without microvascular revascularisation.

The surgical technology is ready for the step beyond replantation, that of transplantation of limbs and limb parts. The remaining obstacle to making transplantation as successful as replantation is immunological rejection of non-host tissues. Immunological rejection is the host's defense against infectious agents and tumours. In the last quarter century, immunologists have made enormous progress in understanding the various immune systems. Delayed hypersensitivity, which is the basis for transplant rejection, has shown to be dependent upon specific cells comprising the defence army. Understanding how these various cells communicate with one another to mobilise the body's defenses is still being studied. Several major humoral factors which turn the rejection system on and off have been discovered. The host's ability to distinguish foreign tissue from its own, and to destroy such foreign tissue through the rejection phenomenon, is a complex process. A simplified view of the rejection phenomenon is depicted in Figure 19.3.

The detailed mechanisms of the rejection phenomenon are not yet fully understood. Macrophages are the host cells predominantly engaged in presenting the antigen of the transplant tissue cells to the T-lymphocytes that participate in cellular immunity. Macromolecules that act as messengers in this process are such substances as interleukins and interferons. The B-lymphocytes participate in the transplantation process to a lesser extent, and thus are not emphasised in this discussion. Cells

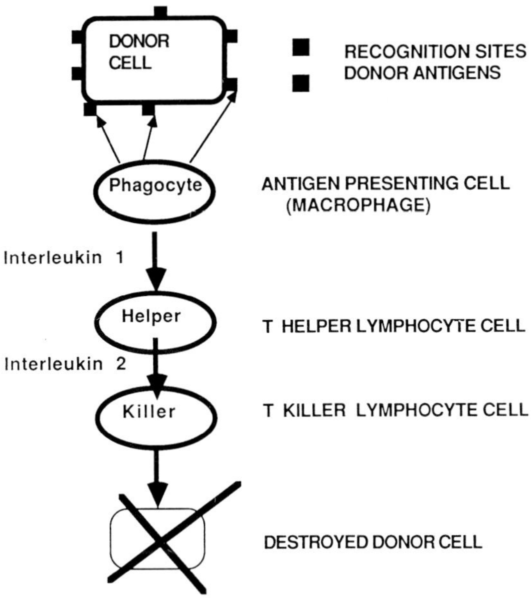

Fig. 19.3 General scheme of immune system for transplantation.

other than macrophages, including dendritic cells, Kupffer's cells, Langerhans' cells, B-lymphocytes, T-lymphocytes and, in some cases, endothelial cells, may present antigens from the transplant donor cells to the T-lymphocytes.

There are two major populations of T-lymphocytes with disparate functions. One of the populations is the T-helper lymphocyte, which helps to initiate the development of the other major population of T-lymphocytes, the T-killer lymphocytes. T-helper lymphocytes also stimulate B-lymphocytes into becoming specific antibody producers.

There is a specific T-lymphocyte which recognises each antigen from the donor cells. Such T-cells form a clone of cells specific to the donor cell antigen. If the T-helper lymphocyte population is depleted, the ability to recognise donor transplant cell antigen markers is diminished and rejection is less likely to occur. This creates a state of tolerance characterised by a host unable to recognise and therefore to reject the donor transplant.

The generic goal in the field of transplantation is to make the host tolerant to a specific donor transplant to negate the rejection phenomenon. Ideally, one would wish to dampen or reverse the host's ability to reject the specific tissue elements within a transplanted part, such as an upper limb.

Present methods of immunosuppression rely on a variety of chemotherapeutic agents, anti-lymphocyte globulin, or total body radiation. Each carries with it a significant risk to the patient, and thus limb transplantation in human beings remains a procedure for the future.

Microarthroscopy

Arthroscopic examination and surgical manipulations using arthroscopy are commonplace when applied to large joints, usually the knee. With continuing refinement of instruments, the techniques are now applicable for medium-sized joints, such as the wrist. The small joints of the hand are likely to be subject to examination and micromanipulation of their component parts in the years ahead.

To achieve this requires only the continuing development of remotely controlled micromanipulators and systems of electronic magnification of images through tiny probes. Microsurgeons, without doubt, will be able to achieve within the metacarpophalangeal joints and the interphalangeal joints what already is being done regularly within the knee.

Newborn and in utero surgery on hands

Raus (1984) has already demonstrated some of the virtues of syndactyly surgery within hours after birth. It is well known that scars generated in newborns and by in utero surgery are less significant, to the point of being nearly nonexistent (Martin 1976, Miller 1976).

With increasing reliability of small vessel anastomoses and nerve junctures, it takes only a little imagination to picture surgery very early after birth for the whole array of congenital limb abnormalities. One, more futuristic, step is the thought of hysterotomy for corrective surgical procedures, and replacement of the fetus in utero for completion of gestation. The technology for such fetal surgery is already in development in animals. The advent of safe imaging techniques using ultrasound and fetoscopy may make it possible to carry out procedures either in utero or through hysterotomy (Christ 1986, Stone 1984).

Lymphatic anastomoses and reconstruction

Although microsurgery on lymphatic vessels is reported and continues to be studied, the results leave a great deal to be desired (O'Brien et al 1978). New and as yet unthought-of techniques using non-biological and biological materials yet to be refined may in the future make lymphatic reconstructive microsurgery more productive. The need is evident, and the problem is in part understood, but the barriers to success in overcoming the tragedy of lymphoedema remain.

Perhaps free block composite transfers including lymphatics will become bridges across areas of blocked lymph flow in obstructive lymphoedema. This might be particularly useful in post-surgical and post-infectious lymphoedema, where blockade is localised and distal lymphatics are normal. The composite bridge might simultaneously carry interposition vascularised vein grafts to treat the venous contributory cause of lymphoedema.

Additional composite transfers

Composite tissue transfers with immediate microsurgical re-establishment of blood supply has been one of the great contributions of microsurgery. Such transfers have carried various combinations of skin with subcutaneous tissue, bone, muscle, tendon, nerve, interpositioned vessels and whole parts, such as digits.

Scanning the anatomy for additional tissues and combinations of tissues is useful in thinking of future initiatives. For example, free endocrine gland transfers or transplants will depend upon microsurgeons. Thyroid and parathyroid, thymus, adrenal, pancreas, ovary, testis and, even, hypophysis should not be ruled out as subject to transfer to a new anatomical venue by microsurgery.

Skin and subcutaneous tissue with special characteristics, such as concentrations of sensory end organs, sweat glands, etc., might find new applications. For example, the use of skin with high level, two-point discrimination potential as a transfer to the residual limb of an amputee for revascularisation and, importantly, re-innervation from funiculi from the amputation neuroma could be very useful. Such a patch of skin with high level perceptive discriminatory capabilities might be used as a port to the central nervous system from a prosthetic arm with sensory stimulators. Even more imaginative would be to innervate the composite patch with afferent nerves which would go to a specific unit, such as the thumb, then to be stimulated by sensors on the thumb substitute of the prosthesis. Similarly, the ulnar finger proximal nerves to a second composite part could be placed in position to be stimulated by sensors in the unit to be opposed by the thumb. This would then require less central re-orientation when a useful sensory prosthesis is developed.

Peacock and Madden (1967) carried out trials of composite tendon, tendon sheath and pulleys as a free composite graft. It is time to consider transfer or transplant of such units as *vascularised* composite transfers. Vascularised small joints, fingernails and intrinsic muscles will be refined and found useful as vascularised composite transfers in the years ahead.

TUMOUR THERAPY

Reliable small vessel anastomoses and small vessel grafting have opened the door to more aggressive treatment of tumours. This is particularly so for haemangiomas and other varieties of arteriovenous malformation. It seems probable that radical excision of intercalated vascular lesions of small but critical vessels can be considered safely with the reality of immediate vascular reconstruction using grafting techniques. For example, arteriovenous malformations in the hand which were previously inoperable because of the prospect of devascularisation, may become operable by radical excision and immediate graft revascularisation of more peripheral parts. The same principle applies to various tumours which can be completely removed only by excision of critical end arteries.

Microsurgery will also make it possible to isolate and cannulate very small tumour vessels for tumour perfusion with chemotherapeutic tumouricidal agents.

MICROSURGERY AND FUTURE PROSTHESES

The prospect of using implantable electronic devices, such as intraneuronal silicon chips, sets the stage for direct nerve to prosthesis linkages. Such linkages may be bidirectional, sending signals peripherally to generate electronically controlled motion, or receiving signals from electronic sensors embedded in the prosthesis. Such bioprostheses will be dependent upon medicine's ability to identify motor and sensory funiculi, and to microsurgically implant microtransducer systems into nerves in continuity or into residual nerve stumps.

Crossing the skin barrier with fine wire leads will continue to be a problem for surgeons to cope with and to solve. Perhaps the solution will be telemetry systems within the body, sending signals to the extracorporeal receivers within a prosthesis.

Various myelo-electric prostheses have been developed and are being improved upon. Such a prosthesis with a dexterous endpiece and sensibility is the goal of prosthesis investigators. Microsurgeons may contribute to the solution by micro-implants as noted above, or by using free transferred composite specialised skin islands as noted in the section on Additional composite transfers.

Micro-implants in proximal muscles may be a viable source of prosthesis switching. Central nervous system control of muscles, and even small parts of muscles, is credible when some feedback, such as that from a prosthesis, is supplied (Close 1973, 1986).

One of the major unsolved problems in upper limb prostheses is the lack of sensory feedback. It is possible to imagine that one might develop a system of tactile stimulators from prosthetic devices that could be fed to the residual limb. The contribution microsurgery conceivably could make would be to transplant to the residual limb an island of tissue, such as the glabrous skin from a toe, to be re-innervated by nerves from the amputation neuroma. In other words, one might then have a patch of highly sensitive discriminatory skin on the residual limb to receive feedback from tactile stimulators within the prosthesis. For example, tactile stimulators receiving impulses from the prosthetic thumb and index finger might then be directed to the microsurgically-transferred free skin island on the residual limb, innervated by nerves that ordinarily would go to the thumb end and index finger. Such possibilities are not far-fetched and seem to have practical value.

REFERENCES

Carrel A 1902 La technique opératoire des anastomoses vasculaires et al transplantation des viscères. Lyon Médecine 98: 859–864

Carrel A 1908 Results of the transplantation of blood vessels, organs and limbs. Journal of the American Medical Association 51: 1662–1667

Christ J E 1986 Fetal surgery: a frontier for plastic surgery. Plastic and Reconstructive Surgery 77: 645–647

Close J R 1973 Functional anatomy of the extremities. Charles C Thomas, Springfield

Close J R 1986 Personal communication

Edell D J 1980 Development of a chronic neuroelectric interface. PhD dissertation, University of California, Davis, Ca

Edell D J 1986 A peripheral nerve transducer for amputees long term multichannel recordings from rabbit peripheral nerves. International Electrical and Electronic Engineering Transactions, Biomedical Engineering 33 (2): 203–214

Jacobson J H, Suarez E L 1960 Microsurgery in the anastomosis of small vessels. Surgical Forum 11: 243

Llinas R, Nicholson C, Johnson K 1973 In: Phillips M I (ed) Brain unit activity during behavior. Charles C Thomas, Springfield, ch 7

Loeb G E, Marks W B, Beatty P G 1977 Medicine Biology Engineering Computers 15: 195–201

Martin L W 1976 Observation of the influence of age on wound healing. In: Longacre J J (ed) The ultrastructure of collagen. Charles C Thomas, Springfield p 10–19

Miller E J 1976 Biochemical characteristics and biological significance of the genetically distinct collagens. Molecular Cellular Biochemistry 13: 165–192

O'Brien B McC, Black M J, Fodestam I 1978 Role of microlymphaticovenous surgery in obstructive lymphedema. Clinics of Plastic Surgery 5: 293

Peacock E E, Madden J W 1967 Human composite flexor tendon allografts. Annals of Surgery 166: 624–629

Raus E E 1984 Repair of simple syndactylism in the healthy neo-newborn. Orthopedic Review 13: 498–502

Rosen J M, Grosser M 1987 Nerve repair at the axon level: a merger of microelectronics and microsurgery. In: J D Andrade et al (eds) Artificial organs. Proceedings of the International Symposium on Artificial Organs, Biomedical Engineering and Transplantation in Honor of the 75th Birthday of William J Kolff. VCH Publishers, New York pp. 583–594

Stone M L 1984 What's new in gynecology and obstetrics? American College of Surgeons Bulletin 69: 19–21

Index